CRIMINAL
Clinical and Forensic Perspectives
POISONING

Edited by

Christopher P. Holstege, MD
Chief, Division of Medical Toxicology
Associate Professor, Departments of Emergency Medicine & Pediatrics
University of Virginia School of Medicine
Charlottesville, VA

Thomas M. Neer, SSA
FBI Supervisory Special Agent
National Center for the Analysis of Violent Crime
Critical Incident Response Group, Behavioral Analysis Unit
FBI Academy
Quantico, VA

Gregory B. Saathoff, MD
Associate Professor of Research
Departments of Psychiatry and Neurobehavioral Science & Emergency Medicine
University of Virginia School of Medicine
Charlottesville, VA

R. Brent Furbee, MD
Medical Director, Indiana Poison Center
Medical Toxicology, Methodist Hospital of Indiana
Indianapolis, IN

JONES AND BARTLETT PUBLISHERS
Sudbury, Massachusetts
BOSTON   TORONTO   LONDON   SINGAPORE

World Headquarters
Jones and Bartlett Publishers
40 Tall Pine Drive
Sudbury, MA 01776
978-443-5000
info@jbpub.com
www.jbpub.com

Jones and Bartlett Publishers
Canada
6339 Ormindale Way
Mississauga, Ontario L5V 1J2
Canada

Jones and Bartlett Publishers
International
Barb House, Barb Mews
London W6 7PA
United Kingdom

Jones and Bartlett's books and products are available through most bookstores and online booksellers. To contact Jones and Bartlett Publishers directly, call 800-832-0034, fax 978-443-8000, or visit our website, www.jbpub.com.

Substantial discounts on bulk quantities of Jones and Bartlett's publications are available to corporations, professional associations, and other qualified organizations. For details and specific discount information, contact the special sales department at Jones and Bartlett via the above contact information or send an email to specialsales@jbpub.com.

Production Credits
Executive Publisher: Chris Davis
Editorial Assistant: Sara Cameron
Production Director: Amy Rose
Associate Production Editor: Jessica deMartin
Senior Marketing Manager: Barb Bartoszek
V.P., Manufacturing and Inventory Control: Therese Connell
Composition: Nicolazzo Productions
Printing and Binding: Malloy, Inc.

Cover Credits
Cover Design: Kristin E. Parker
Cover Printing: Malloy, Inc.
Cover Image: Top background
© maximum/Dreamstime.com;
Bottom © photobank.kiev.ua/
ShutterStock, Inc.

Library of Congress Cataloging-in-Publication Data
Criminal poisoning : clinical and forensic perspectives / Christopher Holstege ... [et al.].
    p. ; cm.
Includes bibliographical references and index.
ISBN-13: 978-0-7637-4463-2
ISBN-10: 0-7637-4463-8
1. Poisoning. I. Holstege, Christopher P.
[DNLM: 1. Poisoning. 2. Crime. 3. Forensic Medicine--methods. 4. Poisons. QV 600 C929 2011]
HV6549.C737 2011
614.13--dc22
                          2009041721

6048

Printed in the United States of America
14 13 12 11 10   10 9 8 7 6 5 4 3 2 1

Dedications

TO MY WIFE, Angela, for your love, grace, and ever-enduring fortitude; to my six children (Erik, Elijah, Benjamin, Samual, Noah, and Annalee) for infusing levity into daily life; and to both my parents, Henry and Lois Holstege, for your selfless sacrifice in providing for my years of valued education.

Christopher P. Holstege

TO MY WIFE, Tip, for your love, patience, and enduring support; to Margaret MacDonald, for your friendship, encouragement, and editing advice; to FBI Special Agent Jim McCarthy, for your insight, humor, and years of partnership...it's been a great run!

Thomas M. Neer

TO MY WIFE, Andrea, and to our children, Graham, Kathleen, and Kenneth. I remain grateful for your love, patience, understanding, and humor. You continue to provide me with what I value most in life.

Gregory B. Saathoff

TO MY WIFE, Esther, for your love, understanding, and assistance in everything I try. You make my life so much better. To my partners and coworkers: Mary, Dan, Louise, Kris, Blake, Jim, Maggie, and the nurses and pharmacists of the Indiana Poison Center for sharing in our vision and making it a reality. Work would just be work if not for people like you. Many thanks.

R. Brent Furbee

Contents

SECTION 2
Agents Used by Past Poisoners

SECTION 3
Specific Classes of Poisoners

About the Editors

Christopher P. Holstege

Christopher P. Holstege, MD, is an associate professor of emergency medicine and pediatrics at the University of Virginia's School of Medicine and chief of the University of Virginia's Division of Medical Toxicology. His clinical practice is associated with the University of Virginia's Center of Clinical Toxicology. He has published extensively in the medical literature with over 100 publications in medical journals, periodicals, and books. Dr. Holstege speaks extensively on various topics in the field of medical toxicology, with a focus on areas such as criminal poisoners and chemical weapons of mass destruction. He has been integrally involved in the diagnosis and management of a number of high profile criminal poisonings, including the dioxin poisoning of the Ukrainian President Viktor Yushchenko.

In appreciation of his work in both education and clinical service, Dr. Holstege received the Dean's Award for Clinical Excellence from the University of Virginia, the National Faculty Teaching Award from the American College of Emergency Physicians, and the Attending Teacher of the Year Award from the University of Virginia's Department of Emergency Medicine. He currently serves on the Board of Trustees of the American Academy of Clinical Toxicology and on the Steering Committee of the University of Virginia's Critical Incident Analysis Group (CIAG). He is a consultant to the Federal Bureau of Investigation (FBI).

Dr. Holstege received his bachelor of science degree in chemistry from Calvin College (Grand Rapids, Michigan) and his doctor of medicine from Wayne State University School of Medicine (Detroit, Michigan); he completed his residency training in emergency medicine at Butterworth Hospital (Grand Rapids, Michigan) and his fellowship training in medical toxicology at Indiana University (Indianapolis, Indiana). He is a diplomate of both the American Board of Emergency Medicine and the American Board of Medical Toxicology.

Thomas M. Neer

Supervisory Special Agent (SSA) Thomas Neer is a 25-year veteran of the FBI with extensive experience in complex criminal and counter-terrorism investigations. Since 1995, he has been assigned to the FBI's Behavioral Analysis Unit in Quantico, Virginia where he provides FBI field offices and state, local, and foreign police with behavioral assessments on cases involving unusual circumstances or serial offenders. Among his many cases, SSA Neer served as the FBI's principal behavioral advisor during the investigation of Michael Swango, a medical doctor who was convicted of murdering several patients in hospitals.

Prior to his career with the FBI, SSA Neer was employed by the Naval Criminal Investigative Service and the Federal Bureau of Prisons. SSA Neer's diverse law enforcement career includes extensive operational travel to Europe, Asia, Africa, and the Middle East.

A 1976 graduate of the University of Florida, SSA Neer pursued graduate studies in 1977 at the Southern Illinois University's Center for the Study of Crime Delinquency and Corrections. A 2001 graduate of the Police Staff College in Bramshill, England, SSA Neer is currently a candidate for a master of arts degree at the Fletcher School of Law and Diplomacy, Tufts University.

Gregory B. Saathoff

Gregory B. Saathoff, MD, is associate professor of research in psychiatry and neurobehavioral sciences, and associate professor of emergency medicine at the University of Virginia's School of Medicine. A veteran of the First Gulf War, he has treated male and female violent and non-violent prison inmates who suffer from mental illness since 1991. He also serves as executive director of the University of Virginia's Critical Incident Analysis Group (CIAG). In this capacity, he directs the group, which operates as a "ThinkNet" that provides multidisciplinary expertise in developing strategies that can prevent or mitigate the effects of critical incidents.

He wrote *The Negotiator's Guide to Psychotropic Drugs* for the FBI's Crisis Negotiation Unit, and he was a co-author of the FBI's threat assessment monograph: *The School Shooter*. In addition to this, he has published in the areas of personality disorders, police psychiatry, post-traumatic stress disorders, public response to weapons of mass destruction, and biologic psychiatry. He assembled and led a University of Virginia medical team that served as the U.S. component of the international medical group charged with diagnosis and treatment of President Viktor Yuschenko who was poisoned in 2004. He has served as an expert witness on espionage- and terrorist-related cases in federal court. Since 1996 he has served as a conflict resolution specialist, and in 2006, he was appointed to the Research Advisory Board of the FBI's National Center for the Analysis of Violent Crime.

Dr. Saathoff earned his MD at the University of Missouri and completed his residency in psychiatric medicine at the University of Virginia in Charlottesville.

R. Brent Furbee

R. Brent Furbee, MD, was trained in medicine at the Indiana University School of Medicine (1977). He completed an emergency medicine residency at Methodist Hospital of Indiana (1980) and a fellowship in medical toxicology at Good Samaritan Hospital in Phoenix, Arizona (1991). He has served as the medical director of the Indiana Poison Center since 1988. In 1992, he started the state's only medical toxicology service followed by a medical toxicology fellowship in 1994. He consults at Methodist, Indiana University, and Wishard hospitals in Indianapolis. He is active in the education of fellows, residents, medical students, and nurses.

Dr. Furbee has served as a consultant in several criminal and civil cases in the United States. He was a member of the investigative team for the Indiana State Police in the *State of Indiana v. Orville Lynn Majors* case, the largest criminal investigation in that state's history. He has authored publications regarding homicidal poisoning and the toxicity of heavy metals, manganese, plants, drugs of abuse, pharmaceuticals, and venomous animals. Dr. Furbee is an associate clinical professor of emergency medicine at the Indiana University School of Medicine and a fellow of the American College of Medical Toxicology.

Contributors

Juan C. Arias, MD
Visiting Professor
Universidad de La Sabana School of Medicine
Bogotá, Colombia

Kevin S. Barlotta, MD
Assistant Professor, Department of Emergency
 Medicine
Medical Director, Department of Critical Care
 Transport
University of Alabama at Birmingham Hospital
Birmingham, AL

Laura K. Bechtel, PhD
Assistant Professor, Department of Emergency
 Medicine
Director of Research, Division of Medical
 Toxicology
University of Virginia School of Medicine
Charlottesville, VA

Stephen W. Borron, MD, MS
Professor of Emergency Medicine and Medical
 Toxicology
Texas Tech University Health Sciences Center
Associate Medical Director, West Texas
 Regional Poison Control Center
El Paso, TX

Jou-Fang Deng, MD
Director, National Poison Center of Taiwan
Division of Clinical Toxicology
Taipei Veterans General Hospital
Taipei, Taiwan

David L. Eldridge, MD
Assistant Professor, Department of Pediatrics
Brody School of Medicine at East Carolina
 University
Greenville, NC

Timothy B. Erickson, MD
Professor, Department of Emergency Medicine
Director, Division of Clinical Toxicology
University of Illinois
Chicago, IL

Blake A. Froberg, MD
Assistant Professor, Department of Pediatrics
Associate Medical Director, Indiana Poison
 Center
Indiana University School of Medicine
Indianapolis, IN

Rachel Haroz, MD
Assistant Professor, Department of Emergency
 Medicine
University of Medicine and Dentistry, New
 Jersey (UMDNJ)
Cooper University Hospital
Camden, NJ

Ashley L. Harvin, BS
Department of Chemical Engineering
University of Virginia
Charlottesville, VA

Bryan S. Judge, MD
Assistant Professor, Michigan State University
Associate Program Director, Emergency
 Medicine Residency
Grand Rapids Medical Education and Research
 Center (GRMERC)
Grand Rapids, MI

Ziad N. Kazzi, MD
Assistant Professor, Department of Emergency
 Medicine
Emory University
Atlanta, GA

Jenny J. Lu, MD
Instructor, Department of Emergency
  Medicine—Division of Toxicology
Cook County-Stroger Hospital
Rush Medical College
Chicago, IL

Paul M. Maniscalco, PhD(c), MPA, MS, EMT/P
President, International Association of EMS
  Chiefs
Senior Research Scientist and Principal
  Investigator, The George Washington
  University
Office of Homeland Security Center for
  Preparedness and Resilience
Deputy Chief, Paramedic FDNY EMS
  Command
Washington, DC

James McCarthy, JD
Special Agent, Federal Bureau of Investigation
Melville, NY

Susan Ney, MD
Department of Emergency Medicine
Cooper University Hospital
University of Medicine & Dentistry of New
  Jersey
Camden, NJ

Ayrn D. O'Connor, MD
Instructor, Department of Medical Toxicology
Banner Good Samaritan Medical Center
Phoenix, AZ

Kelli D. O'Donnell, MD
Instructor, Department of Emergency
  Medicine
Albert Einstein Medical Center
Philadelphia, PA

Gerald F. O'Malley, DO
Associate Professor, Department of Emergency
  Medicine
Thomas Jefferson University Hospital
Director of Research, Department of
  Emergency Medicine
Albert Einstein Medical Center
Faculty Consultant, Department of Pediatrics,
  Division of Emergency Medicine
Children's Hospital of Philadelphia and the
  Philadelphia Poison Control Center
Philadelphia, PA

Rika N. O'Malley, MD
Instructor, Albert Einstein Medical Center
Department of Emergency Medicine
Philadelphia, PA

Bernard Postles
Detective Chief Superintendent, Retired
Lancashire, England

William H. Richardson, III, MD
Instructor, Palmetto Health Richland,
  Department of Emergency Medicine
Medical Director, Palmetto Poison Center
South Carolina School of Pharmacy
University of South Carolina
Columbia, SC

Adam K. Rowden, DO
Assistant Professor, Department of Emergency
  Medicine
Jefferson Medical College
Director, Division of Toxicology, Department
  of Emergency Medicine
Albert Einstein Medical Center
Philadelphia, PA

Daniel E. Rusyniak, MD
Associate Professor, Departments of
  Emergency Medicine and Pharmacology &
  Toxicology
Adjunct Associate Clinical Professor of
  Neurology
Indiana University School of Medicine
Indianapolis, IN

Matthew Salzman, MD
Instructor, Department of Emergency
  Medicine—Division of Medical Toxicology
Albert Einstein Medical Center
Philadelphia, PA

Kahoko Taki, MD
Instructor, Department of Emergency
  Medicine
Saga Medical School
Saga, Japan

Foreword

*C*riminal Poisoning: Clinical and Forensic Perspectives, edited by Dr. Holstege, Agent Neer, Dr. Saathoff, and Dr. Furbee, is to our knowledge the most comprehensive book written to date specifically addressing the subject of criminal poisoning. This text will provide a valuable resource for any medical or law enforcement personnel evaluating a potential criminal poisoning.

Historically, criminal poisoning cases have often proved difficult to diagnose, investigate, and prosecute. The delivery methods employed can be markedly sophisticated and subtle. The deviousness associated with criminal poisonings is manifest in such notorious cases as the 1982 Chicago Tylenol Cyanide Murders and the 2006 Alexander Litvinenko Polonium-210 Poisoning. The criminals behind such acts may be able to avoid detection for decades and until caught may even be viewed as model citizens, as exemplified by the medical serial killer Dr. Harold Shipman, who is estimated to have murdered some 250 of his patients in the 1980s and 1990s in Britain. This book is timely not only because of the increased range of poisons now available for the more "common criminal" contexts and in family and domestic crimes, but also because the use of poisons has even extended in recent times to attempts to change high-level political leadership, exemplified by the 2004 dioxin poisoning of the current Ukrainian president Viktor Yushchenko.

This book combines the expertise found within the fields of law enforcement, toxicology, and psychiatry to give a unique perspective on criminal poisoning. All of the four editors have not only recognized expertise in their respective fields, but also extensive personal experience investigating criminal poisoning cases, and each has worked closely with both medical and law enforcement systems to bring criminal poisoners to justice.

The time and resources necessary to medically detect, formally investigate, and legally prosecute a criminal poisoning can be substantial. We commend the editors, authors, and publisher on the extensive work needed to produce this important book. There is no doubt that *Criminal Poisoning: Clinical and Forensic Perspectives* is a major step forward in assisting our medical and law enforcement personnel with criminal poisoning cases.

The Lord Alderdice, FRCPsych
Consultant Psychiatrist
House of Lords, London, UK

Honorable Edwin Meese, III
Former United States Attorney General
1985–1988

Preface

Throughout history, poisons and their effects have been well described. Paracelsus (1493–1541) correctly noted that "All substances are poisons; there is none which is not a poison. The right dose differentiates a poison...." As life in the modern era has become more complex, so has the use of numerous poisons by criminals.

A criminal poisoning occurs when an individual or group of individuals deliberately attempts to inflict harm on others through the use of a toxin. Such acts can be performed by an individual working alone (e.g., medical murderer Michael J. Swango), by a specific group (e.g., Aum Shinrikyo attacks on the Tokyo subway system), or through government sponsorship (e.g., the Soviet-Bulgarian poisoning of Georgi Markov). Innumerable potential toxins can inflict harm on humans. Such toxins can include pharmaceuticals, herbals, household products, environmental agents, occupational chemicals, drugs of abuse, and chemical warfare agents.

The detection and prosecution of criminal poisoning cases has become more challenging. The emergence of the Internet has allowed a wealth of information on poisoning to become more accessible. That free flow of information, coupled with the emergence of a host of new chemicals, has made the job of detecting and prosecuting criminal poisonings more difficult.

This book, *Criminal Poisoning: Clinical and Forensic Perspectives*, is intended for use by law enforcement, attorneys, and medical providers when investigating a criminal poisoning. It is divided into three sections: 1) Introduction to Poisoning; 2) Agents Used by Past Poisoners; and 3) Specific Classes of Poisoners. The agents chosen for inclusion were chosen either because they have been frequently encountered in past criminal poisonings (e.g., cyanide) or have been infrequently encountered but have been recently present in actual prominent cases (e.g., dioxin) or highlighted in the media due to the potential concern of use (e.g., sodium monofluoroacetate).

Each chapter that is dedicated to a specific toxin is divided into 6 sections: Case, History, Potential Delivery Methods, Toxicologic Mechanisms, Analytical Detection, and the Conclusion. The intention of providing a case at the beginning of each toxin's chapter is to reinforce the difficulty in medically diagnosing and legally evaluating a criminal poisoning. Much can be learned from past criminal poisonings to both help detect future poisonings and prevent perpetuation of errors that can occur during the investigation. Many different delivery methods have been devised by past poisoners, some quite unique to avoid detection by both the victim and the investigative team. When considering a criminal poisoning, the investigative team must realize that some poisoners have devised sophisticated and unique methods in which to administer toxins. Because the intention of this book is not to fully educate the general law enforcement community and basic medical providers into the biochemical mechanisms and analytical detection techniques, these sections were written with the intent to give a basic overview. This book is not intended to be a comprehensive resource for laboratory analysis of criminal poisoning.

This book is written by skilled clinicians engaged in the diagnosis and treatment of poisoned patients and by law enforcement officials experienced in investigating criminal poisonings. This diverse group of professionals brings unique clinical expertise to each area, many with past research and publications within their respective areas. It is the intent of the editors to provide the reader with unique insight into the realm of criminal poisoning.

Acknowledgments

We are indebted to Research Strategies Network for their support and guidance in the completion of this book. It is the tireless dedication of such exemplary foundations that enables diverse disciplines (i.e., law enforcement, academicians, clinicians) to assemble in neutral settings. These assemblies allow experts with unique skills and experience to learn from each other and subsequently pass those lessons on to others through venues such as this book.

We also appreciate the grammatical and literary critique provided by Ms. Sabrina N. Rissing. Her rapid and thorough reviews of each chapter helped to keep the book focused in a standard and appropriate style.

Introduction to Poisoning

1 | History of Criminal Poisoning

Bryan S. Judge

"The forcible administration of poison is by no means a new thing in criminal annals."

—SHERLOCK HOLMES
A STUDY IN SCARLET, *SIR ARTHUR CONAN DOYLE, 1887*

INTRODUCTION

The above quote was aptly spoken by arguably the greatest fictional sleuth. However, the contents of this chapter are not of fiction. This chapter will summarize the real-life attempts by individuals to eradicate their victim(s) through poison. One of the earliest recorded criminal poisonings occurred in ancient Rome when Locusta, at the behest of Nero's mother, poisoned Claudius and then Britannicus so that Nero could ascend to the throne.[1] While ancient and medieval history is replete with anecdotes of infamous poisoners, much of this chapter will focus on poisoners of the 19th, 20th, and 21st centuries—the so-called "modern criminal poisoners"—the methods they employed, their underlying motives, and the often unsuspecting victims.

CRIMINAL POISONING STATISTICS

Accurate compiled data regarding homicidal poisonings in the U.S. and abroad are sparse.[2] Two studies by Westveer and colleagues have analyzed data from the Federal Bureau of Investigation's Uniform Crime Report (UCR) in an attempt to better characterize poisoners and their victims.[3,4] Combining the data from these studies results in a total of 389,756 homicides in the United States from 1980 through 1999; only 638 (0.16%) homicides during this period were ascribed to poisoning. Although the total number of homicides declined almost 8% from the 1980–1989 UCR to the 1990–1999 UCR, the number of homicidal poisonings during the 1990s increased 18%.[4]

While the UCR reports that homicidal poisoning accounts for a small fraction of all murders committed in the United States, the true incidence is probably much higher because cases are often unrecognized. Poisoning cases may go undetected for several reasons. For example, (1) the victim may have died with symptoms that mimic another disease,[3] (2) the victim's death might not have been unanticipated,[5] and (3) an autopsy or toxicologic analysis may not have been performed. Suspicion for criminal poisoning should arise when a person's death occurs abruptly or is unexplained.

FACE OF THE MODERN-DAY POISONER

Forming a typical profile for poisoners has been a challenge because each modern poisoning case is unique. No rigorous scientific study has been performed that has analyzed the psychopathology of the modern poisoner. Sometimes the poisoner and his or her motive remain unknown, as seen in the Extra Strength Tylenol tampering case that resulted in the death of seven individuals in 1982.[6] Finally, much of what is known about poisoners stems from media sources, which may aggrandize their traits, perpetuate myths, or provide inaccurate information.

Several demographic factors regarding modern-day poisoners and their victims have been identified (Table 1.1).[3] Although analyzing data from the UCR may aid in an investigation, it does not provide a detailed profile about each poisoner, affords almost no insight into their thoughts, and cannot predict who will become a poisoner. The UCR data are hindered because many poisoners have unknown characteristics[4] and because the UCR does not include potentially helpful information about poisoners such as their criminal background, education level, employment history, psychiatric history, personality traits, or socioeconomic status.

History may shed some light on the question of who will become a future poisoner. Although historic information cannot be utilized to categorically identify future poisoners, it can provide a framework to build upon when investigating homicidal poisonings. Daniel Bondeson is an example of a seemingly normal individual who unexpectedly poisoned members of his community. Bondeson was a 53-year-old bachelor farmer, high school ski coach, and part-time nurse from New Sweden, Maine, who in April 2003 poisoned fellow church members with arsenic and committed suicide.[7] His exact motive remains a mystery; one theory is that he was

TABLE 1.1 Demographics of 292 Homicidal Poisonings in the United States, 1980–1989

Variable	Poisoner	Victim
Age	35% were 20–34 years of age	48% were 20–34 years of age
Motive	Indeterminable in 62% of cases	
Race	58% White 12% Black 30% Other/unknown	83% White 16% Black 1% Other
Relationship	34% of poisoners were related to the victim	
Sex	49% Male 22% Female 29% Unknown	50% Male 50% Female

Data from Westveer AE, Trestrail III JH, Pinizzotto AJ. Homicidal poisonings in the United States: an analysis of the Uniform Crime Reports from 1980 through 1989. *Am J Med Forensic Pathol.* 1996;17:282 (with permission).

disturbed because a communion table donated by his family was not being used. Acquaintances described Bondeson as quiet, friendly, and helpful to parishioners.

CHOICE OF POISONS

The ideal poison for homicides would be lethal in minute quantities, inconspicuous to the victim, slow-acting so as not to arouse suspicion,[1] readily available, difficult to identify through laboratory testing, and similar to natural illness in signs and symptoms. Very few substances match this description. There are certain poisons that have become "classics" (such as arsenic, cyanide, and strychnine) because they have been used by numerous individuals since the 19th century.[8] Over the past few centuries, however, a diverse array of toxins—disguised and distributed in many ways—have been used to attempt or commit murder (Table 1.2).

The Internet has made it easier to gain knowledge about poisonous substances and has provided a realm in which to buy and sell them. In 2005, Cantrell published a study documenting auctions of poisons on eBay.[9] Over a 10-month period, 121 poisonous products were identified. Almost 20% of the products contained ingredients deemed "super toxic," (e.g., arsenic trioxide, cyanide, nicotine, pilocarpine, strychnine) as defined by lethality in oral doses of 5 mg/kg or less. Just over 50% of the products were comprised of "extremely toxic" ingredients (including antimony, arsenates, atropine, inorganic mercury, picrotoxin, scopolamine, soluble barium, and thallium) that would probably cause death if 5–50 mg/kg of the substance were ingested. Many of the product containers were full or partially full. The potency of the ingredients, however, was not tested. This study illustrates that the previous safeguard of a pharmacy log is no longer available; now poisoners can simply buy on the Internet in relative anonymity.

The possible impact that media outlets have on homicidal poisonings should be considered. Television series such as *CSI: Crime Scene Investigation, House, Quincy, M.E., Crossing Jordan, Diagnosis Murder, E.R., Star Trek,* and *Murder, She Wrote* have "educated" viewers about the dangerous effects and homicidal potential of a variety of toxins.[10] Watching television programs that mention poisons also has had an influence on deliberate self-poisonings.[11,12] Individuals

TABLE 1.2 Poisons Used to Attempt or Commit Murder from a Sample of Cases Mentioned in Newspaper Articles Dating from the Mid-19th Century to Present Day

Poisons used	Poisoning victims	Deaths
Arsenic	214	97
Unspecified	139	137
Sodium fluoride	59	47
Brodifacoum	34	0
Cyanide	24	23
Thallium	18	11
Strychnine	16	12
Mercury	5	4
Compound 1081	4	4
Paris green	4	2
Antimony	2	2
Ethylene glycol	3	3
Ricin	2	2
Succinylcholine	2	2
Atropa belladonna	1	0
Dioxin	1	0
Polonium 210	1	1
Quinine	1	1

Note: In this sample of poisons used to attempt or commit murder, 530 individuals were poisoned, and 66% died as a result of the poisoning. An unspecified poison was used in 26% of cases. Newspaper articles dating from the mid-19th century to present day were arbitrarily selected after using the search term "murder by poison" on NewspaperARCHIVE.com, a subscription database that provides access to newspaper stories from more than 2,500 titles in 700 cities over the past 239 years. Almost 170,000 results were obtained using this search strategy; not all of the results were reviewed, and several of the articles that were did not necessarily involve a poison used to attempt or commit murder.

clearly can obtain ideas about poisons and homicidal poisoning from television, but the influence that such programming has on the behavior of viewers requires further evaluation.

INFAMOUS MODERN CRIMINAL POISONERS

Reviewing the details of notable criminal poisoning cases from the past few centuries can provide some insight into poisoners. The cases chosen for discussion are categorized chronologically and were selected on the basis of interest factor, impact on society, or use of a particular poison. The intent of this overview is to emphasize patterns, peculiarities, personalities, or poisons so that medical professionals and investigative law enforcement personnel involved with potential homicidal poisonings have a heightened awareness when dealing with such cases.

19th Century

Dr. Thomas Neill Cream—Strychnine

Although not as infamous as his contemporary Jack the Ripper, Dr. Thomas Neill Cream was one of the most audacious serial killers during 19th century Victorian England.

After graduating in 1876 from McGill University Medical School in Montreal, Quebec, Cream began his career.[13,14] Shortly after graduation, Cream became involved with Flora Brooks, who nearly succumbed to a botched abortion. Cream was forced to marry Brooks on September 11, 1876. The morning after his wedding, however, Cream fled to London where he served as an obstetrical clerk at St. Thomas' Hospital. In Canada, Brooks had become gravely ill; she confided to her doctor that she had been taking medicine sent to her by her husband, and she died mysteriously in August of 1877.

After Brooks's death, Cream moved to London, Ontario to practice medicine and soon another mysterious death occurred. In 1879, the body of Kate Gardener, a pregnant chambermaid, was discovered in a shed behind the doctor's office with a bottle of chloroform beside her. Her cause of death was deemed to be an overdose of chloroform. Cream was considered a suspect in her death. He avoided indictment due to lack of evidence, but his reputation in the community was sullied, and he relocated to Chicago.

Cream set up practice near Chicago's redlight district where he performed abortions and marketed an elixir for epilepsy. He also developed an addiction to morphine and cocaine. Two prostitutes died in 1880 while under Cream's care; Mary Faulkner died from a septic abortion, and Ellen Stack was prescribed pills later discovered to be strychnine. Although authorities were suspicious of Cream, they could not positively link him with the intent to commit murder.

Cream's first conviction for murder occurred in 1881. Daniel Stott believed in the healing powers of Cream's remedy for epilepsy and often sent his attractive wife to pick up the elixir. She and Cream began an affair, and it is believed that when Stott became suspicious of the affair, Cream poisoned him by adding strychnine to the elixir. Stott died in June 1881, and his death was initially attributed to epilepsy. A pharmacist, however, insisted in letters to both the coroner and the district attorney that an exhumation be performed, citing that Cream was responsible for Stott's death. After an exhumation was granted, strychnine was found in Stott's body. Cream was found guilty of second-degree murder and sentenced to life inprisonment in the Illinois State Penitentiary. After less than 10 years, Cream was released from prison on July 31, 1891.

Cream returned to England in October 1891 and posed as a physician, Dr. Thomas Neill, at St. Thomas' Hospital. Soon after his arrival, two prostitutes, Ellen Donworth and Matilda Clover, died in similar manners 1 week apart. Donworth had seizure-like activity, and her autopsy confirmed strychnine poisoning. Clover had experienced the same convulsions and confided on her deathbed that she had been poisoned by a man named "Fred." A postmortem was not initially performed, and Clover's death was attributed to alcoholism; later her body would be exhumed to prove that she had died from strychnine. Another prostitute, Lou Harvey, avoided death by disposing of some pills that a "Dr. Neill" had given her to cure her pale complexion. In April 1892, two more women, Alice Marsh and Emma Shrivell, died within hours of each other, both suffering from convulsions. They had been entertaining a man known as "Fred" who presented himself as a doctor. Before departing their company, he provided each woman with three long, thin pills that they obediently swallowed.

The details leading to Cream's arrest vary, but Cream's arrogance likely gave him away. One account describes how Cream befriended former detective John Haynes who was trying to obtain a position at Scotland Yard. Haynes was impressed by Cream's knowledge of the victims, demonstrated while on a tour of the Clover, Donworth, Marsh, and Shrivell murder sites. Haynes, however, was perplexed by Cream's claims that Clover and Harvey had been murdered because Clover's death was attributed to alcohol and he was unaware of Harvey's death. Haynes contacted a colleague, Inspector Patrick McIntyre of Scotland Yard, who helped spearhead an investigation of Cream. Authorities discovered that Cream had forged documents claiming that he was Thomas Neill. Many prostitutes gave details of being approached by a man fitting Cream's description, and when Harvey was found, she was able to provide incriminating evidence against "Dr. Neill." With evidence mounting, Cream was arrested in June 1892.

Throughout his incarceration and trial, Cream maintained his innocence. Prostitutes who saw him with Clover, however, were able to identify him; a witness recognized him as the man whom Shrivell had let out of her house on the night of her death. Harvey identified him as the man who had tried to make her take capsules. It has been reported that Cream was stoic during his trial except when the bailiff introduced Harvey to the courtroom and he appeared startled. It was proved that Cream had written letters saying that Clover died by strychnine when nobody knew the real etiology of her death. In addition he was found in possession of strychnine. The jury deliberated for only 10 minutes before finding him guilty for the murders of Clover, Donworth, Marsh, and Shrivell. He was sentenced to death and was hanged on November 15, 1892.

20th Century

Nannie Doss—Arsenic

For over 20 years, Nannie Doss concealed her murderous nature with her penchant for romance magazines and "lonely hearts" ads.[15] She was found guilty of poisoning four husbands and her mother, but several other close relatives, including two of her children and a grandson, are thought to have perished at Doss's hands as well.

Nancy "Nannie" Hazle married Charley Braggs in 1921. They raised their four daughters in the rural town of Blue Mountain, Alabama. The marriage was tumultuous; both drank alcohol in excess and were unfaithful. In 1927, two infant daughters died mysteriously within a matter of hours; their deaths were attributed to food poisoning. Relatives and neighbors reportedly said that "there was something funny about the way they died because they turned black so

quick."[16] After their daughters' deaths, Braggs said "when she got mad I wouldn't eat nothing she fixed or drink nothing around the house." They divorced in 1929. Braggs was Doss's only husband who lived.

Doss met Frank Harrelson through a "lonely hearts" ad, and they married in 1929. Their blissful marriage turned sour as Harrelson's fondness for alcohol took precedence. Doss endured Harrelson's drunken brawls and abuse for 16 years. In 1945, at the age of 38, he died writhing in pain. Doss later explained why she put rat poison containing arsenic into his whiskey: "He'd been on a bender all day. He tried to force me to go to bed with him. I decided I'd teach him and I did. I poisoned his rotgut."

Husbands three and four, Arlie Lanning and Richard Morton, and Doss's mother, Loulisa Hazle, met similar fates a few years later. Lanning and Morton's philandering apparently irked Doss. Lanning died suddenly after eating a bowl of prunes and drinking a cup of coffee that Doss had prepared; his last words were, "It must have been the coffee." Loulisa died in 1953, shortly after moving in with Doss and Morton, with debilitating abdominal pains. Several months later, Morton died with symptoms akin to those of Loulisa.

Doss's last husband, Samuel Doss of Tulsa, Oklahoma, was different from the others because he led a relatively ordinary life. Doss, however, soon became frustrated with his frugality, stubbornness, disapproval of her romance magazines, and rules forbidding radio or television. She left Oklahoma and returned to Alabama, but Samuel Doss wooed her back by giving her access to his bank account and by purchasing a life insurance policy with Doss as the beneficiary. In September 1954, Samuel Doss started retching and developed excruciating abdominal pain after eating Doss's prune cake. He was hospitalized and treated for over 3 weeks for a severe gastrointestinal infection. Upon returning home in early October, Doss wasted no time and gave him coffee laced with rat poison. Samuel Doss died on October 6, 1954, from the toxic effects of arsenic.

Because of Samuel Doss's rapid and unexplained death, an autopsy was performed, which showed lethal levels of arsenic in his system. Doss was taken in for questioning but proved to be "difficult" to interrogate. Initially she denied any involvement in Samuel Doss's death and giggled in response to the investigator's questions. Doss's behavior earned her the monikers "The Giggling Granny" and "The Jolly Widow" in the press. After several hours of denial, she relented and admitted to killing Samuel Doss and husbands two, three, and four. The bodies of Harrelson, Lanning, Morton, and Loulisa were exhumed, and all contained significant amounts of arsenic. In 1955, Doss pled guilty to the murder of Samuel Doss and was sentenced to life in prison. While incarcerated, she died in 1965 from leukemia.

David Richard Davis—Succinylcholine

After poisoning his wife of a year, Shannon Mohr, in 1980, David Richard Davis avoided justice for almost a decade by assuming another identity and hiding on a tropical island.[17] Davis thought he had committed a perfect murder and might have gotten away with it had an observant tipster not revealed his whereabouts after seeing a television program profiling the murder of Shannon Mohr.

Davis, a former pharmacology student, had dated Kay Kendall and Jeanne Hohman prior to Mohr. He mentioned to Kendall how succinylcholine would be the perfect murder weapon. Davis wanted to marry Kendall, but the relationship ended in April 1979, around the time he became involved with Hohman. He was quick to discuss marriage with Hohman, but she was hesitant. Before marrying Mohr, Davis confided in Hohman that he was going to perform dangerous work and would be unable to see her for a year. Hohman believed that Davis worked for a government agency.

Davis and Mohr met in August 1979 and were married in Las Vegas on September 24, 1979. In October of that year, the couple purchased life insurance policies. Each policy had a face value of $110,000, named the other person as primary beneficiary, and contained a double indemnity clause for accidental death. A few weeks after his marriage, Davis resumed his relationship with Hohman and told her that the government would pay him about a quarter of a million dollars for his work. In June 1980, Hohman asked Davis how much longer his project would continue; he indicated another month.

On July 23, 1980, Davis and his wife rode horses from their Michigan farm to their neighbor's farm. After visiting their neighbors, the couple headed home and rode through a small wooded section. A half-hour later, Davis rode back to his neighbor's farm; he was soaked with perspiration, had a blood-stained shirt, and exclaimed that his wife had fallen from her horse, was gravely injured by striking her head on a rock, and needed immediate medical attention. Davis and his neighbor drove to the wooded area and found Mohr positioned on the ground with a cyanotic appearance, her shirt undone, and her shoes off. She was transported to a local hospital where she was pronounced dead. At the hospital, Davis stated that Mohr's body would be cremated, but her parents vehemently objected. According to witnesses, Davis informed them shortly after Mohr's death that she had no life insurance, and many people noticed abrasions on Davis's face, which he credited to brushing against tree branches during his horse ride.

About a week after the tragic death, Davis and Hohman departed for Florida. Davis never divulged to Hohman any information pertaining to his marriage or Mohr's death. Hohman flew back to Michigan after a week. In the meantime, Mohr's parents were suspicious of her death because Davis was trying to collect on a $220,000 life insurance policy when previously he had said that no policy existed. Mohr's body was exhumed in August 1980, and an autopsy was performed. A comprehensive drug screen was performed on tissue samples and demonstrated a significant unidentifiable peak on gas chromatography. Sergeant Dan Brooks from the Michigan State Police who was investigating Mohr's death theorized that she had been chemically paralyzed prior to death. A cousin of Mohr's testified that in the summer of 1980 she had visited Mohr's farm and noticed about 12 syringes fastened together in the refrigerator and several bottles labeled Anectine, the trade name for succinylcholine, in the freezer.

When Sergeant Brooks suggested the possibility of succinylcholine as a possible murder weapon, the toxicologists were skeptical because the pharmacologic properties of the compound make it difficult to detect. To eliminate succinylcholine as a possibility for producing the unknown peak, the toxicologists tested succinylcholine on the gas chromatographer and found that it was an identical match with the peak. Another autopsy was performed that revealed multiple contusions and an injection site. Large concentrations of succinylcholine were detected in tissues surrounding the contusions.

In October 1981, Davis was indicted for the murder of Shannon Mohr. At that time, he had last been seen in Haiti. His whereabouts remained unknown until an anonymous viewer of *Unsolved Mysteries* contacted police in December 1988. In January 1989, Mohr was arrested in Pago Pago, American Samoa, where he was using the alias David Myer Bell, posing as a doctor, nurse, and harpsichord player. Davis was extradited to Michigan where he stood trial and was found guilty of first-degree murder. He is now serving a life sentence without the possibility of parole in a federal prison in Michigan.

The Tylenol Tamperer—Cyanide

On September 29, 1982, four people died in Chicago within moments after ingesting a commonly used over-the-counter analgesic, Extra Strength Tylenol.[6, 18, 19] The first victim was 12-year-old Mary Kellerman who had taken the medication to help relieve her sore throat. A few hours later in a nearby suburb, a young postal worker, Adam Janus, took Tylenol for chest discomfort, collapsed, had a seizure, and died. His family gathered that evening to mourn. His wife, Theresa, and brother, Stanley, complained of headaches and took Tylenol from a bottle on the kitchen counter. Within minutes, both collapsed and later died. Officials linked the deaths to Tylenol after two firefighters, discussing the day's unfortunate events, recalled that paramedics had indicated that all of the victims had taken the analgesic. Tests performed the following day found that the capsules—all from lot number MC 2880—had been laced with potassium cyanide. By October 1, Tylenol tainted with cyanide would claim the lives of three more Chicago-area residents, Mary McFarland, Mary Reiner, and Paula Prince.

A large-scale investigation was launched across the Chicago metropolitan area in an attempt to determine the source of contamination. Poison centers nationwide were flooded by panic-stricken callers as officials warned against the use of Tylenol. Days after the poisonings, McNeil Consumer Products issued a nationwide recall of Tylenol products and offered a $100,000 reward for information leading to the arrest and conviction of whoever was responsible. Shortly after the poisoning murders, officials at Johnson & Johnson, the parent company of McNeil Consumer Products, received a handwritten letter demanding $1,000,000. The letter was linked to James Lewis who was later arrested and convicted of extortion but not the deaths. To date, the poisoner(s) who killed seven innocent individuals remains unknown and at large.

In November 1982, Johnson & Johnson reintroduced Tylenol with tamper-resistant packaging and launched an aggressive "Trust Tylenol" campaign. The homicidal poisonings that occurred over a 3-day period had a significant impact on consumer confidence in nonprescription medication safety and changed the way consumer products are packaged in the United States.[20] As a result of the tragedy, Congress passed the Federal Anti-Tampering Act in 1983, which made tampering with consumer products a federal offense; the pharmaceutical industry shifted away from capsules, which are easier to contaminate; and the Food and Drug Administration introduced regulations requiring that most over-the-counter products have tamper-resistant packaging.

Julia Lynn Womack—Ethylene Glycol

Maurice Glenn Turner married Julia Lynn Womack in 1993, and prior to their marriage, he named her the beneficiary of both his life insurance policy and retirement accounts.[21] Soon after they married in Georgia, Womack began an affair with Randy Thompson. Turner became ill in March 1995 and went to the emergency department complaining of nausea and vomiting; he was treated with intravenous fluids and discharged. Womack fed him Jell-O in the morning and found him dead in bed that afternoon. The medical examiner determined Turner's death was from natural causes due to a cardiac dysrhythmia. He was buried on March 6, 1995; Womack collected over $150,000 in death benefits and moved in with Thompson less than a week after his burial.

Over the next few years, Womack and Thompson were seemingly happy and had two children. In 1998, Randy increased his life insurance coverage to $200,000 after the birth of his son. Womack was a prodigal spender, which caused their relationship to deteriorate. After Thompson moved out, he remained in contact with Womack. After having dinner with her, Thompson developed nausea, vomiting, and disorientation on January 20, 2001. He was treated at the hospital with intravenous fluids, released, and died at home the following day. Of note, Womack fed Thompson Jell-O the day he was released from the hospital. The medical examiner determined that his cause of death was a cardiac dysrhythmia. Womack collected $36,000 in benefits.

Turner's mother knew something was amiss when she read about Thompson's death. She contacted his mother, and they brought the similarities of the two cases to the deputy chief medical examiner of the Georgia Bureau of Investigation. Upon autopsy, calcium oxalate crystals were discovered in Thompson's kidneys, but blood and urine tests performed by the Georgia State crime lab were negative for ethylene glycol. The deputy chief medical examiner sent findings to an independent laboratory, which confirmed his suspicions: Levels of ethylene glycol were elevated in Thompson's blood and tissues. The technician who performed the initial tests later testified that he had made a mathematical error in determining the presence of ethylene glycol.[22] Turner's remains were exhumed and were found to have ethylene glycol. With this new forensic evidence, the medical examiner changed the causes of death for both men to ethylene glycol poisoning.

Womack was indicted for the murder of her husband and stood trial in 2004. During her trial, damaging testimony was heard from several witnesses. Turner's close friend testified that Turner had told him 2 months before his death that if anything happened to him "to look at Lynn." A nurse who cared for Turner in the emergency department described how Womack seemed unconcerned about her husband. An insurance agent recalled how persistent Womack was in having herself named the beneficiary on Turner's life insurance policy. An employee from an animal shelter testified that 4 years after Turner's death Womack had inquired about the effects of antifreeze on cats. On May 14, 2004, Womack remained emotionless as the jury read the verdict: guilty of malice murder with life imprisonment.[23] Womack maintains her innocence, and prosecutors are currently seeking the death penalty.[24]

21st Century
Poisoning of a Ukrainian Presidential Candidate—Dioxin

Poisoners have become more sophisticated in their choice of weapon by selecting esoteric or infrequently used toxins, making detection and diagnosis difficult. But history has a way of repeating itself, and like many before him, Viktor Yushchenko was poisoned for political reasons. Because the toxin used on Yushchenko has been used so rarely, it was difficult for healthcare providers to diagnose his condition until telltale signs from his exposure occurred. Sophisticated testing later confirmed their suspicions.[25]

In September 2004, Yushchenko, Ukraine's oppositional presidential candidate, fell ill after attending a dinner with Ukrainian security officials. His wife reported that when he returned from the dinner, she "kissed him as usual and tasted something medicinal on [her] lips."[26] Yushchenko was admitted to an Austrian hospital. He later developed chloracne. Although Yushchenko survived, the etiology of his illness remained a mystery. Subsequent tests confirmed that he had been exposed to a potent dioxin—TCDD (2,3,7,8-tetrachlorodibenzo-*p*-dioxin).[27] His dioxin levels were reported to be more than 6000 times higher than what would be expected in a normal human sample.[28] No individual has been formally prosecuted for the poisoning; however, Yushchenko blames his attempted murder on supporters of his Kremlin-backed opponent, Prime Minister Viktor Yanukovych. After his poisoning diagnosis in December 2004, Yuschenko defeated Yanukovych in a runoff election.

The Toxic Teacup—Polonium 210

On November 23, 2006, Alexander Litvinenko, a former officer in Russia's Federal Security Service, became the first known person in history to be murdered with polonium 210.[29] Litvinenko became ill on November 1, 2006, after meeting with Andrei Lugovoi and other associates at a hotel bar in London. He was hospitalized and developed alopecia, bone marrow suppression, and gastrointestinal symptoms. As Litvinenko lay dying, tests to detect a toxicologic etiology were unrevealing; early tests demonstrated the presence of thallium, but not in quantities typically associated with toxicity. Authorities sent a sample of Litvinenko's urine to a laboratory with special equipment that detected a large quantity of alpha particles, a type of radiation. Postmortem analysis of Litvinenko's tissues demonstrated significant levels of polonium 210.

While on his deathbed, Litvinenko accused Lugovoi of poisoning him and Vladimir Putin of ordering his death. Both denied involvement. The hotel rooms where Lugovoi had stayed prior to meeting with Litvinenko, however, were contaminated with polonium 210 as was the aircraft that he had traveled on. Litvinenko's colleagues maintain that the tea he drank during his meeting with Lugovoi was laced with the deadly isotope.[30,31]

CONCLUSION: WHAT WE HAVE LEARNED

Poisoning continues to be an unusual but effective way to commit murder. The cases discussed illustrate that poisoners can use many substances, from mundane to unusual, as a means to harm or kill their victim(s). Although this chapter has only provided a brief overview of criminal poisonings, knowledge of those cases and others will help investigators and healthcare providers recognize and better comprehend future cases. Unfortunately, there is little that can be done to predict with any certainty who will become a poisoner because each killer is unique in terms of motive, choice of poison, and victim(s).

REFERENCES

1. Moog FP, Karenberg A. Toxicology in the Old Testament. *Adv Drug React Toxicol Rev.* 2002; 21:151–156.
2. Watson K. Medical and chemical expertise in English trials for criminal poisoning, 1750-1914. *Med Hist.* 2006;50:373–390.
3. Westveer AE, Trestrail JH III, Pinizzotto AJ. Homicidal poisonings in the United States: an analysis of the Uniform Crime Reports from 1980 through 1989. *Am J Forensic Med Pathol.* 1996;17:282–288.
4. Westveer AE, Jarvis JP, Jensen CJ III. Homicidal poisoning: the silent offense. *FBI Law Enforcement Bull.* August 2004:1–8.
5. Furbee RB. Criminal poisoning: medical murderers. *Clin Lab Med.* 2006;26(1):255–273.
6. Dunea G. Death over the counter. *BMJ.* 1983; 286: 211–212.
7. Alexander M. The killer among us. *Reader's Digest.* January 2004:98–104.
8. Blyth AW. *Poisons: Their Effects and Detection.* New York: William Wood; 1885:134–136.
9. Cantrell FL. Look what I found! Poison hunting on eBay. *Clin Toxicol.* 2005;43:375–379.
10. Chyka PA, Banner W. The history of poisoning in the future: lessons from *Star Trek. J Toxicol Clin Toxicol.* 1999;38:793–799.
11. Krishnakumar P, Geeta MG, Gopalan AV. Deliberate self-poisoning in children. *Indian Pediatr.* 2005; 42:582–586.
12. Hawton K, Simkin S, Deeks JJ, et al. Effects of a drug overdose in a television drama on presentations to hospital for self poisoning: time series and questionnaire study. *BMJ.* 1999;318:972–977.
13. Pearson EL. Doctor Cream. In: Jones RG, ed. *Poison! The World's Greatest True Murder Stories.* Secaucus, New Jersey: Lyle Stuart Inc; 1987;143–149.
14. Geringer J. Dr. Thomas Neill Cream. Serial killers: killers from history. In: Bardsley M, ed. *Crime Library.* Court TV; 2007.
15. Geringer J. Nannie Doss: Lonely hearts lady loved her man to death. Serial killers: killers from history. In: Bardsley M, ed. *Crime Library.* Court TV; 2007.
16. International News Service. Murder charged to 4-time widow. *The Charleston Gazette.* November 30, 1954:17.
17. *State of Michigan v David Richard Davis.* Docket Nos. 132398, 138005. Court of Appeals of Michigan; Submitted January 6, 1993. Decided May 3, 1993.
18. Malcolm AH. 100 agents hunt for killer in 7 Tylenol deaths. *New York Times.* October 3, 1982:1–2
19. Tifft S, Griggs L. Poison madness in the Midwest. *Time Magazine.* October 11, 1982: 1–2.
20. Murphy DH. Cyanide-tainted Tylenol: what pharmacists can learn. *Am Pharm.* 1986;S26:19–23.
21. Ramsland K. Forensic toxicology. Criminal mind: forensics & investigation. In: Bardsley M, ed. *Crime Library.* Court TV; 2007.
22. Sweetingham L. Expert: second dose of poison killed firefighter [transcript]. Court TV; May 13, 2004.
23. Sweetingham L. Wife found guilty of killing husband with antifreeze [transcript]. Court TV; May 14, 2004.
24. Associated Press. Lawyer seeks death for woman who poisoned husband with antifreeze [transcript]. Court TV; December 7, 2004.
25. Rosenthal E. Liberal leader from Ukraine was poisoned. *International Herald Tribune.* New York Times Company. December 12, 2004.
26. Stoyanova-Yerburgh Z. Who poisoned Yushchenko? *Worldpress.org.* December 13, 2004.
27. Yushchenko poisoned by most harmful type of dioxin [transcript]. *CBC News.* CBC television. December 17, 2004.
28. Yuschenko dioxin levels off charts. CBS News. CBS television. December 15, 2004.
29. McAllister JFO. The spy who knew too much. *Time Magazine.* December 18, 2006:30–38.
30. Cowell A, Myers SL. Britain charges Russian in poisoning case. *New York Times.* May 22, 2007.
31. Spy death: Russia blocks handover. *CNN.com.* CNN. May 22, 2007.

2 | Poisoners and Their Relationship with Victims: The Need for an Evidence-Based Understanding

Gregory B. Saathoff

To cook a cake quite large
and fill each layer in between
with icing mixed with poison
til it turns a tempting green

(icing mixed with poison
til it turns a tempting green)

we'll place it near the house
just where the boys are sure to come
and being greedy they won't care to
question such a plum

(the boys who have no mother sweet)
no one to show them their mistake
(won't know it's dangerous to eat)
so damp and rich a cake—

and so before the winking of an eye
those boys will eat that poison cake
and one by one they'll die—

(they'll die, they'll die, they'll die,
they'll die, they'll die! olé!)

—Captain Hook (and pirates)[1]

INTRODUCTION

In the last half of the 20th century, any American with a television had an opportunity to see and hear Cyril Ritchard as Captain Hook in the televised stage version of *Peter Pan*. Through YouTube, one can reexperience Hook's morbid tango. Although the production is dated and rarely shown, the underlying themes are as meaningful as when it first aired in 1960. Superficially, the portrayal succeeds in part because it is deliberately exaggerated. On a deeper level, however, some essential truths about those who choose to kill with poison are revealed: Poisoners often have dual roles in the life of a victim, thereby masking their intent. For them, the plan is critical to the process—a way to make murderous fantasy operational. Poisoners succeed when they exploit their victims' trust and naïveté. Therefore, a discussion of Hook serves as a good entry to this chapter on the psychology of poisoning.

In the televised production of *Peter Pan*, Ritchard plays two roles: the protective father and the dastardly pirate Hook. Although these roles are markedly different, they share at least one similarity—they both maintain power over the lives of others. Even his choice of song reveals the dyadic nature of the act of poisoning. Just as the tango is a dance of love and passion, the deliberate process of poisoning is often one of intimacy and obsession. Capitalizing on the vulnerabilities of his victims, Hook details a plot that has the precision of a blueprint. The cunning plan itself is clearly half the fun.

To be most effective, the plan requires a degree of anonymity. Although the victims often know their poisoners, they do not know the poisoner's plan. Thus, the true nature of the poisoner and poison remains concealed. Unlike a crime of passion, this crime is one of stealth, as calculated as it is cowardly. Rather than confronting the victim, most poisoners distance themselves by duping their prey. The vehicle for the poison—whether it is food, drink, or medication—serves as a Trojan horse. Once the victim discovers the attack, it is often too late.

The only thing easier than taking candy from a baby is giving candy to a baby. Poisoners know this and, whenever possible, seek to exploit an existing relationship of trust. In addition to his almost obsessive attention to detail, Hook takes special pleasure in the fact that the children themselves will unwittingly be the instruments of their own deaths. Trust is the vulnerable point of entry for most successful poisonings.

Perhaps less clear from this example, but of vital importance, is the actual poison chosen. Those poisons that occur in nature are easily accessible to the general public. Their administration does not require the stealth, intelligence, expertise, and skills of a poisoner who resorts to rare and difficult-to-obtain poisons. Depending upon the poison, its successful administration requires a greater or lesser combination of abilities, including meticulous planning, patience, experience, and often fine motor skills. For each poisoner, murderous fantasy must be matched by capability; fantasy alone is insufficient for a successful poisoning.

BACKGROUND ON POISONERS

Poisoners are a compelling group of criminals because their relationships to their victims are often complex. One need only read Shakespeare's *Hamlet* to see the myriad ways that poison can be used to provoke and enact revenge.[2] The crime of poisoning is at the same time intimate (in that the victim ingests and incorporates the weapon) and distant (in that the assailant may never even touch the victim or even be seen near the poison). In fact, the victim may die while seeking solace from a perpetrator who feigns concern, even to the point of assuming the role of caretaker. If there were Academy Awards for compelling criminal theatrics, successful poisoners would likely receive a large number of nominations.

Compelling mythical and real stories present problems for forensic science because disparate narratives, no matter how dramatic, are also anecdotal. Consider the difficulty in extracting meaningful conclusions from these wide and varied poisoning cases: Michael Swango, the physician who poisoned his patients[3]; Ronald Clark O'Bryan, who poisoned his own son for insurance money[4]; Nannie Doss, who murdered four husbands and six others[5]; the Nazi-obsessed British teenager Graham Young, who poisoned family members and coworkers[6]; the umbrella-wielding enemy who injected Georgi Markov with ricin[7]; or even James Lewis, who was convicted of writing the extortion letter for the 1982 Tylenol killings.[8] Like the Tylenol cyanide poisonings, poisoners and poisonings can inspire copycat crimes that are just as deadly as the originals.[9,10]

As demonstrated by these cases, it is clear that no single profile exists for those who poison or are poisoned. With countless poisons, cultures, personality types, and motives, an investigator can feel overwhelmed when faced with a poisoning case. There are, however, aspects of criminal poisonings that can inform the investigative process.

Poisoning requires stealth and secrecy. The poisoner observes the victim and may even titrate dosing unbeknownst to the victim. Poisonings, in fact, share similarities with bombings in that material must be procured, prepared, transported, and delivered. The victim's ingestion of poison is just the final step, like the lighting of a fuse.

There are also striking differences between a poisoning and a bombing. In a bombing, the crime scenes are clearly the sites of assembly and the explosion. In contrast, a poisoning crime scene is ultimately the human body, a moving target both physically and physiologically. While most explosions are easily recognized as unnatural events, illness and death are commonplace, making it difficult to discriminate between the symptoms of those who are poisoned and those who are ill from natural causes. A bomb explosion is readily identifiable for all who witness it; in contrast, even highly trained experts may disagree as to whether a poisoning has occurred. The victim may even be unsure as to whether symptoms originated naturally or not. For all of these reasons, poisonings can be the most difficult crimes to investigate.

A poisoner's stealth not only minimizes the opportunity to examine the crime, but if undetected, also limits the potential for that particular poison to be included in any research. Compared to other homicides, quantitative and even qualitative research in poisoning are limited. The investigator is often left with single case reports and narrative literature that limits an evidence-based approach to the process.

Poison is a multipurpose tool that can accomplish goals related to different motivations. Although the ultimate goal can be death of the victim, poisons can also be designed to disable, as in the case of chronic poisoning, or temporarily impair, as in the case of a "date-rape" drug. Whether the poisoner is motivated by financial gain, political ambition, jealousy, lust, revenge, or delusion, the ultimate method requires control of the poison and usually prediction of the behavior of the victim. What makes poisons unique is that they are tools that require control over time. Control, therefore, is central to understanding the poisoner and his or her environment.

What then of the random poisoner who engages in product tampering? Douglas and Olshaker liken random poisoners to the person who throws rocks from an overpass onto cars below.[11] Such a person is more concerned with acting out anger than targeting a particular type of victim. While the motive can be financial, such crimes terrorize in a way that gains notoriety. As more terror is created in the community, the poisoner's sense of omnipotence increases.

CHARACTERISTICS OF THE POISONER AND VICTIM

As noted previously, compelling stories of poisoners and their victims can inspire others' creativity, in literature and within the minds of future poisoners. While often dramatic, they are of limited value to professionals who seek to understand the forest that is forensic toxicology (and not the "trees" represented by the individual poisoning cases). Retrospective in nature, the content of these cases is often presented without systematic comparison. Today's mobile society, with its global delivery networks, offers increased and more accessible information to more people. As a result, there is a larger web of poisoners who now have the actual capability to perpetrate their crime.

Existing literature has provided myriad personality characteristics of poisoners. Rowland describes poisoners typically as being vain, spoiled, unsympathetic, unimaginative, and often connected with the medical community.[12] Perhaps not surprisingly, such people were also found to have unhappy marriages. In contrast, Wilson describes poisoners as artistic daydreamers who could also be cowardly and avaricious.[13]

Why is empirical research rare in this field? An obvious explanation is that these crimes are prosecuted infrequently, whether because of the rarity of the events or because of the difficulty of detection. While firearms, knives, and blunt objects are the most common homicidal weapons, poison is one of the least common, ranked with drowning, arson, and explosives.[14] The low reported frequency of poisoning clearly does not reflect actual poisonings that masquerade as natural death. As a consequence, statistics underestimate the actual prevalence of the crime.

Empirical study of poisoners requires data collection where poisoning agents are reported as a cause of death. These data can be found in the Uniform Crime Reporting (UCR)

Supplementary Homicide Reports (SHR).[14, 16] A review of reported poisonings from 1980 to 2000 reveals a 35% increase in the rate that these cases were referred to law enforcement.[16]

There is often a dyadic nature in poisoning that indicates a relationship between offender and victim. Notably, offender characteristics are dictated in part by the characteristics of the victims. Therefore, when considering the profile of the poisoner, the demographic characteristics of the victim are useful. Unfortunately, much more is known about victims than poisoners. Almost 20% of verified poisonings are perpetrated by offenders who have eluded detection. Other homicidal victims, by contrast, are likely to be linked with known offenders. This distinction is in large part due to the dearth of witnesses in the often covert crime of poisoning. Westveer et al.[14] note that when victims are female, offenders are predominately male. In contrast, male victims are poisoned by either males or females in equal percentages.

Gender is not the only determinant in the relationship. Race has historically been a factor, as poisoners rarely cross racial lines. Whites are predominately the victims of male offenders, while African Americans are equally poisoned by male and female offenders. When looking at other characteristics, Westveer and his colleagues[16] found that in the 1990s victims ranged in age from a single victim less than 1 week old to 13 victims 75 years or older. More than one-third of the victims ranged in age from 24 to 44 years. Notably, poisoners are usually somewhat younger than their victims, ranging, on average, from 20 to 34 years of age with victims who were 5 to 10 years older. In general, victims were divided similarly between males and females. In addition, 75% of victims were poisoned with drugs or narcotics, and almost two-thirds of these victims were poisoned by someone who was not a family member.

In a more recent study, Shepherd and Ferslew examined more than 500 poisoning deaths from 1999 through 2005.[15] A total of 523 homicidal poisoning deaths were identified. Males were significantly more likely to be victims than females. In their study, death was more likely at extremes of age, and medications were the most common type of poison. They also noted a geographic disparity, with increased rates in the western compared to the northeastern United States.

Because these crimes are often undiscovered initially, poisoners can be emboldened to commit more and more poisonings. For serial poisoners, each success increases confidence that they can commit another undetected murder. When the crimes are undetected, there is an opportunity to gain even more intimacy with the victim by acting as caregiver. The victim is not only injured but also continues to be invaded psychologically through intimate duplicity. Power and control are paramount, and when poisonings are undetected, those attributes are fueled by continued successes.

For those who are narcissistic and easily wounded, fantasies of revenge can be fulfilled by poisoning—a silent weapon that can be used at a precise time. This method is similar to serial bombers who collect grievances and exact revenge on their own timetables. Poisoners and bombers are capable of exacting revenge while maintaining a veneer of passivity.

Although biologic weapons such as the human immunodeficiency virus, anthrax, and smallpox are distinct from poisons, it can be useful to consider the person who poisons in conjunction with the person who uses biologic attacks. In my work, I have interviewed prisoners who have been convicted for using their human immunodeficiency virus as a purposeful weapon against others. Like many poisoners, these biologic attackers exploit intimacy to exact revenge and fulfill fantasies of rage. In doing so, they are able to transform themselves psychologically from a state of illness to omnipotence. It is striking that some of these perpetrators fantasize about and are equally comfortable with the use of poison and biologic weapons. Preliminary understanding would suggest that people who attack with poisons or biologic weapons have psychological similarities. After all, the road of stealth, intimacy, and duplicity leads to the same final destination—the human body.

THE FUTURE POISONER

How will poisoning be shaped over time? What can be said of the future poisoner? If the past is any guide, we know that dramatic developments in information, transportation, communication, medicine, and technology will be paralleled by an evolution of criminality and investigative processes. As a consequence, the successful poisoner will integrate these changes to his or her advantage. As noted earlier, greater mobility within society, delivery networks, education, and information accessibility have increased total numbers, diversity, and capabilities of poisoners. Investigators will need to be increasingly open to considering a variety of suspects who span a range of ages and backgrounds.

In addition to the availability of searchable information, transportation is remarkably easy, as seen in the flow of illegal drugs from country to country. By merging national boundaries through the European Union, the governments of Europe have encouraged not only the free flow of commerce but also the greater flow of criminals and their resources.

Transportation infrastructure has advanced, and with it, our ability to track movement. While poisoners of the past were limited in their ability to monitor their victims before and after the crime, our expanding surveillance culture can provide sophisticated, real-time information in the form of video monitoring and even tracking devices. As a consequence, technology will expand our concept of poisoning as well as our definition of these crimes.

Physicians have been implicated in poisoning over the centuries. Perhaps the most concerning was the recent case of Dr. Harold Shipman in the United Kingdom.[17] As medical knowledge becomes more accessible and prescription medications more available from international sources, there will likely be a corresponding increase in poisonings by individuals in nonmedical fields relative to medical fields. Although the medical and paramedical environment will always attract some who are prone to poisoning, available medical information should serve to "level the playing field" for those poisoners who have not had the benefit of medical training.

THE FUTURE VICTIM

The Internet is a friend to poisoner and victim alike. The public is much more knowledgeable about medications and medical help. Adding to this, the pharmaceutical industry has developed a direct connection with consumers through sophisticated marketing. Health sites have proliferated on the Internet, circumventing the informational role that doctors played in the past. Greater public access to drug information and symptom description may promote

greater awareness. It is difficult to know whether federal laws such as the Health Insurance Portability and Accountability Act of 1996 have had an effect, positive or negative, on the process of poisoning. We do know that it increases confidentiality by limiting the sharing of information regarding symptoms and diagnoses, arguably limiting the ability for patterns to readily emerge. On the other hand, the poisoner who previously could call a hospital anonymously or casually inquire about the health of a stricken colleague is now forced to reveal an interest that ultimately betrays his or her real intent.

THE RELATIONSHIP OF POISONING AND CYBER CRIME

Access to information via the Internet is perhaps the most profound change affecting both poisoners and those who investigate poisoning; thus it creates a conundrum. The Internet can be both the solution and the problem, as in a recent heavily publicized case in which traces of chloroform were reportedly discovered in the trunk of the suspect's car, along with DNA evidence of the suspect's missing child. While certainly suspicious, this evidence became highly relevant after investigators examined the hard drive of the suspect's computer, revealing evidence that an Internet search using the word "chloroform" had been completed shortly before the disappearance of the child.[18] In this way, ready availability of searchable information is critical not only for the commission of a crime but can also be a clue to its solution. In parallel to this, access to increased information also facilitates a greater availability of many toxins, particularly those that are used in the development and manufacture of products.

To the extent that poisoners are patiently obsessive, the increased availability of information will provide even greater access to the myriad ways that poisoning can be accomplished. In an age when al Qaeda manuals are accessible to all, the process of poisoning can be examined throughout the supply chain. Importantly, we know much more about poisons than the individuals who use them. Despite the diagnostic wonders of science, we learn from the Internet and mainstream media that poisons ranging from dioxin to polonium may leave few fingerprints. The unsolved case provides a welcome "teachable moment" for any potential poisoner.

It is clear that current and expanding Internet capabilities provide a ready means for a poisoner to "name his poison" through research of instruments. What may be less clear is that the Internet will continue to challenge our concept of poisoning in another way, providing an opportunity to meet and identify those who may ultimately become future victims. The extraordinary revolution in social networks allows a poisoner in one country to survey the field to identify and befriend a future unsuspecting victim in another country. The Internet allows this poisoner to possess expertise in poisons and to shape relationships with unsuspecting victims.

While physical appearance, personal characteristics, and traditional interpersonal abilities were once necessary for poisoners to form intimate relationships with their victims, the Internet environment is tailor-made for poisoners who value stealth and duplicity. An obvious example would be the poisoner who harbors fantasies of exacting revenge against a former lover or superior. Even though the future victim moves away and establishes a new life in a different place, social networking sites provide the opportunity to reacquaint the predator with his or her prey.

CONCLUSION

Poisoners are often strongly identified with their victims. Because there is no single profile of the poisoner, we can understand these individuals better when we look at the company they keep, including the victim(s) and even the poison. Narrative histories reveal a rogue's gallery of killers but are limited in their ability to provide the investigator with a conceptual framework to narrow the forensic investigation. Empiric research, such as that made possible by the Uniform Crime Reports, complements and even trumps the narrative approach; it is absolutely necessary for any real understanding of these offenders as a group.

As the face of society changes, so does the face of the poisoner. This person is more likely to conduct research on the Internet, which can also leave electronic fingerprints. As medical information and prescription medications from international resources become more available for the nonmedical public, the percentage of these nonmedical poisoners will likely grow. Although there are a limited number of cases of biologic attack, there are similarities in the personalities of perpetrators who use biology and toxicology as a means of gaining power over victims.

REFERENCES

1. Donehue, V [director]. *Peter Pan.* Music Charlap and Leigh. National Broadcasting Company; 1960.
2. Shakespeare W. *Hamlet.* New York: Bantam; 1980.
3. Stewart JB. *Blind Eye: How the Medical Establishment Let a Doctor Get Away with Murder.* New York: Simon & Schuster; 1999.
4. Babineck M. O'Bryan's deed haunts Halloween. *Laredo Morning Times.* October 31, 1999:7A.
5. Manners T. *Deadlier Than the Male.* London: Pan Books; 1995.
6. Bowden P. Graham Young (1947-90): The St. Albans poisoner: his life and times. *Crim Behav Ment Health.* 1996;6:17.
7. Crompton R, Gall D. Georgi Markov—death in a pellet. *Med Leg J.* 1980;48(2):51–62.
8. Saltzman J. Fatal tampering case is renewed. *Boston Globe.* February 5, 2009.
9. Ruling on Japan poison-diary girl [transcript]. *BBC News.* BBC. May 1, 2006.
10. Varnell RM, Stimac GK, Fligner CL. CT diagnosis of toxic brain injury in cyanide poisoning: considerations for forensic medicine. *Am J Neuroradiol.* 1987;8(6):1063–1066.
11. Douglas J, Olshaker M. *Mindhunter: Inside the FBI's Elite Serial Crime Unit.* New York: Scribner; 1995.
12. Rowland J. *Poisoner in the Dock.* London: Arco; 1960:230–237.
13. Wilson C. *The Mammoth Book of True Crime.* New York: Carroll Graf; 1988:476–484.
14. Westveer AE, Trestrail JH, Pinizzotto AJ. Homicidal poisonings in the United States: an analysis of the Uniform Crime Reports from 1980 through 1989. *Am J Forensic Med Pathol.* 1996:17(4);282–288.
15. Shepherd G, Ferslew BC. Homicidal poisoning deaths in the United States 1999-2005. *Clinical Toxicol.* 2009;47(4):342–347.
16. Westveer AE, Jarvis JP, Jensen CJ. Homicidal poisonings: the silent offense. *FBI Law Enforcement Bull.* August 2004:1–8.
17. Kinnell, H. Serial homicide by doctors: Shipman in perspective. *BMJ.* 2000;321:1594.
18. Caylee Anthony. *OrlandoSentinel.com.* http://www.orlandosentinel.com/topic/crime-law-justice/crimes/crime-victims/caylee-anthony-PECLB004332.topic. Accessed January 21, 2009.

3 | Evaluating a Potential Criminal Poisoning

Thomas M. Neer

CASE STUDY

A 62-year-old man arrived at a local hospital emergency department with dehydration, hypotension (74/60 mm Hg), diarrhea, and vomiting. The cause of his distress was not immediately determined. Laboratory tests revealed abnormal liver function, metabolic acidosis, elevated bilirubin, and low platelet count. As his condition worsened, his personal physician (who had treated him and followed similar symptoms and numerous hospitalizations for several years) advised the hospital that a test conducted the previous summer had revealed the presence of arsenic. This revelation came a day before the man expired. Although the man's wife initially refused to authorize an autopsy, with encouragement she eventually relented, and an examination revealed high concentrations of arsenic and multiple organ failure.

A police investigation ensued, and an exhumation of the decedent confirmed arsenic poisoning. Evidence implicated his wife: she had been married on four previous occasions; she had an acrimonious relationship with her husband and his family; she had isolated her husband from his family, thus making herself the sole preparer of his food; she had persuaded him to name her as sole beneficiary of his estate; and she gave neighbors conflicting explanations of the toxicologic findings of arsenic. Investigation showed that when the decedent was hospitalized with similar symptoms, the hospital informed his wife that lab results showed high levels of arsenic. When she was unable to account for this finding, the hospital decided that the lab had made a mistake. The hospital asked the wife to bring in a new urine specimen from her husband, which was found to be normal at that time.

Police could never locate the source of the arsenic used nor prove that the wife had access to it, but rat poison containing arsenic could have been purchased locally. A trial was held based on the findings of medical experts and on compelling circumstantial evidence. Prosecution and defense experts, however, disagreed over whether the death resulted from Guillain-Barré syndrome or chronic arsenic poisoning. They also disagreed as to whether the decedent was suicidal. Citing these disagreements and the absence of specific evidence against the wife, the court issued a directed verdict of not guilty.[1]

Whether or not the decedent's wife got away with murder, this case highlights the difficulty of detecting and proving homicides by poisoning and underscores the need for collaboration among police, toxicologists, pathologists, mental health professionals and prosecutors.

HISTORY

Since ancient times, people have used poisons such as arsenic, strychnine, and antimony to kill enemies, competitors, and even family members. Motives for poisoning others were personal (e.g., anger, jealousy, revenge), financial, and political. The frequency with which poisonings occurred was due not only to the availability of toxic substances, but also to the ease with which they could be administered. Toxicology was in its infancy, so fear of detection and prosecution was minimal. Because everyone must eat, food became a natural medium through which poisons were often dispensed, and because women had the primary responsibility for meal preparation, they perpetrated many of these misdeeds either for personal reasons or on behalf of others. So frequent were murders of this type that members of royal families often employed food tasters to sample their dishes.

Today, homicidal poisonings occur for many of the same reasons as in the past but have become less common as methods to detect poisons improve and as perpetrators are increasingly brought to justice. Despite this progress, or perhaps because of it, criminal poisoning has evolved. There are instances of poisoning in cases of child abuse, product tampering, and drug-facilitated sexual assaults. Detecting and proving criminal poisoning remains a considerable challenge, but as healthcare professionals and police share information, there is a greater chance for successful resolution.[2]

DEFINITION

The Centers for Disease Control and Prevention (CDC) defines a poison as any substance harmful to bodies when ingested, inhaled, or absorbed.[3] Almost any substance, including salt and water, can be lethal if introduced into a body in high concentrations. A major premise in the field of toxicology is that dose determines toxicity. For example, most people have small concentrations of toxins such as lead in their bodies, but these do not cause clinically significant damage unless the concentration reaches a specific level.[4] When a criminal poisoning is suspected, it is the responsibility of the toxicologist to identify the poison involved and to demonstrate that its concentration was sufficient to cause death.

CLASSIFICATION

The CDC maintains a comprehensive database of diseases and injuries, including poisonings. They classify poisonings as either *intentional* (excessive use of drugs or chemicals for recreational purposes or purposely taking/giving substances to cause harm) or *unintentional* (excessive use of drugs, chemicals, medications, or nonmedicinal substances for nonrecreational purposes).[3,5-9]

AVAILABILITY OF POISONS

Poisons are readily available. For example, in most homes there are ample numbers of medications and herbal remedies that, when used in high doses or mixed with other substances, can become lethal. Kitchens, bathrooms, and garages usually contain products that contain potential poisons, including disinfectants, sanitizers, pesticides, rodenticides, and various other chemicals. All of these products contain potentially toxic substances that when ingested, inhaled, or absorbed under the right circumstances can cause serious injury or death.[10] The ease of availability of toxins is highlighted by the CDC when, in 2006, they reported 32,691 poisoning deaths in the United States. Of these, 18% were determined to be intentional (including 5744 suicides and 89 homicides).[11]

RESEARCH

Medical research on poisoning tends to focus on specific toxins, antibodies, infections, and immunologic factors or on broader issues, such as detecting and managing occupational and environmental risks or minimizing risks to specific populations such as children, drug users, the elderly, or people with certain diseases. Research on criminal poisoning is less common and tends to focus on specific categories of criminal poisoning such as drug-facilitated sexual assault (DFSA)[12,13] or Munchausen by proxy (MBP).[14-22] A review of the literature revealed two recent studies on homicidal poisoning.

Using data collected from FBI Uniform Crime Reports (UCR) and accompanying Supplementary Homicide Reports (SHR) from 1990 through 1999, the FBI found that of 186,971 total homicides committed in the United States during this period, 346 were poisonings involving a single victim and single offender or a single victim and an unknown number of offenders. On average, this represents approximately 34 homicidal poisonings per year, a rate of 1.9 per 100,000 homicides. Types of poisons were not identified because the UCR does not collect this finding. The study revealed that victims of homicidal poisonings were nearly equally divided between males and females, with most victims being between the ages of 25 and 44 years of age. By race, white victims were divided equally between males and females. Black males poisoned victims twice as often as did black females. When victims were females, the offender was almost always a male. When victims were

males, however, the offenders were equally divided between the sexes.[23]

In 2006, researchers at the University of Georgia Department of Emergency Medicine conducted a trend analysis of 523 homicidal poisonings occurring between 1999 and 2005. On average, this study represents approximately 87 homicidal poisonings per year. Conclusions regarding the age and sex of the victims differed significantly from those in the FBI study. Using data from the CDC's National Mortality Statistics Database, they found that males were nearly 1.5 times more likely to be the victims of homicidal poisonings than females. They determined that medications (65%) were the most common poison, followed by gasses and vapors (28%), and then chemicals, corrosives, and pesticides (7%). Death was more likely to occur at extremes of age, especially in children less than a year old and in the elderly. The authors concluded that the poisonings of children were less a function of premeditation and more a consequence of negligence and poor parenting/coping skills on the part of the offender. They opined that the death of elderly victims was more likely a result of their living in abusive environments.[24]

One of the limitations in trying to compare these studies is that they rely on different ways in which homicides are defined or characterized. The FBI defines homicide as "murder and non-negligent manslaughter: the willful (non-negligent) killing of one human being by another."[25] Deaths caused by negligence, attempts to kill, assaults to kill, suicides, and accidental deaths are excluded from their definition. In contrast, the CDC compiles data from certificates of death submitted by individual states, which rely on coroners or medical examiners to list the manner of death. Due to a lack of uniformity in the process, one state may label the death of a child "accidental" while another may consider it a "negligent homicide." In the latter case, the death is reported as a "homicide" even if the child's death was unintentional. This difference may explain the higher number of homicidal poisonings of small children found in the University of Georgia study.

Another limitation of these studies is the lack of qualitative data to help in understanding poisoners. Although both the UCR and CDC collect a wealth of demographic data, neither requires contributing agencies to submit information about the circumstances surrounding criminal poisonings. Without important contextual information, researchers are unlikely to develop a comprehensive understanding of the motivations and thought processes of offenders. Future research should focus on the backgrounds of offenders and victims, their behavioral characteristics, their interpersonal dynamics, the events that precipitated the poisonings, the reasons offenders chose to use poisons instead of other weapons, how offenders were discovered, whether they have committed other poisonings, and steps they may have taken to avoid detection.

INITIAL ROLE OF THE MEDICAL COMMUNITY

Presentation of Poisoning Cases

In most serious poisoning cases, a victim either dies at home or appears at a hospital emergency room complaining of nonspecific symptoms such as nausea, vomiting, and diarrhea. Victims typically do not know what caused their distress and often attribute it to an etiology other than poisoning. For example, the initial signs and symptoms of arsenic poisoning can look identical to infectious gastroenteritis, strychnine poisoning looks identical to tetanus with both mimicking seizures,[2] and opioid toxicity with its associated central nervous system depression and small pupils can look identical to a brain pontine infarction.[26]

If there is doubt about a patient's condition, medical personnel should request a toxicology screening to evaluate the possibility of accidental or intentional poisoning. Screening can consist of a single test capable of detecting multiple drugs, or it can be a panel of individual tests. A negative routine toxicologic screen, however, does not exclude poisoning because many substances often go undetected.[27] It is imperative that the clinicians clearly document the clinical effects and if a poisoning is suspected relay this information to the laboratory personnel. In addition, early involvement of a medical toxicologist should be sought and can easily be obtained by contacting the local poison center if the healthcare facility does not have one on staff.

In acute poisonings, the activities and eating habits of the patient shortly before the onset of symptoms often provide clues as to what occurred. When there is evidence of chronic poisoning, clinicians should try to determine a patient's pattern of behavior and the associated progression of symptoms.[28]

Conditions That Should Raise Suspicion

If a poisoning is suspected but cannot be detected readily, a medical toxicologist should be contacted and told about the circumstances surrounding a patient's hospitalization so that he or she can decide what additional tests are warranted. If there are any suspicions that the poisoning was intentional (i.e., suicide or homicide) and if any of the following factors are present, the police should be notified immediately[2,24]:

- Death of an individual who was previously in good health
- Doctors unable to determine cause of illness
- Associates of victim overly involved in his or her treatment (e.g., feeding the victim)
- Family refuses to authorize an autopsy (exclusive of religious reasons)
- Recently acquired life insurance or enhancement to existing policy
- Protracted and intense domestic conflicts between victim and others
- Unexplained death of pets in household or neighborhood
- Prior hospitalizations of victim with similar symptoms
- Detection by toxicologists of uncommon poisons
- Access by victim or close associate to substances that could cause the distress
- Spouse or relative of victim is a nurse or doctor
- Evidence of prior abuse, especially for children or the elderly

This list is intended only as a guide, not as a definitive catalogue, and should serve merely as a starting point for assessing the need for continued investigation or referral to police.

INVESTIGATION OF POISONING CASES

Initiation of Criminal Investigations

A problem in many poisoning cases is that referral to the police is delayed. The longer the police must wait to commence an investigation, the greater the likelihood that important evidence may disappear or be destroyed. In poisoning cases, time is of essence. As they do in other criminal investigations, the police must (1) prove that a crime was committed, (2) identify who was responsible, and (3) obtain supporting evidence. However, in cases of suspected poisonings, the police must consult with appropriate healthcare specialists early in their investigation.

Criminal poisoning investigations can be extremely challenging. The very nature of a criminal poisoning is that offenders use stealth and deception to perpetrate and conceal their crimes. Preplanning is common; perpetrators may obtain poisons that are not easily detectable, create cover stories and alibis, destroy evidence, and feign concern (often exaggerated) for their victims.

In criminal poisoning cases, the investigators must identify the substance used, be prepared to demonstrate its toxicity, and prove that a particular subject knowingly introduced the substance into the victim. To accomplish this, the police and health care workers must work closely together even though their interests and responsibilities may be quite different. The benefit of interdisciplinary collaboration is that it can strengthen an investigation by encouraging objectivity and allow for greater exchange of information. Experience has shown that some criminal poisoning cases are misidentified because of false assumptions and/or lack of accurate medical information.

Every year there are cases in which one spouse kills the other using poison. The spouse who intends to poison his or her mate is sometimes reluctant to administer a one-time lethal dose for fear of causing instant death and inviting unwelcome suspicion. Thus, spouses may choose to poison their mates slowly in the hopes that their actions will not be noticed. Fear of being discovered motivates them to plan their murders carefully. When their spouses begin to react to the poisoning, the perpetrators will often exaggerate their concern. Therefore, healthy skepticism is a virtue for police, especially in domestic poisoning cases where there may be conflicts between husband and wife.

Police should remain open-minded during their investigations, as poisoning cases can be highly unusual. In two unrelated cases, wives planned to kill their husbands (one succeeded) and make it appear that the deaths were the result of the husband ingesting tainted over-the-counter medication. To make the ruse more credible, the wives added poison to pills, which they repackaged and placed on store shelves. Their hope was that random deaths in the community would help divert suspicion away from them.[29,30]

The list of questions in Table 3.1 can help investigators of possible poisoning cases direct their investigation and obtain better results. In order to corroborate statements and to clarify possible inconsistencies, the police must question not only victims (assuming they are still alive), but also others who had or have access to them. For legal and practical reasons, these interviews should almost always be conducted privately. In cases where police suspect that someone close to the victims may have poisoned them, care should be given to how this information is presented to a victim. Reactions can range from disbelief to a desire for revenge. Victims are often in denial that a loved one or a caregiver could be capable of intentionally hurting them. Rather than keeping an open mind, some may become preoccupied with defending their mates' reputation. Spouses who poison their mates often feign emotions and spend inordinate amounts of time with the victim. They want this access in order to determine the effectiveness of the poison they have administered, to deliver stronger doses if necessary, and to demonstrate how much they care.[30] Such charades have fooled not only spouses but also families, neighbors, and healthcare professionals.[31]

Suspect Identification

Before the police begin to search for a suspect, they should have obtained from the doctor and toxicologist details about the type of poison used, the amount of concentration, and how it was introduced into the victim. This information will help the police plan the direction for their investigation.[2]

To help identify potential suspects, police should focus primarily on those who have had access to the victim, particularly ones who have something to gain. In cases of assisted suicide (which some states regard as murder), what is often gained is a peaceful death for a terminally ill patient. Excluding these cases and those that are considered negligent homicides, the

TABLE 3.1 **Questions to Consider when Investigating a Possible Poisoning**

- Where was the victim when symptoms first appeared?
- Does the victim's occupation place him or her near poisons?
- Who called for help? (When and how?)
- What was the victim doing prior to onset of the symptoms?
- What did the victim eat or drink prior to the symptoms?
- Who prepared or served the food?
- Did others consume the same items?
- Is the victim experiencing problems in his or her marriage?
- Is the victim involved in illegal or immoral behavior?
- Is the victim experiencing problems with neighbors or colleagues at work?
- Does the victim have legal or financial problems?
- Who would profit from the victim's illness or death?

motivations for homicidal poisonings may be financial (insurance or inheritance), personal (revenge for a perceived wrong), or psychological (a desire for power and control).[32]

Most poisoning cases require that an offender have access to the victim. Thus, investigation should focus on those within close proximity. All family and friends having access should be viewed as potential suspects regardless of their age, occupation, or status. Experience has consistently shown that even the most trusted members of families and communities may have a "secret" side. While this does not make them a murderer, it means that police should explore the backgrounds of all potential suspects, looking for motive, means, and opportunity. An example of an unlikely suspect was Dr. Michael Swango, a U.S. medical school graduate who charmed people with his humor and intellect while maintaining a secret life as a serial poisoner.[33] In another case, an investigation of the arsenic poisoning of a preacher in North Carolina revealed an unlikely suspect: his genteel, well-spoken girlfriend, who concealed her true identity and was found to have killed two other people with poisons.[31]

Evidence Considerations

There are two types of evidence that police will gather—direct and indirect (circumstantial). Direct evidence stands on its own, such as laboratory findings, fingerprints, DNA, and eyewitness accounts. Circumstantial evidence is implied or inferred. For example, if an investigation reveals that a poisoning suspect hated the victim, this, by itself, does not mean that he or she committed the act. It merely suggests a possible motive. As an investigation progresses, circumstantial evidence may (or may not) assume greater importance. Although direct evidence is preferred for criminal prosecutions, in reality, both direct and circumstantial evidence can demonstrate someone's guilt.

Evidence in Drug-Facilitated Sexual Assault (DFSA) Cases

Obtaining evidence in DFSAs is difficult; victims usually have great difficulty recalling what happened, and traces of drugs that offenders gave them may only be detected within a couple days of the assault.[12] If the victim waits to report the crime, as many do, physical evidence may be lost. In these cases, the police should be knowledgeable about drugs used in DFSA cases. With limited evidence, police must not only be knowledgeable about these types of crimes, but they must be persistent. In the absence of tangible physical evidence, they should consider using proactive investigative measures including the use of informants and undercover officers. (*See* Chapter 28).

Evidence in Munchausen by Proxy (MBP) Cases

In cases of suspected MBP where caregivers (usually mothers) intentionally fabricate or induce illnesses in a child, evidence may be elusive. More than any other criminal poisoning, MBP cases require ongoing dialogue between police and healthcare specialists. Research and experience has shown that information sharing is the key to successful resolution.[21] Evidence in MBP will usually consist of nurses' documentation of their observations and interactions with MBP patients. If a decision is made to install covert video surveillance, someone will have to review the tapes and later store them using a chain of custody.

Documentary evidence will include medical histories, laboratory findings, records of prior hospitalizations, notes regarding treatment regimens (some of which are very technical in nature), observations by medical staff, and statements made by the offender.[14,18,21,22] Because MBP is a disorder characterized by fabrication, neither healthcare professionals nor the police can afford to accept statements by the caregiver as being necessarily true. All information must be independently corroborated.

Because of the complexity of MBP, only the most experienced of police and hospital staff should be assigned to these cases. These professionals should possess strong knowledge of this disorder to avoid losing objectivity and being inadvertently pulled into the mother's drama. Two problems can occur if inexperienced practitioners are assigned to manage these cases. First, they may completely disbelieve that the illness exists or that a caregiver (most commonly the mother) is capable of harming her child. Second, they may be manipulated by the MBP offender. Because MBP offenders often have backgrounds in nursing, they are comfortable in hospital environments, know how to ingratiate themselves with staff, and can use both of these capabilities to convince staff of the legitimacy of their child's illness (See Chapter 27).[14,18,20,21]

MBP skeptics believe that rigorous studies of MBP are lacking and that some mothers have been unfairly stigmatized.[15,16]

Jurisdictional Issues

Poisoning cases often involve multiple jurisdictions, which can present a host of problems (especially to law enforcement agencies) in terms of conducting interviews, collecting and preserving evidence, issuing subpoenas, avoiding duplication of effort, building investigative expertise, and maintaining investigative continuity. In criminal law, jurisdiction generally attaches to the location where a crime has occurred. However, this can be complicated. For example, where would the jurisdiction be if a suspect procures a poison in one state, carries it to another, administers it in a third, the victim dies in a fourth, and the suspect moves to a fifth?

Under law, police are not authorized to conduct investigations outside their designated areas (i.e., state, county) of jurisdiction. Instead, they must rely on the assistance of police in other jurisdictions. Considering how frequently people travel and that some poisons act slowly,

a scenario involving multiple jurisdictions is possible and must be addressed early in an investigation. One possible solution is to create a multi-agency task force that would include the Federal Bureau of Investigation (FBI), whose jurisdiction extends through all 50 states. In cases involving an international murder investigation where there are U.S. subjects involved, the FBI would work with foreign police through coordination with the Department of State, Interpol, and the U.S. Attorney's Office.

Search Considerations[2]

Searches of homes, vehicles, and storage lockers of possible suspects should be undertaken carefully to avoid exposure to toxins and to minimize the inadvertent destruction of evidence. Sterilized containers should be used to collect evidence. When deciding what evidence should be seized, police should keep in mind that anything that helped a suspect plan, prepare, or conceal a crime will be of evidentiary value. If a search reveals questionable substances, a toxicologist and/or hazmat team should be on hand.

As cunning as many poisoners seem, they often find it difficult to part with poisons or related materials. Dr. Swango had a virtual laboratory with recipes for making deadly poisons. Notebooks, letters, diaries, or financial documents should all be seized. Even if such documents do not contain information about poisons, they may contain information concerning motives. In some case, offenders have actually created evidence (e.g., forged suicide notes for victims), which ultimately helped convict them.[34,35] Police should not assume that all poisoners will get rid of incriminating evidence. When police searched the garage of thallium killer George Trepal in Florida, they discovered a bottle of thallium and a bottle-recapping machine that he is believed to have used during his crime.[36] Table 3.2 provides a list of items that may have clear evidentiary value.

Poisonings in Hospitals

Many criminal poisonings occur in hospitals where drugs are readily available and access to patients is practically limitless. During the past two decades, there have been numerous examples of healthcare workers committing murders of multiple patients using a variety of drugs.

TABLE 3.2 **Items to Carefully Consider when Investigating a Possible Poisoning**

- Medications (container may specify one drug but contain another)
- Herbal remedies (labels may be in a foreign language)
- Illegal drugs and drug paraphernalia
- Unusual potions (should be handled with care)
- Sponges, syringes, vials, burners, utensils
- Books, diagrams, videos
- Diaries, address books, recipe cards, mail (note return address)
- Maps, passports
- Checkbook, credit card receipts, telephone bills
- Telephone, computers, PDAs
- Employment applications
- Food and drinks on counter and in refrigerator
- Glasses, dishes, can openers
- Cooked food
- Bottle resealers, tape to reseal
- Vomitus and feces (have appropriate container to store)
- Clothing and shoes (particularly those recently worn)

Note: If a suspect is to be searched, the investigator should ensure that the search warrant covers seizure of hair, nails, and fingerprints (same for victim or roommates). Certain poisons such as arsenic may be detected in these locations.

Searches in these environments can be difficult because there are so many potential lethal substances. Evidence against suspects usually comes from witnesses who consistently observe the same person in a patient's room before a code or before the patient is found dead. Nursing charts and pharmaceutical inventories should be seized. Suspect vials and syringes should be handed over to supervisors who should maintain the items in a special storage locker with controlled access. Maintenance of a chain of custody is essential. Police should be notified early and if a formal investigation is initiated, arrangements should be made between the hospital and the police that will enable the latter to have complete access to relevant information.

Following searches, if items are found that need to be tested in a laboratory, a chain of custody should be prepared, and the items should be sent via courier or registered mail. One of the responsibilities of the toxicologist, besides identifying poisonous substances, is to determine their concentration and lethality.[28] Because the recovery of toxicologic substances may become an issue at trial, police should be extra careful in maintaining a proper chain of custody.

CONTINUED ROLE OF THE MEDICAL COMMUNITY

Pathology

In cases of unusual or unattended deaths, autopsies should be conducted so a medical examiner can collect postmortem specimens of body fluids and tissues where poisons reside. Hair, nails, bones, and vitreous humor are all locations where poisons may be detected. Drugs and intoxicants have been found in maggots attached to bodies. Unabsorbed poisons may be found among gastrointestinal contents. Analysis may be complicated by postmortem changes. When the toxicologist receives these samples, he or she will want to know what poison is being sought so tests can be focused accordingly. Under ideal circumstances, the toxicologist will be able to determine the route in which the poison was administered and the dose given, and he or she will offer an opinion as to whether the concentration was sufficient to cause death.[28] Again, because the handling, transferring, and transportation of samples may eventually become the subject of legal scrutiny, a chain of custody should be maintained.

Exhumations

Periodically, criminal investigations require exhumations. In these cases, either an initial autopsy found no evidence of a homicide or an autopsy was never conducted. Whatever the case, exhumations may be ordered after new information surfaces suggesting a victim's death was the result of a homicide. In addition to taking soft tissue samples, the pathologist may take vitreous humor from the eyes as well as hair and fingernail clippings to be tested for poisons. Depending on the degree of decomposition, samples may be taken from remaining organs.[37] In exhumations, maintaining a proper chain of custody remains vitally important.

Anyone who reads about exhumations and the resultant discovery of new findings, particularly cases in which the manner of death is changed to homicide, must wonder how often a cause of death is misdiagnosed. A study carried out in Germany in 2004 evaluated 155 consecutive forensic exhumations on the basis of inconclusive police and autopsy reports and death certificates. In 103 cases, the cause of death could be clearly determined. In 57 cases, there were major deviations between the causes of death listed on the death certificate and that diagnosed after autopsy. Three cases of homicidal poisoning (parathion, clozapine, diazepam) were discovered. Of 51 suspicious nonpoisoning cases, 19 were confirmed as homicides, including 15 patients killed by injections of air by a serial killer. The two most common reasons for overlooking these cases were superficial external examinations and low autopsy rate.[38]

MOTIVATION AND INTENT

There is a difference between motivation and criminal intent. Motivation speaks to the purpose behind an offender's desire to poison someone, which may relate to underlying psychological needs of which the offender may or may not be aware. Intent refers to one's willingness to carry out the deed. Earlier we spoke of the need to prove that the suspect had guilty knowledge about the poison used, knew it could cause harm, and used it for that purpose. There are many ways to find evidence to prove intent, but the best way to start is for the investigating officer to avoid rushing to judgment and to keep an open mind while interviewing witnesses and conducting searches.

Intent can be established by demonstrating the suspect had prior knowledge that a substance was potentially lethal. This information is sometimes provided by witnesses who recall sinister comments made by an offender, or it may be found in poisoning literature the offender accessed or ordered on the Internet. Suspects who decide to procure poisons covertly may unintentionally reveal their identity when they purchase the poison, or they may try to conceal their identity, a sure sign of guilty knowledge.

Establishing the motive for a criminal poisoning can help investigators determine the extent of how many victims an offender has poisoned and where evidence of these crimes may be found. Understanding what drives an offender can help police formulate investigative strategies and guide the search for relevant evidence. Prosecutors may use this information when deciding how to present their case in court. Investigators should be careful to avoid rushing to judgment about motivation. Sometimes, the motivation for a poisoning may appear obvious, but investigation is needed to ascertain the true reason(s) the crime was committed. Investigators should be careful not to accept at face value explanations provided by a suspect regarding his or her motivation, as this might be an attempt to mislead the investigation.

Examples of Different Motivations in Criminal Poisonings

Personal Vindication

In one case motivated by revenge, a jilted lover stole dimethylnitrosamine (a carcinogen) from his employer, broke into his ex-lover's home, and poured the substance into lemonade, causing two deaths.[39]

In another case, a man broke into the house of a neighbor with whom he had been arguing, added thallium to soda bottles, and resealed them.[40]

Punishment (Battered Child Syndrome)

In several documented cases, mothers forced pepper down children's throats as punishment. The children's deaths were due to asphyxia and ruled as homicides.[41-43]

Financial Gain

In 1991, Joann Curley killed her husband using thallium in order to collect $287,000 in insurance money. She had previously collected over $1 million in a settlement from an auto accident.[44]

Facilitation of Another Crime

Elderly men were intentionally administered a combination of benzodiazepines and opiates to suppress consciousness so that a group of criminals could carry out robberies.[45]

Travel-related poisoning was studied following several reports of tourists being offered food and drinks containing benzodiazepines to induce drowsiness before they were robbed.[46]

Excitement/Thrill-Seeking/Relief of Boredom

A 14-year-old student lined her teacher's coffee mug with strawberry-flavored lip gloss, knowing the substance would cause an allergic reaction that would compel the teacher to leave the classroom.[47] In a separate case, students baked brownies with laxatives and left them in the faculty lounge as a prank.[48]

Sadistic Pleasure and Money

A minister's girlfriend "comforted" him during multiple hospitalizations that she had caused and continued to cause by feeding him poisonous concoctions even as his painful and debilitating condition worsened. Despite mounting evidence, the minister had difficulty believing that this woman intended to kill him. She was easily able to access the victim alone and could roam the hospital ward almost freely after having devoted considerable time to ingratiating herself with hospital staff. She had secretly purchased a sizeable insurance policy on him and had poisoned two others for insurance money.[31]

Terrorism (Cult)

A cult in Oregon intentionally contaminated self-service salad bars with salmonella to change the regional vote, causing gastrointestinal distress to over 700 people.[49]

Terrorism (Political)

The Japanese cult/terrorist group Aum Shinrikyo attacked the Tokyo subway system using highly lethal sarin gas. Thousands were hospitalized, and 12 people died.[50]

Investigation revealed that the level of dioxin in the blood of Ukrainian presidential candidate Viktor Yushchenko was more than 6000 times higher than normal, suggesting an intentional poisoning.[51]

Murder Concealment (Product Tampering)

A woman killed her husband with cyanide and tried to disguise the crime as product tampering by putting cyanide in aspirin bottles and placing them on store shelves. She hoped to collect an insurance premium that would have paid more if her husband's death was the result of product tampering by a serial killer.[52]

Attention (Munchausen by Proxy)

A mother repeatedly brought her infant son to the hospital with a variety of symptoms. Doctors determined that he had high levels of bacteria in his blood but puzzled over the cause. During hospitalizations with the mother at his side, the child had several respiratory arrests and eventually could not be revived. The mother later was observed by a hidden camera blowing into her son's gastrostomy tube. She later told her husband that she had intentionally contaminated her son's stool specimen because she

did not believe the normal results and wanted to trap the testers. She was diagnosed as having Munchausen by proxy and referred for psychiatric evaluation.[53]

MURDERS BY MEDICAL PROFESSIONALS

Case 1: A nurse gave his wife a fatal injection of insulin. She died later while taking a bath. Vomitous found near her body suggested that the victim had experienced GI distress prior to her death by drowning. The husband's explanation that injection sites on her buttocks resulted from the couple's attempt to abort a fetus were not believed, and he was convicted.[34]

Case 2: A nurse brought her healthy husband to the emergency department with hypoglycemia, suggesting a newly diagnosed insulinoma. Tests revealed severe brain damage. Insulin tests suggested exogenous rather than endogenous insulin excess as the cause. She prepared a suicide note after her husband's hospitalization, forged a deed of gift transferring his property, and provided inconsistent statements to police.[54]

Case 3: A registered nurse called 911 to report the death of her 59-year-old cardiac surgeon husband, who was a diabetic attached to an insulin pump to control glucose. Before responders arrived, the wife disconnected the insulin reservoir, tubing, and battery from the pump and discarded them. Unbeknownst to her, the pathologists drew a toxicology screen. Three weeks later when the descendents called for a death certificate she was surprised to learn that the screening revealed an unexplained anesthetic induction agent, etomnidate. The body was exhumed and an autopsy found etomidate in the decedent's liver as well as laudanosine, a metabolite of a neuromuscular blocking agent used in anesthesia. The wife, who denied complicity, worked in a hospital endoscopic suite where these drugs were available. During the investigation, police found a witness to whom the wife had shared her plans. Removing the reservoir and battery was an effort to conceal her actions, as without a battery, data stored in the pump's microprocessor are lost within 2 hours.[55]

Case 4: A respiratory nurse, initially referred to as "The Angel of Death," injected hospital patients with pancuronium bromide, a muscle relaxant, to kill them. He was subsequently convicted of six murders, although the numbers were probably much higher considering the 8 years he worked at the hospital.[56] A search of his possessions revealed morphine and the paralytic succinylcholine.[57]

Case 5: A doctor who worked in several hospitals in the United States killed patients by injecting them with various substances such as succinylcholine, epinephrine, and air. When dismissed from one hospital, he would apply to work in another, and the killings continued until he was finally caught returning from Africa where he was committing similar murders in hospitals. Before becoming a doctor, he had served time in prison for poisoning fellow paramedics with arsenic.[33]

CONCLUSION

As toxicology has evolved, so has the nature of criminal poisoning. Rather than being simply a means to kill someone quickly, anonymously, and without confrontation, it has become a means to satisfy other, more selfish and pathological desires. In ancient times, science and technology helped slow the epidemic of domestic poisonings. Today, with more poisonous substances available to potential poisoners, the police and medical community must rely not only on science but also on effective information sharing. This can best be accomplished through cultivating and maintaining collaborative partnerships. Only by exchanging information on a regular basis will the two disciplines be able to develop the core of expertise necessary to detect and successfully prosecute poisoning cases.

One of the goals of a future partnership would be to create joint training initiatives to help increase internal awareness about the cases. For there to be effective treatment, prevention, and enforcement, there must be education. Although available statistics indicate that homicidal poisoning is a relatively rare event, there is still much to learn. Future research on the behavioral and psychological aspects of criminal poisonings will fill a gap in our understanding of the motivation and methodologies of those who use poisons.

REFERENCES

1. Poklis A, Saady JJ. Arsenic poisoning: acute or chronic? Suicide or murder? *Am J Forensic Med Pathol.* 1990;11(3):226–232.

2. Trestrail JH. *Criminal Poisoning: Investigational Guide for Law Enforcement, Toxicologists, Forensic Scientists, and Attorneys.* Totowa, NJ: Humana Press Inc. 2007.

3. Poisoning in the United States: Fact Sheet. Centers for Disease Control and Prevention Web site. http://www.cdc.gov/HomeandRecreationalSafety/Poisoning/poisoning-factsheet.htm. Accessed September 2, 2009.

4. Mutschler E, Derendorf H. *Drug Action-Basic Principles and Therapeutic Aspects.* Boca Raton, FL: CRC Press; 1995:615.

5. Arsenic. ToxFAQs. Department of Health and Human Services Agency for Toxic Substances and Disease Registry (ASTDR) Web site. http://www.atsdr.cdc.gov/tfacts2.html. Accessed September 2, 2009.

6. Thallium. ToxFAQs. Department of Health and Human Services Agency for Toxic Substances and Disease Registry (ASTDR). http://www.atsdr.cdc.gov/tfacts54.html. Accessed September 2, 2009.

7. Facts About Strychnine. Centers for Disease Control and Prevention Web site. http://emergency.cdc.gov/agent/strychnine/basics/pdf/facts.pdf. Accessed September 2, 2009.

8. Facts about ethylene glycol. Department of Health and Human Services, Agency for Toxic Substances and Disease Registry (ASTDR) Web site. http://www.atsdr.cdc.gov/tfacts96.html. Accessed November 17, 2009.

9. Facts about ricin. Centers for Disease Control and Prevention Web site. http://emergency.cdc.gov/agent/ricin/facts.asp. Accessed September 2, 2009.

10. Pesticides. National Safety Council Web site. http://www.nsc.org/news_resources/Resources/Documents/Pesticides.pdf. Accessed November 17, 2009.

11. Poisoning in the United States: fact sheet. Centers for Disease Control and Prevention Web site. http://www.cdc.gov/ncipc/factsheets/poisoning.htm. Updated March 13, 2008. Accessed September 2, 2009.

12. Hazelwood R, Burgess AW. *Practical aspects of rape investigation.* Boca Raton, FL: CRC Press; 2008.

13. Bechtel LK, Holstege CP. Criminal poisoning: drug-facilitated sexual assault. *Emerg Med Clin North Am.* 2007;25(2):499–525.

14. Bartsch C, Risse M, Schütz H, et al. Munchausen syndrome by proxy (MSBP): an extreme form of child abuse with a special forensic challenge. *Forensic Sci Int.* 2003;137:147.

15. Rand DC, Feldman MD. Misdiagnosis of Munchausen syndrome by proxy: a literature review of four new case studies. *Harvard Rev Psychiatry.* 1999;7:94–101.

16. Butz MR, Evans FB, Webber-Dereszynski RL. A practitioner's complaint and proposed direction: Munchausen syndrome by proxy, factitious disorder by proxy, and fabricated and/or induced illness in children. *Professional Psychol.* 2009;20(1):31–38.

17. Allison DB, Roberts MS. Disordered mother or disordered diagnosis? Munchausen by proxy syndrome (Review). *Psychoanalytic Studies.* 2000;2(2).

18. Fulton DR. Early recognition of Munchausen Syndrome by Proxy. *Crit Car Nurs Q.* 2000;23(2):35–42.

19. Makar AF, Squier PJ. Experience and reason briefly reported: Munchausen syndrome by proxy; father as perpetrator. *Pediatrics.* 1990;85(3):370–373.

20. Tannay Z, Akcay A, Kilic G, et al. Corrosive poisoning mimicking a cicatricial pemphigoid: Munchausen syndrome by proxy. *Child: Care Health Dev.* 2007;33(4):496–99.

21. Horwath J. Interagency practice in suspected cases of Munchausen syndrome by proxy (fictitious: illness by proxy). *Child Fam Soc Work.* 1999;4:109–118.

22. Holstege CP. Criminal poisoning. *Clin Lab Med.* 2006;1:243–53.

23. Westveer EA, Jarvis PJ, Jensen JC. Homicidal poisoning: the silent offense. *FBI Law Enforcement Bull.* August 2004:1–8.

24. Shepherd G, Ferslew B. Homicidal poisoning deaths in the United States 1999-2005. *J Clin Toxicol.* 2009;47(4):342–347.

25. Uniform crime reports (UCR). Crime in the United States. Department of Justice. http://www.fbi.gov/ucr/ucr.htm. Accessed November 17, 2009.

26. Poklis A. Forensic toxicology. In: Eckert W, ed. *Introduction to Forensic Science.* Boca Raton, FL: CRC Press; 1996.

27. Rainey PM. Laboratory principles in toxicologic emergencies. In Goldfrank L, Hoffman R, Lewin N, Flomenbaum N, Howland M, Nelson L, eds. *Goldfrank's Toxicologic Emergencies.* 8th ed. New York: McGraw-Hill; 2006:100.

28. Poklis A. Analytic/forensic toxicology. In Klassen C, ed. *Casarett and Doull's Toxicology: The Basic Science of Poisons.* New York: McGraw-Hill; 2007.

29. Fisher D. Hard Evidence: *How Detectives Inside the FBI's Sci-Crime Lab Have Helped Solve America's Toughest Cases.* New York: Dell; 1995.

30. *United States of America v Joseph Melling,* 47F3rd 1546; 41 Fed. R Evid Serv 593 (United States Court of Appeals for the 9th Circuit, February 22, 1995).

31. Schutze J. *Preacher's Girl: The Life and Crimes of Blanche Taylor Moore.* New York: William Morrow; 1993.

32. Douglas JE, Burgess AW, Burgess AG, Ressler RK. *Crime Classification Manual: A Standard System for Investigating and Classifying Violent Crimes.* Hoboken, NJ: John Wiley & Sons; 2006.

33. Stewart JB. *Blind Eye: How the Medical Establishment Let a Doctor Get Away with Murder.* New York: Simon & Schuster; 1999.

34. Birkenshaw VJ. Investigation in a case of murder by insulin. *BMJ.* 1958;2:463–468.

35. *Berrie v State,* CR 20; 29 P 2nd 979; 55Okl.Cr.302 (Oklahoma Court of Criminal Appeals, February 2, 1934).

36. Good J, Goreck S. *Poison Mind: The True Story of the Mensa Murderer and the Policewoman Who Risked Her Life to Bring Him to Justice.* New York: William Morrow; 1995.

37. Breitmeie D, Graefe-Kirci U, Albrecht K, et al. Evaluation of the correlation between time corpses spent in in-ground graves and findings at exhumation. *Forensic Sci Int.* 2005;154(2-3):218–223.

38. Karger B, Lorin de la Grandmaison G, Bajanowski T, et al. Analysis of 155 consecutive forensic exhumations with emphasis on undetected homicides. *Int J Legal Med.* 2004;118(2):90–94.

39. Harper v Grammer, 895 F. 2nd 473. No. 87-278 (US Court of Appeals 1990).

40. Johll ME. *Investigating Chemistry: A Forensic Science Perspective.* New York: Freeman; 2006.

41. Cohl S. Homicidal asphyxia by pepper aspiration. *J Forensic Sci.* 1986;31(4):1475–1478.

42. Cohl S, Trestrail JD III, Graham MA, et al. Fatal pepper aspiration. *Am J Dis Child.* 1988;142(6):633–636.

43. Adelson L. Homicide by pepper. *J Forensic Sci.* 1964;9(3):391–395.

44. Wecht CH, Saitz G, Curriden M. *Mortal Evidence: The Forensics Behind Nine Shocking Cases.* Amherst, NY: Prometheus; 2003.

45. Stankova E, Gesheva M, Hubenova A. Age and criminal poisonings. *Przeglad Lekarski.* 2005;62(6):471–474.

46. Majumber B, Basher A, Faiz MA, et al. Criminal poisoning of commuters in Bangladesh: prospective and retrospective study. *Forensic Sci Int.* 2008;180(1):10–16.

47. Rowe C, Harrell DC. Girls, 12, allegedly poison teacher at school. *Seattlepi.com.* March 31, 2007.

48. Hunte M. Students expelled in laxative cupcake cape. *Times-Picayne.* Sep 16, 2008.

49. Torak TJ, Tauxe RV, Wise RP, et al. A large community outbreak of salmonellosis caused by intentional contamination of restaurant salad bars. *JAMA.* 1997;278(5):389–395.

50. Olsent K. Aum Shinrikyo: once and future threat? *Emerging Infectious Diseases* 1999;5(4):513–516.

51. Cosgrove-Mather B. Yushenko dioxin levels off charts. *CBSNews.com.* 2004.

52. *United States v Stella Nickel,* 883 F. 2nd 824 (Court of Appeals, 9th Circ).

53. Fulton DR. Early recognition of Munchausen's syndrome by proxy. *Crit Care Nurs Q.* 2000;23(2): 35–42.

54. Koskine PJ, Nuutinen HM, Laaksonen H, et al. Importance of storing emergency serum samples for uncovering murder with insulin. *Forensic Sci Int.* 1999;105:61–66.

55. Benedict B, Keyes R, Sauls FC. The insulin pump as a murder weapon—a case report. *Am J Forensic Med Pathol.* 2004;25(3):159–60.

56. Ramsland K. *Inside the Minds of Healthcare Serial Killers.* Santa Barbara, CA: Greenwood; 2007:85–90.

57. Furbee RB. Criminal poisoning: medical murderers. *Clin Lab Med.* 2006;26(1):255–273.

Agents Used
by Past Poisoners

4 Acids and Alkalis

Matthew Salzman and Rika N. O'Malley

CASE STUDY

In 1979, in an inpatient setting for dementia patients in Sweden, a resident claimed that she had been given a medication that was too strong. A nurse noticed that the patient's breath smelled strongly of Gevisol, a commercial cleanser known to contain phenol, a caustic with a pH of 12. A 19-year-old man employed by the nursing home subsequently confessed to murdering 27 residents and to having tried to kill an additional 15 residents over a period of 3 months by having them drink Gevisol, Ivisol (another commercial cleaner that contains potassium hydroxide and that has a pH of 13), or Desderman (a highly concentrated alcohol solution).

Of the patients who died, autopsies demonstrated findings that could be normal in dementia patients, including esophageal epithelial cells aspirated into the lungs. After reexamining and reviewing the medical records, however, many of these patients were found to have swollen lips with small tears in the mucosa. Further, patients were found to have reddish stripes running from the corners of the mouth and down the neck. These were initially thought to be funga infections but were later found to be due to chemical burns. One patient, an 83-year-old woman who died 5 hours after receiving a dose of Gevisol, at autopsy was found to have tears in the mucosa of her stomach and esophagus, as well as a perforation of the stomach wall. In order to confirm poisoning with Gevisol or Ivisol, patients' organs, blood, and/or urine were analyzed for the presence of parachlorcresol, a component of both cleansers. By finding this chemical in various samples, combined with physical findings and microscopic tissue analysis, police believed they had enough evidence to substantiate murder in 11 cases.[1] The suspect was found to be insane and was subsequently sent to a mental hospital. He allegedly killed the patients to alleviate their suffering. Other staff initially thought the causes of these deaths were due to various infections. He was released several years later and was never heard from again.

HISTORY

A caustic, also known as a corrosive, is a chemical capable of causing injury upon tissue contact. Caustics are divided into two categories: acids and alkalis (bases). Generally, strong acids with a pH of less than 3 and strong bases with a pH of greater than 11 are of the greatest concern in regard to human exposure. Many household and industrial products contain caustic chemicals, including hydrochloric acid, potassium hydroxide, sodium hydroxide, sulfuric and phosphoric acids, as well as many others. Hydrofluoric acid—a strong acid in its anhydrous state, but a weak acid in its aqueous form—causes distinct injuries from those caused by other common acids and alkalis, and it therefore warrants separate discussion.[2]

POTENTIAL DELIVERY METHODS

Caustics can be delivered to unsuspecting victims in a variety of ways. Because these chemicals are often in either liquid or crystalline states, they can be added to beverages. Such an instance was reported by the *Milwaukee Journal Sentinal* on November 12, 2005, when a man in Mequon, Wisconsin, was charged with first-degree reckless injury after paying a woman $20 to drink an unknown liquid because it excited him to watch women drink dangerous things. He allegedly took 30 to 40 pellets of sodium hydroxide from his work place and mixed them with water, which the unsuspecting victim then consumed. Caustics can also be poured over a victim's body. In Queensland, Australia, in 2007, a man was convicted of grievous bodily harm to his stepdaughter after he gave her caustic soda (lye or sodium hydroxide) to drink and then spilled the strong alkali on her groin.

Further, a caustic could be placed into an incendiary device designed to detonate and spray its contents over unsuspecting passersby. A homicide investigation was launched in November 1996 in Brooklyn, NY, when one sanitation worker was killed and another injured after being exposed to hydrofluoric acid fumes. According to the *New York Times* on November 14, 1996, a 1-gallon container of hydrofluoric acid stored inside a garbage bag was placed at a curbside for routine garbage pick-up. When the truck crushed the container, one of the sanitation workers inhaled hydrofluoric acid fumes, leading to the man's death while the other sustained cutaneous burns.

Finally, there have been reports of caustic agents being administered as an enema in an attempt to commit serious bodily harm or homicide.[3]

TOXICOLOGIC MECHANISMS

Acids and alkalis are known to produce different types of tissue damage. Acids generally cause coagulation necrosis, with eschar formation that may limit substance penetration and injury depth.[4] Alkalis, in contrast, combine with tissue proteins and cause liquefactive necrosis and saponification. Additionally, alkali absorption leads to clot formation in blood vessels, impeding blood flow to already damaged tissue.[5] After caustic ingestion, esophageal injury mechanisms, however, may be more complicated than the chemical burns previously described. Reactive oxygen species generation with subsequent lipid peroxidation has been implicated as contributing to initial esophageal injury. Investigators have measured concentrations of malondialdehyde, a known end product of lipid peroxidation, as well as glutathione, a known endogenous free-radical scavenger, in esophageal tissue exposed to sodium hydroxide. The investigators found significantly higher malondialdehyde concentrations, indicating the presence of reactive oxygen species 24 hours after exposure. These concentrations remained high for 72 hours after exposure compared with noninjured controls. Moreover, significantly lower glutathione concentrations in tissue exposed to sodium hydroxide were found in injured esophageal tissue compared with controls, further supporting the presence of reactive oxygen species and free-radical damage.[6] Tissue injury may begin within minutes after corrosive exposure and may persist for hours thereafter if the corrosives are left in place without decontamination.[7]

Although a weak acid in its aqueous state, hydrofluoric acid acts more like an alkali. After contact with human tissue, it slowly dissociates into hydrogen and fluoride ions, resulting in tissue penetration by way of a nonionic diffusion gradient that can potentially cause extensive liquefaction necrosis.[8] Additionally, fluoride ions penetrate tissues and form insoluble salts with positively charged ions such as calcium and magnesium, causing tissue injury, hypocalcemia, hypomagnesemia, and pain that is often out of proportion to visible tissue injury.[9]

CLINICAL EFFECTS

Patients seeking medical care following caustic ingestion may have varied presentations, ranging from asymptomatic to premorbid states. Death may occur immediately after caustic ingestion.[10] Signs and symptoms may include abdominal pain, chest pain, nausea, vomiting (bloody or nonbloody), dysphagia, odynophagia, drooling, or stridor.[11,12] Hemolysis, disseminated intravascular coagulation, renal failure, and liver failure have all been reported following caustic ingestion.[13] Death may result from internal bleeding leading to cardiovascular collapse. Patients may also die from severe infections as a result of a perforated esophagus or stomach, leading to either peritonitis or mediastinitis.

Patients presenting after rectal caustic administration may have varied symptoms, including anorectal pain, abdominal pain, and tenesmus. In one report, a 5-year-old boy who had inadvertently received an acetic acid enema presented with lethargy and cyanosis.[14] Clinical findings may include hematochezia, hypotension, hypogastric tenderness, flank tenderness, and a hyper- or hypotonic anal sphincter.[3,14] Frank peritonitis has never been reported immediately following rectal caustic administration, although delayed bowel perforation with peritoneal findings is not uncommon. Death

after caustic enema may result from sepsis, renal failure, or multisystem organ failure.[3]

Hydrofluoric acid (HF) acts more like an alkali than an acid. Dermal contact with HF is the most common route of exposure; hand injuries from using low-concentration rust remover and aluminum cleaning products are especially common.[15] After HF skin contact, symptoms may be immediate or delayed up to 24 hours if solution concentration is less than 20%.[16] Exposure to HF may cause immediate or delayed pain that can be severe and throbbing; this pain can be accompanied by a whitish discoloration of the skin. Aqueous HF solutions are highly volatile and produce vapors that are lighter than ambient air, often resulting in concomitant inhalational and dermal injury, especially with head and neck exposures.[8] Pulmonary effects include upper airway irritation and narrowing, swelling, and obstruction of the upper airway that may be immediate or delayed up to 36 hours.[16] Physical findings may include stridor, wheezing, or rhonchi, as well as erythema and ulceration of the upper respiratory tract.[17] Inhalation of high-concentration HF may result in rapid onset of noncardiogenic pulmonary edema and death.[18]

Ocular exposure to HF may be the result of aqueous or HF vapor contact. Eye contact may result in pain, corneal sloughing, revascularization, corneal opacification, and occasionally keratoconjunctivitis sicca as a long-term complication.[19]

Ingestion of HF can cause gastritis while sparing the remainder of the gastrointestinal tract. After ingestion, patients may present with nausea, vomiting, or abdominal pain. Systemic absorption is rapid and usually fatal within the first 30 minutes after ingestion but potentially as long as 7 hours after ingestion.[9]

Death following HF exposure is often a result of cardiac dysrhythmias, most notably ventricular fibrillation.[19] These cardiac dysrhythmias are most likely multifactoral, secondary to electrolyte abnormalities, acidosis, or hypoxia.[15] Hypocalcemia alone is probably insufficient to explain the dysrhythmias because rats exposed to sodium fluoride still died of cardiovascular failure despite calcium replacement.[20] Some authors postulate that hyperkalemia precipitates cardiac toxicity because fluoride ions increase intracellular calcium concentration, subsequently causing potassium efflux and systemic hyperkalemia.[21]

ANALYTIC DETECTION

Routine laboratory testing is unlikely to be helpful after caustic poisoning. The diagnostic study of choice after either caustic ingestion or enema is endoscopy with a flexible endoscope.[2] Esophageal endoscopy is considered to be safe up to 96 hours after ingestion and may reveal a range of findings from a normal esophagus to extensive tissue necrosis.[22] Sigmoidoscopy or colonoscopy after caustic enema may reveal a range of injury, from none to friable mucosa to extensive full thickness necrosis that extends as far proximally as the terminal ileum.[2] An increase in ionized serum fluoride and decrease in total and ionized serum calcium, hyponatremia, and hyperkalemia can occur following moderate HF exposure.[23] Therefore electrolyte analysis after HF poisoning may also be crucial, as electrolyte alterations may contribute to a victim's death. No routine laboratory testing, however, is available to definitively diagnose caustic poisoning.

In the case study described at the beginning of this chapter, specific testing was done postmortem that helped determine a cause of death for a number of victims. Unfortunately, this type of testing is not available in most hospitals and will require a forensic laboratory's expertise and results may not be available immediately. Certainly, should the actual poison be found, pH testing could be done easily to determine whether the substance is a strong alkali or base.

CONCLUSION

Caustic chemicals are readily available in many household and industrial products, and they can be delivered to victims in a variety of surreptitious ways. Results of caustic poisoning can be devastating, ranging from gross disfigurement and lifelong disability to death. Physical findings can be variable among victims, and testing victims' blood is unlikely to be helpful. In the setting of caustic ingestion or enema, endoscopy or postmortem examination may be the most useful tool in confirming a diagnosis. Testing the poison itself, if available, is likely to be the most useful.

REFERENCES

1. Jonsson J, Voigt GE. Homicidal intoxications by lye- and parachlorcresol-containing disinfectants. *Am J Forensic Med Pathol.* 1984;5(1):57–63.
2. Salzman M, O'Malley RN. Updates on the evaluation and management of caustic exposures. *Emerg Med Clin North Am.* 2007;25(2):459–476.
3. Diarra B, Roudie J, Ehua Somian F, Coulibaly A. Caustic burns of rectum and colon in emergencies. *Am J Surg.* 2004;187(6):785–789.
4. Havanond C. Is there a difference between the management of grade 2b and 3 corrosive gastric injuries? *J Med Assoc Thai.* 2002;85(3):340–344.
5. Mamede RC, de Mello Filho FV. Ingestion of caustic substances and its complications. *Sao Paulo Med J.* 2001;119(1):10–15.
6. Gunel E, Caglayan F, Caglayan O, Akillioglu I. Reactive oxygen radical levels in caustic esophageal burns. *J Pediatr Surg.* 1999;34(3):405–407.
7. Satar S, Topal M, Kozaci N. Ingestion of caustic substances by adults. *Am J Ther.* 2004;11(4):258–261.
8. Kirkpatrick JJ, Enion DS, Burd DA. Hydrofluoric acid burns: a review. *Burns.* 1995;21(7):483–493.
9. Kao WF, Dart RC, Kuffner E, Bogdan G. Ingestion of low-concentration hydrofluoric acid: an insidious and potentially fatal poisoning. *Ann Emerg Med.* 1999;34(1):35–41.
10. Katzka DA. Caustic injury to the esophagus. *Curr Treat Options Gastroenterol.* 2001;4(1):59–66.
11. Zwischenberger JB, Savage C, Bidani A. Surgical aspects of esophageal disease: perforation and caustic injury. *Am J Respir Crit Care Med.* 2002;165(8):1037–1040.
12. Jain AL, Robertson GJ, Rudis MI. Surgical issues in the poisoned patient. *Emerg Med Clin North Am.* 2003;21(4):1117–1144.
13. Poley JW, Steyerberg EW, Kuipers EJ, et al. Ingestion of acid and alkaline agents: outcome and prognostic value of early upper endoscopy. *Gastrointest Endosc.* 2004;60(3):372–377.
14. Kawamata M, Fujita S, Mayumi T, Sumita S, Omote K, Namiki A. Acetic acid intoxication by rectal administration. *J Toxicol Clin Toxicol.* 1994;32(3):333–336.
15. Caravati EM. Acute hydrofluoric acid exposure. *Am J Emerg Med.* 1988;6(2):143–150.
16. Medical management guidelines for hydrogen fluoride. Agency for Toxic Substances and Diseases Registry Web site. http://www.atsdr.cdc.gov/MHMI/mmg11.html. Accessed September 3, 2009.
17. Wing JS, Brender JD, Sanderson LM, Perrotta DM, Beauchamp RA. Acute health effects in a community after a release of hydrofluoric acid. *Arch Environ Health.* 1991;46(3):155–160.
18. Dote T, Kono K, Usuda K, Shimizu H, Kawasaki T, Dote E. Lethal inhalation exposure during maintenance operation of a hydrogen fluoride liquefying tank. *Toxicol Ind Health.* 2003;19(2–6):51–54.

19. Rao RB, Hoffman RS. Caustics and batteries. In: Goldfrank L, Hoffman R, Lewin N, Flomenbaum N, Howland M, Nelson L, eds. *Goldfrank's Toxicologic Emergencies.* 7th ed. New York: McGraw-Hill; 2002.

20. Strubelt O, Iven H, Younes M. The pathophysiological profile of the acute cardiovascular toxicity of sodium fluoride. *Toxicology.* 1982;24(3–4):313–323.

21. Cummings CC, McIvor ME. Fluoride-induced hyperkalemia: the role of Ca2+-dependent K+ channels. *Am J Emerg Med.* 1988;6(1):1–3.

22. Zargar SA, Kochhar R, Mehta S, Mehta SK. The role of fiberoptic endoscopy in the management of corrosive ingestion and modified endoscopic classification of burns. *Gastrointest Endosc.* 1991;37(2):165–169.

23. Murano M. Studies of the treatment of hydrofluoric acid burn. *Bull Osaka Med Coll.* 1989;5:39–48.

5 | Animals

Blake A. Froberg

CASE STUDY

A 14-year-old boy was brought to the hospital for persistent vomiting. On arrival in the emergency department (ED), he admitted that he cut the head off a western diamondback snake *(Crotalus atrox)*, milked the venom from the fangs, and then used a syringe to inject the venom into his right antecubital vein. Shortly after arrival at the hospital he developed swelling of his lips and tongue, hypotension, thrombocytopenia, and a coagulopathy. He required endotracheal intubation, intravenous fluids, dopamine, and four vials of Crotalidae Polyvalent Immune Fab (Ovine) antivenin. The patient's hypotension resolved rapidly, his thrombocytopenia and coagulopathy corrected 48 hours after admission, and he was extubated 3 days after admission. He recovered completely and never developed any tissue destruction at the site of venom injection.[1]

HISTORY

Poisonous animals have been used by various cultures throughout history. While not necessarily considered criminal activity, the earliest documented use of poisonous animals was to enhance projectiles in hunting and warfare. Alexander the Great encountered the use of putrefied snakes on arrowheads during his conquest of Asia in 326–325 BC.[2,3] The Scythians applied a mixture of putrefied snakes and human blood to the tips of their arrows used in warfare. In southern Africa, Bushman tribes still coat their arrows with the innards of leaf-eating beetle pupae. Groups in southern and eastern Africa added scorpion venom to the mixtures used in their arrow poisons. In North America, certain native tribes applied venom from rattlesnakes along with crushed bees, scorpions, and centipedes to their arrows. The Choco tribe of western Columbia used *Phyllobates* sp. poison on blowgun darts.[4]

The exact components of many of the past poisons for projectiles are difficult to determine. The predominate toxicity of some arrow poisons may be the result of bacteria-contaminated putrefied flesh instead of the animal poison itself. Some animal poisons that were used may have become ineffective during preparation, such as snake venom that was boiled before application.[3]

Along with the use of animal poisons on projectiles, there are other historic accounts of knowledge and intentional use of animal poisons. The ancient Greeks revered animal poisons and classified the known poisons as mineral, plant, or animal based on origin. Opponents of the occupation in Asia by Rome hurled clay pots filled with venomous scorpions at Roman troops. The use of scorpions in this way probably served as an ineffective weapon but an effective means of terrorism.[5] One of the most famous intentional uses of an animal poison is the suicide of Cleopatra, who was allegedly envenomated by an asp.

Criminal incidents using animal poisons are rare in the modern world. The rarity of these events is likely due to the availability of other poisons, the difficulty in obtaining animal poison, and the unreliable effects of animal poison. There may be undetected cases of the criminal use of animal poison because of the difficulty in detecting the use of such poisons.

In October 1978, Joseph Musico and Lance Kenton, members of the Synanon religious group, were arrested in connection with using a snake to harm attorney Paul Morantz, who had recently won a $300,000 case against the Synanon religious group. Morantz was bitten by a diamondback rattlesnake that was placed in his mailbox. The snake's rattle had been cut off so that he would not be warned of the strike. Morantz survived the snakebite.[6,7]

Snake-handling as a religious practice occurs in some Pentecostal churches. These churches are located predominately in the southeastern United States, although churches that perform snake-handling have been identified in Indiana and Michigan and in the Canadian provinces of Alberta and British Columbia. George Hensley, the founder of the present-day snake-handling movement, died in 1955 from a snakebite. In 1998, the Reverend John Wayne "Punkin" Brown, Jr., died after receiving 23 bites from a timber rattlesnake during a ceremony.[8] In 2006, a 48-year-old woman died after she was bitten by an unidentified snake during a church service in Kentucky.[9] In 1992, Reverend Glenn Summerford, a pastor at the Church of Jesus with Signs Following, was convicted of attempted murder for making his wife place her hand in a cage full of agitated venomous snakes; although she was bitten, she did not die.[10] Some states have laws about using poisonous animals in places that endanger others, owning poisonous animals without a license, or handling snakes during church services. The consequence of breaking these laws is often minimal, usually with a classification of a misdemeanor and a $50 to $150 fine. The laws are also difficult to enforce.

Snakes have been used as weapons and in attempts to create hysteria. In two instances, snakes have been swung at police officers. In both cases the officers were unharmed, but the attackers were envenomated as they swung the snakes.[11,12] In South Africa, an individual emptied a bag of five venomous puff adder snakes onto a bank's floor for revenge. One bank worker was bitten while trying to catch these snakes. The man who released them faced charges of assault with intent to cause grievous bodily harm.[13,14]

The medical literature reports several cases of intentional use of snake venom. The majority of these cases are suicide attempts. The first documented case of suicide by snake venom was in 1977. Which snake venom was used remains unclear.[15] In 1980, a snake farm employee committed suicide using venom from a viper of African origin.[16] In 1986, a 23-year-old man injected himself with the venom from an eastern diamondback rattlesnake. He became critically ill with a coagulopathy but received antivenin and survived.[17]

Exotic animals, including venomous and nonvenomous snakes, have been linked to illegal drug trafficking. Exotic animals have been used as a form of currency to trade for illegal drugs, as a way to smuggle illegal drugs, and as a way to protect caches of illegal drugs. Heroin wrapped in condoms has been found in the gastrointestinal tract of boa-constrictors in a failed smuggling attempt.[18] Venomous snakes have been used as a deterrent for proper searching of a cage that contained heroin as well as a security measure for protecting a cache of methamphetamine.[18,19] There are no well-documented historic cases of criminal use of scorpion venom. Envenomations have occurred in areas where scorpions are not endemic; these have been traced back to scorpions that have been stowaways on airplanes.[20]

Two cases in the literature describe the intentional use of black widow venom. The first case was reported in 1976 and involved an attempted suicide by a 36-year-old man. He reportedly agitated the spider until it envenomated him. He suffered pain and muscle cramping but survived the event.[21] In 1996, a case report was published of an intravenous drug user who injected a crushed black widow spider in an effort to "get high"; despite anaphylaxis, pain, and muscle cramping, she survived the injection.[22]

There are no described cases of homicide/suicide using Bufo sp. toad toxin. There are, however, many cases of this toxin's misuse. Dried venom from species of these toads has been used for centuries in a traditional Chinese medicine called chan su. In other Asian countries, a traditional medicine called kyushin also contains this toxin. In the United States, similar formulations have been sold as aphrodisiacs under the names "Love Stone," "Black Cube," and "Rock Hard." In the 1990s, several deaths were caused by ingesting alternative medicines that contained Bufo sp. toad toxin.[23] There is also a practice of licking Bufo sp. toads or smoking the dried poison for hallucinogenic effects, only

the Bufo alvarius species secretes a poison with known hallucinogenic effects. There are reported cases of toxicity from mouthing or licking Bufo sp. toads.[24]

There are no well-documented cases of human toxicity from Phyllobates sp. toxins. In 2002, a criminal was convicted of soliciting murder after attempting to obtain poison from an Amazonian frog, to cause a heart attack without a trace. It is unclear to which frog he was referring, although a Phyllobates sp. would fit this description. The criminal was unsuccessful because he was trying to obtain this poison through an undercover police officer.[25]

In 1954, Arthur Kendrick Ford killed two female coworkers using cantharidin, also known as "Spanish fly." Ford erroneously believed that cantharidin would act as an aphrodisiac. He placed the cantharidin in "coconut ice," a type of candy. After eating the candy, the two women became ill and later died while in hospital care. Ford developed blistering on his face from cantharidin exposure. Cantharidin was detected in both victims during postmortem analysis. Ford served 5 years in prison for manslaughter.[26,27]

In 1998, a 2-year-old boy died after an estimated 432 yellow jacket stings. The child was not brought immediately to medical attention because his parents' religious beliefs opposed the use of modern medical care. Although the boy's death was not an intentional poisoning, it did raise questions of child abuse/neglect and medico-legal ramifications.[28]

POTENTIAL DELIVERY METHODS

There are two manners in which animal poisons have been delivered to victims of poisoning. First, the animal's natural mechanism of envenomation may be used (i.e., bite or sting). There are, however, problems with administering the poison in this manner: The animal may not become agitated enough to strike; the animal may strike the victim on a part of the body that results in no or minimal toxicity; and even if a venomous animal strikes, it may not deliver a harmful amount of venom. For instance, it is estimated that 25% of Crotalinae snake bites are "dry bites" (i.e., bites without venom release).[29]

The second delivery method involves extracting the animal poison and delivering it by another method. Examples include milking of snake venom and injecting it with a syringe and needle, crushing a black widow spider for injection, administering crushed blister beetles orally, drying *Bufo* sp. toad poison and administering it in a pill form, and wiping frog poison onto the surface of a dart.[30]

TOXICOLOGIC MECHANISMS

Snake venom varies from species to species; within species it can vary depending on age, size, diet, and climate. Snake venoms are a solution containing many different components, making it difficult to define the mechanism of action. *Crotalinae* sp. venom often has proteolytic components that cause local tissue destruction and hemotoxins that can cause blood coagulation abnormalities and thrombocytopenia (Figure 5.1). The Mojave rattlesnake *(Crotalus scutulatus)*, located in California, also has a neurotoxic component to its venom. This venom, called Mojave toxin, prevents the presynaptic release of acetylcholine at the neuromuscular junction, resulting in paralysis and respiratory arrest.[29] The venom of *Elapidae* sp. is comprised mainly of neurotoxins. The elapid α-neurotoxin antagonizes the neuromuscular junction nicotinic receptor leading to weakness and paralysis. In contrast to *Crotalinae* venom, the *Elapidae* venom has few local tissue destructive properties.[31]

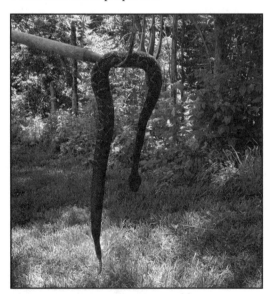

FIGURE 5-1   **Timber rattlesnake (*Crotalus horridus horridus*)**
(See Color Plate 1.)

The venom of the bark scorpion *(Centruroides sculpturatus)* is predominately neurotoxic

(Figure 5.2). The venom acts by opening sodium channels on neurons. This causes a release of neurotransmitters including acetylcholine and catecholamines in both the sympathetic and parasympathetic nervous system.[32]

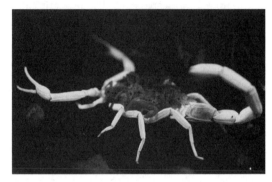

FIGURE 5-2   **Bark scorpion (*Centruroides sculpturatus*)**
(See Color Plate 2.)

Black widow spider *(Latrodectus genus)* venom contains α-latrotoxin, which is toxic to humans (Figure 5.3). α-Latrotoxin enhances calcium influx in presynaptic neurons, resulting in increased release of acetylcholine from presynaptic neurons.[33]

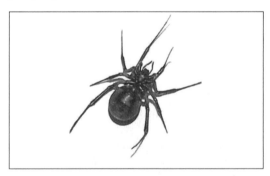

FIGURE 5-3   **Black widow (*Latrodectus mactans*)**
(See Color Plate 3.)

The composition of the poison excreted by the *Bufo* sp. toad varies among the over 200 species in the genus. Some toads in the genus *Bufo* sp. secrete a poison on their skin called bufadienolide, also named bufotalin. Bufadienolide is a cardiac glycoside and has an effect similar to that of digoxin.[23] Bufadienolide inhibits the potassium–sodium ATPase pump that is found on cardiac cells. The inhibition of this pump results in slower activity of the sodium–calcium exchange pump and an increase in intracellular calcium. Excessive intracellular calcium interferes with the contraction and conduction of the heart and can lead to dysrhythmias. Many of the *Bufo* sp. toads secrete epinephrine, dopamine, and serotonin. The substance bufotenine is secreted by many *Bufo* sp. toads, and because of its reported hallucinogenic effects, it is classified as a Schedule I substance by the U.S. Drug Enforcement Administration. It appears, however, that bufotenine does not cross the blood–brain barrier and likely has no hallucinogenic effects in humans. The *Bufo alvarius* toad secretes 5-methoxydimethyltryptamine, a known hallucinogen.[34]

Poison-dart frogs (*Phyllobates* sp.) have a poison that contains several alkaloids, the most potent of which is batrachotoxin (Figure 5.4). Batrachotoxin acts on sodium channels located on the outer membrane of neurons and cardiac cells. In the presence of batrachotoxin, there is an increase in sodium influx into neurons and cardiac cells and a resulting depolarization. As a result, neural cells are not able to propagate impulses, and cardiac cells are left in a continuously contracted state.[4]

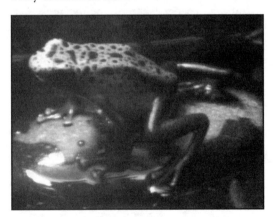

FIGURE 5-4   **Poison-dart frogs (*Phyllobates*)**
(See Color Plate 4.)

Blister beetles (*Cantharis vesicatoria*) secrete a substance called cantharadin through their leg joints. Cantharadin disrupts the integrity of endothelial cells and leads to tissue destruction. Cantharadin binds to albumin and is excreted in the urine.

Honeybees and bumblebees (*Apidae* sp.) as well as yellow jackets, hornets, and wasps (*Vespidae* sp.) have venoms with similar components and mechanisms of action. The *Apidae* sp. venom has three main proteins: melittin, hyaluronidase, and phospholipase A$_2$. Melittin hydrolyses cell membranes, leading to histamine and biogenic amine release. Hyaluronidase alters cell membranes, allows the dispersion of other venom factors, and acts as an allergen. Phospholipase A$_2$ is the main allergen in *Apidae* sp. venom and can cause hemolysis particularly in the presence of melittin. *Vespidae* sp. venom also contains hyaluronidase and phospholipase A$_2$ as two of its major components. Another protein found in *Vespidae* sp. venom is antigen 5, which has predominately allergen effects. Both *Apidae* sp. and *Vespidae* sp. contain mast cell degranulating peptides that are responsible for histamine release.[35,36]

CLINICAL EFFECTS

Clinical effects from snakebite vary greatly depending on the species involved. If the species is unknown, knowledge of local indigenous snakes is helpful. Investigators, however, must be aware that there is a worldwide distribution of exotic snakes.

Local and systemic clinical findings can help establish that a snakebite has occurred and can possibly help define the circumstances and species involved in the attack. Local findings may be obscured by outdated attempts at first aid, including incision, suction, and tourniquet placement at the site of the bite. Local effects should be apparent before systemic effects with subcutaneous or intramuscular envenomation by a *Crotalinae* sp. Systemic effects may be the presenting symptoms with *Elapidae* sp. envenomation or envenomation by any species that occurs intravascularly.[29]

Typical bites from a *Crotalinae* sp. result in two fang marks, although clothing or victim movement during the bite may result in only one fang mark. Local tissue damage from a *Crotalinae* sp. envenomation usually appears within minutes of the bite. Swelling and pain around the site of the bite is the first sign and is often followed by blistering, ecchymosis, and eventually necrosis of the skin. Swelling frequently progresses proximally to the bite and can involve an entire extremity within a few hours. Cases of *Crotalinae* sp. venom injected into a vein using a syringe and needle have resulted in minimal to moderate local tissue damage. Within the *Crotalinae* family, rattlesnake (*Crotalus* and *Sistrurus* species) venom is the most potent, often causing local and systemic effects. Water moccasin or cottonmouth *(Agkistrodon piscivorus)* venom is less potent than rattlesnake venom and, in comparison, causes less severe local and systemic effects. Copperhead *(Agkistrodon contortrix)* venom is the least potent and usually will only cause local effects (Figure 5.5).[29]

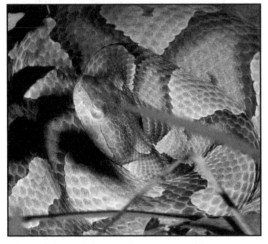

FIGURE 5-5   **Copperhead**
(*Agkistrodon contortrix*)
(See Color Plate 5.)

Systemic effects that have been reported with *Crotalinae* sp. envenomation include vomiting, respiratory distress, hypotension, anaphylaxis/ anaphylactoid reactions, hematologic toxicity, and neurotoxicity. The hematologic toxicity can be profound. Although bleeding, bruising, and hemorrhage can occur because of the hematologic toxicity, the majority of patients with these lab abnormalities do not have severe bleeding. The two cases of intentional intravascular administration of rattlesnake venom reported in the literature resulted in thrombocytopenia, coagulopathy, and gastrointestinal bleeding. Anaphylaxis, characterized by pruritis, urticaria, wheezing, and hypotension, can occur after intravascular envenomation and may be more likely with a history of previous envenomation. Neurotoxic effects are observed with some *Crotalinae* sp., particularly the western-most population of

Mojave rattlesnakes. Mojave rattlesnake envenomation can cause generalized weakness, respiratory failure, and cranial nerve dysfunction.

In contrast to *Crotalinae* sp. envenomation, *Elapidae* sp. envenomation results in subtle local effects. The bite of an *Elapidae* sp. can cause minor pain, but local swelling is usually minimal or absent.[37] It has been estimated that less than 40% of *Elapidae* sp. bites result in envenomation.[31] Systemic signs of *Elapidae* sp. envenomation may be delayed more than 12 hours after the bite. Symptoms include muscle weakness, slurred speech, diplopia, and respiratory distress. The most severe effect is paralysis, which can last up to 5 days. Deaths from *Elapidae* sp. envenomation are usually from respiratory arrest.[31,37]

Bark scorpion envenomation usually results in only local pain and parasthesias. These local symptoms can be increased by tapping over the site of envenomation. Pain and parasthesias may spread to areas away from the envenomation site. Systemic effects from the bark scorpion are rarely seen in healthy adults but may be apparent in children 6 years old and younger, adults with comorbid medical conditions, and the elderly. Possible systemic symptoms include ataxia, wandering eye movements, muscular fasciculations, sweating, tachycardia, hypertension, fever, and respiratory distress.[32] Scorpion species indigenous to countries outside of the United States can cause severe symptoms such as myocarditis, myocardial ischemia, coagulopathy, and pancreatitis.[38]

The two intentional envenomations in the literature involve agitating a black widow spider to provoke a bite and crushing a whole black widow spider and then injecting it into a vein using a needle and syringe. Local symptoms from a black widow bite include a pinprick sensation at the time of the bite. The classically described, but not always seen, "halo rash" at the site of envenomation has central blanching surrounded by erythema. Systemic effects do not always occur, but when they do, they usually appear within an hour of the envenomation. Systemic effects include muscle pain, spasm, and cramping predominately in proximity to the bite. Black widow envenomation can also cause sweating, tachycardia, hypertension, and vomiting.[38] Laboratory findings of elevated white blood count and creatinine phosphokinase may be present.[39] The case of intravenous administration of a crushed black widow spider resulted in generalized muscle pain and cramping, hypertension, tachycardia, and respiratory distress attributed to an anaphylactoid reaction.[22] Despite large numbers of reported envenomations, there are very few well-documented cases of death caused by black widow spiders or other *Latrodectus* sp. There is a reported death in Greece secondary to myocarditis attributed to a *Latrodectus* sp. envenomation.[40]

Toads from the genus *Bufo* have neurotoxic and cardiotoxic poisons. Seizures have been reported after ingestion of poison from *Bufo* sp. toads. Hallucinations may occur after consumption of the poison from *Bufo alvarius* species.[34] Cardiac effects are similar to those found with other cardiac glycosides. Cardiac arrhythmias, premature ventricular contractions, atrial fibrillation or flutter, ventricular tachycardia or fibrillation, and atrioventricular node and sinoatrial node conduction abnormalities may be recorded on electrocardiogram after cardiac glycoside poisoning. Hyperkalemia after acute cardiac glycoside poisoning indicates severe poisoning and a greater chance of morbidity and mortality. *Bufo* sp. toad poison can also cause hypersalivation and vomiting.[24] Deaths have been reported after ingestion of bufotoxin.[23]

Data are limited regarding the clinical effects of *Phyllobates* sp. poison on humans. The expected effects are extrapolated from the research that has been done on batrachotoxin. The two organ systems most likely to be affected are the cardiac and the nervous. Cardiac arrhythmias and arrest are potential effects of batrachotoxin poisoning. Weakness and paralysis are also possible effects from batrachotoxin.[4] Without adequate medical care, death would be an expected outcome of batrachotoxin toxicity.

Cantharadin, or "Spanish fly," causes local blistering and irritation. Clinical effects of ingestion occur in the gastrointestinal and genitourinary tracts. Symptoms include oral pain and ulceration, gastrointestinal pain, gastrointestinal bleeding, blistering of the urinary tract, genital pain and swelling, and kidney damage. Laboratory findings include hematuria, proteinuria, and heme-positive stool. Endoscopy may show severe hemorrhage within the gastrointestinal tract. Death has occurred from gastrointestinal hemorrhage.[26,27,41]

The normal reaction to an *Apidae* or *Vespidae* sp. sting is localized and consists of edema and a wheal-and-flare response. More severe symptoms can be seen with three different scenarios: sting in a critical area, multiple stings, or anaphylaxis. Stings in a critical area such as the oropharynx have led to airway compromise and require intensive medical care to prevent death. Multiple stings can cause vomiting, diarrhea, headache, syncope, and fever. Extremely large numbers of stings (>400), particularly in children, can cause rhabdomyolysis, seizures, renal failure, and death. Anaphylaxis from stings can cause urticaria, pruritis, respiratory failure, and cardiovascular failure. Anaphylaxis accounts for the highest number of deaths from these species.[36,42]

The clinician and investigator must be aware that the antidotes sometimes given for certain snake, scorpion, and spider envenomations may have clinical effects as well. Many of these antidotes are capable of causing anaphylaxis immediately and serum sickness several days after administration.[43] Documented deaths have occurred from anaphylaxis after receiving some of these antidotes.[39] Antidotes that contain whole immunoglobulin have a higher side effect profile than many of the newer antidotes that only contain the less allergenic Fab fragment of the immunoglobulin.[44]

ANALYTIC DETECTION

Confirmation of animal poisoning may be difficult to obtain. Data collection should include photographs of any bites, stings, or other skin lesions. If available, the animal itself or photographs of the animal that was used to intentionally poison should be taken for possible species identification. Laboratory testing for specific animal venoms and poisons is usually not readily available and may require a specialty research laboratory for proper identification.

Snake venom can be detected in blood, urine, and tissue. Tissue near the envenomation site is ideal for testing. Radioimmunoassay has been used to detect snake venom in victims. Radioimmunoassay is effective if proper serum and tissue samples are used but is ineffective if antivenin has been administered.[45] While radioimmunoassay may be the most specific test, ELISA (enzyme-linked immunoassays) testing is quicker, less expensive, and more likely to be available. ELISA testing has been used to detect the venom of many species of snakes, including several that are found in the United States.[46] The CSL pharmaceutical company manufactures a product called the snake venom detection kit that can detect the venom from common Australian venomous snakes. The kit can be used in the field and is most often used to test a cotton-swabbed sample from the envenomation site or a urine sample in an envenomated individual. With all forms of snake venom detection, there may be some cross-reactivity among similar species. Snake venom has been detected in blisters formed around the envenomation up to 48 hours after the bite and in tissue samples up to 2 weeks after a bite. In postmortem cases, regional lymph nodes may contain the highest levels of snake venom, and vitreous humor may be the most appropriate sample from a body with marked decomposition.[46,47] The majority of snake venom testing is available through a research laboratory and is not readily available in the healthcare setting.

Although research laboratories have identified several of the components of bark scorpion and black widow spider venom, there are no readily available tests for the detection of these venoms.

The cardiac glycoside bufadienolide, which is a component of the poison of the *Bufo* sp. toad, can cross-react with a serum digoxin assay. Bufadienolide has variable cross-reactivity with the digoxin assay, and digoxin levels in a human with bufadienolide exposure may be in the therapeutic range even when toxicity is present. Hyperkalemia and electrocardiogram findings may serve as clues of bufadienolide toxicity.[23]

Batrachotoxins as well as other toxins from the *Phyllobates* sp. have been identified by research laboratories.[4]

Cantharadin from the blister beetle can be detected by gas chromatography-mass spectrometry (GC-MS) or high-performance liquid chromatography.[48] Cantharadin has been identified in blood, urine, and gastric fluid.

There are laboratory and pathology tests that may provide data after *Apidae* or *Vespidae* sp. envenomation. Skin in an area of a suspected sting site can be sent to pathology for evaluation. The barbs of these species may be found in the superficial tissue where the sting occurred. Barbs are more likely to be found after envenomation by the *Apidae* sp. because they lose their barb in the process of stinging. In the cases of fatalities, further pathologic evaluation can concentrate on the search for and evaluation of signs of anaphylaxis, including laryngeal edema and pulmonary congestion.

If anaphylaxis is suspected, RAST (radioallergosorbent test) testing and serum tryptase levels should be done. Serum can be sent for RAST testing for bee or wasp venom. This test detects IgE antibodies to bee or wasp venom and confirms prior exposure to bee or wasp venom, which is usually necessary for anaphylaxis to occur. RAST testing has been successfully performed postmortem. A serum tryptase level should only be elevated after anaphylaxis in living humans. Peak serum tryptase levels occur 1 to 2 hours after anaphylaxis. In a postmortem analysis, serum tryptase may be a clue that anaphylaxis occurred, although postmortem serum tryptase has also been elevated in cases of trauma, drug overdose, and ischemic heart disease. If toxicity is suspected from venom alone, some specialty laboratories have performed serum assays for bee venom and phospholipase A_2.[36]

CONCLUSION

Since ancient times, humans have recognized that certain animals possess potent toxins. The difficulty in obtaining and using these toxins has likely prevented their common use in crime. There are well-documented cases of criminal use of animal poisons, and there are other animal poisons that have not been reported in criminal activity but have a high potential for future criminal use.

Investigators and healthcare workers must use historic and clinical clues to determine if a poisoning using an animal poison has occurred. Unfortunately, supporting laboratory data may be difficult or impossible to obtain depending on the type of animal poison used. Suspicion that individuals have used an animal poison to commit a crime may be increased if they have access to poisonous animals—for example, if they are exotic animal venders, researchers who work with poisonous animals, members of snake-handling churches, zoo personnel, or members of organized drug trafficking rings.

During a criminal or medical investigation, care must be taken not to misdiagnose a victim who has been exposed to animal poison.

Snakebite marks have been initially misdiagnosed as thorn punctures, rodent bites, or knife blade incisions. The later signs of *Crotalinae* sp. envenomation (i.e., soft-tissue swelling and bleeding disorders) may be mistaken for cellulitis and sepsis. The finding of paralysis after exposure to Mojave rattlesnake venom, *Elapidae* envenomation, or batrachotoxin poisoning will present in a similar manner to poisoning by the neuromuscular paralytics or curare. Bark scorpion envenomation has been erroneously identified as methamphetamine poisoning and as a psychiatric disorder. Black widow spider bite can cause a rigid abdomen and can be misdiagnosed as peritonitis or appendicitis. *Bufo* sp. toad toxin can cause symptoms that are identical to poisoning by other cardiac glycosides; thus the source may be mistaken as the medication digoxin or a plant-derived cardiac glycoside. The cardiac effects from batrachotoxin may be difficult to distinguish from a cardiac arrhythmia from a preexisting medical cause. Cantharadin poisoning may mimic exposure to a caustic substance such as hydrochloric acid or lye. Milder cases of cantharadin exposure may be similar in presentation to a urinary tract infection. Anaphylaxis secondary to a wasp or bee sting may be difficult to distinguish from anaphylaxis from another source.

Another pitfall may be the misinterpretation of the outcome of a victim of animal poisoning who has received an antidote. It may be the antidote itself and not the animal-derived poison that is responsible for severe symptoms such as anaphylaxis and death.

A thorough knowledge of poisonous animals and the expected clinical symptoms that they cause remains essential when investigating a suspicious criminal case.

REFERENCES

1. Morgan DL, Blair HW, Ramsey RP. Suicide attempt by the intravenous injection of rattlesnake venom. *South Med J.* 2006;99(3):282–284.
2. Bisset NG, Mazars G. Arrow poisons in south Asia. Part 1. Arrow poisons in ancient India. *J Ethnopharmacol.* 1984;12(1):1–24.
3. Bisset NG. Arrow and dart poisons. *J Ethnopharmacol.* 1989;25(1):1–41.
4. Myers CW, Daly JW. Dart-poison frogs. *Sci Am.* 1983;248(2):120–133.
5. Mayor, A. *Greek Fire, Poison Arrows and Scorpion Bombs: Biological and Chemical Warfare in the Ancient World.* Woodstock, NY: Overlook Duckworth; 2003:75–97, 176-86.
6. Rattlesnake tale. *Time.* Dec 18, 1978.
7. The Snake in the Mailbox. *Time.* Oct 23, 1978.
8. Faulk, K. Snake kills snake handling evangelist. *Hidden Mysteries: Religion's Frauds, Lies, Control.* Oct 6, 1998.
9. Woman dies after snakebite during church service. *WBIR.com.* November 8, 2006. http://www.wbir.com/news/local/story.aspx?storyid=39406. Accessed September 3, 2009.
10. Goeringer, C. Trouble for a snake-handling sect. *Hidden Mysteries: Religion's Frauds, Lies, Control.* Dec 8, 1996.
11. Woman Threatens Cops With Poisonous Snakes. *northcountygazette.com.* March 7, 2007. http://www.northcountrygazette.org/articles/2007/030707PoisonousSnakes.html. Accessed October 1, 2009.
12. Man attacked cops with snakes. *News24.com.* September 9, 2004. http://www.news24.com/Content/World/News/1073/b7653d14571246a6adeb8632a1758606/20-09-2004-01-56/Man_attacked_cops_with_snakes. Accessed September 3, 2009.
13. Snake panic in South Africa bank [transcript]. BBC News. *BBC.* Jan 30, 2004.
14. Snake case: bank client pleads not guilty. iol.co.za. May 16, 2005. http://www.iol.co.za/index.php?set_id=1&click_id=13&art_id=qw1116256684982B263. Accessed October 1, 2009.
15. Knight B, Barclay A, Mann R. Suicide by injection of snake venom. *Forensic Sci.* 1977;10(2):141–145.
16. Yadlowski JM, Tu AT, Garriott JC, et al. Suicide by snake venom injection. *J Forensic Sci.* 1980;25(4):760–764.
17. Weston MW. Lovelorn and snakebit. *Hosp Pract (Off Ed).* 1986;21(3A):140–143.
18. Drugs fuel illegal animal trade. *BBC News.* BBC. June 17, 2002.
19. Meth linked to deaths, shootings, other crimes in NW area. *Arkansas-Democrat Gazette.* June 6, 1999.
20. Gram D. Scorpion on a plane bites Vermont man [transcript]. *CourtTV Crime Library.* CourtTV. 2006.
21. Fisher DP. Letter: attempted suicide by black widow spider bite. *JAMA.* 1976;235(25):2718–2719.
22. Bush SP, Naftel J. Injection of a whole black widow spider. *Ann Emerg Med.* 1996;27(4):532–533.
23. Brubacher JR, Lachmanen D, Ravikumar PR, Hoffman RS. Treatment of toad venom poisoning with digoxin-specific Fab fragments. *Chest.* 1996;110(5):1282–1288.
24. Hitt M, Ettinger DD. Toad toxicity. *N Engl J Med.* 1986;314(23):1517–1518.
25. Poison frog murder plot. *St. Albans & Harpenden Review.* Dec 23, 2002.
26. Craven JD, Polak A. Cantharidin poisoning. *BMJ.* 1954;2(4901):1386–1388.
27. Nickolls L.C, Teare D. Poisoning by cantharidin *BMJ.* 1954;2(4901):1384–1386.
28. Herdy A, Danielson R. Parents' religious group disdains medical care. sptimes.com. Oct 1, 1998. http://www.sptimes.com/TampaBay/100198/Parents__religiou6.html. Accessed October 1, 2009.
29. Holstege CP, Miller MB, Wermuth M, et al. Crotalid snake envenomation. *Crit Care Clin.* 1997;13(4):889–921.

30. Suchard JR, LoVecchio F. Envenomations by rattlesnakes thought to be dead. *N Engl J Med.* 1999;340(24):1930.

31. Norris RL, Dart RC. Apparent coral snake envenomation in a patient without visible fang marks. *Am J Emerg Med.* 1989;7(4):402–405.

32. Curry SC, Vance MV, Ryan PJ, et al. Envenomation by the scorpion Centruroides sculpturatus. *J Toxicol Clin Toxicol.* 1983;1(4-5):417–449.

33. Rosenthal L, Zacchetti D, Madeddu L, Meldolesi J. Mode of action of alpha-latrotoxin: role of divalent cations in Ca2(+)-dependent and Ca2(+)-independent effects mediated by the toxin. *Mol Pharmacol.* 1990;38(6):917–923.

34. Lyttle T, Goldstein D, Gartz J. *Bufo* toads and Bufotenine: fact and fiction surrounding an alleged psychedelic. *J Psychoactive Drugs.* 1996;28(3):267–290.

35. Hoffman DR. Hymenoptera venom proteins. *Adv Exp Med Biol.* 1996;391:169–186.

36. Riches KJ, Gillis D, James RA. An autopsy approach to bee sting-related deaths. *Pathology.* 2002;34(3):257–262.

37. Kitchens CS, Van Mierop LH. Envenomation by the Eastern coral snake (Micrurus fulvius fulvius). A study of 39 victims. *JAMA.* 1987;258(12):1615–1618.

38. Allen C. Arachnid envenomations. *Emerg Med Clin North Am.* 1992;10(2):269–298.

39. Clark RF, Wethern-Kestner S, Vance MV, Gerken R. Clinical presentation and treatment of black widow spider envenomation: a review of 163 cases. *Ann Emerg Med.* 1992;21(7):782–787.

40. Pneumatikos IA, Galiatsou E, Goe D, et al. Acute fatal toxic myocarditis after black widow spider envenomation. *Ann Emerg Med.* 2003;41(1):158.

41. Polettini A, Crippa O, Ravagli A, et al. A fatal case of poisoning with cantharidin. *Forensic Sci Int.* 1992;56(1):37–43.

42. Gayer KD, Burnett JW. Hymenoptera stings. *Cutis.* 1988;41(2):93–94.

43. Bond GR. Antivenin administration for *Centruroides* scorpion sting: risks and benefits. *Ann Emerg Med.* 1992;21(7):788–791.

44. Dart RC, Seifert SA, Boyer LV, et al. A randomized multicenter trial of *Crotalinae* polyvalent immune Fab (ovine) antivenom for the treatment for crotaline snakebite in the United States. *Arch Intern Med.* 2001;161(16):2030–2036.

45. Sutherland SK, Couter AR, Broad AJ. Human snake bite victims: the successful detection of circulating snake venom by radioimmunoassay. *Med J Aust.* 1975;1(2):27–29.

46. Minton SA. Present tests for detection of snake venom: clinical applications. *Ann Emerg Med.* 1987;16(9):932–937.

47. Sutherland SK, Coulter AR. Comments on "suicide by injection of snake venom." *Forensic Sci.* 1978;11(3):241–243.

48. Hundt HK, Steyn JM, Wagner L. Post-mortem serum concentration of cantharidin in a fatal case of cantharides poisoning. *Hum Exp Toxicol.* 1990;9(1):35–40.

6 | Arsenic

Ashley L. Harvin and Christopher P. Holstege

CASE STUDY

A 62-year-old man was hospitalized 10 times during a 5-year period before his death in 1986. Six of these hospitalizations occurred between 1985 and 1986. From 1981 to 1984, he was treated for cardiomyopathy, leukopenia, gastrointestinal disturbances, and paresthesia ("pins and needles" feeling) of his toes. A commercial toxicology laboratory performed a full urine drug screen and Reinsch test for heavy metals, and the results were all normal. In 1985, he was hospitalized again for severe gastroenteritis and dehydration. The patient complained of a mild stomach ache and diarrhea that had steadily worsened until he returned to the hospital. He was rehydrated and discharged after 2 days. Prior symptoms from his previous hospitalizations were present, but their cause was still unknown. Records note a "diffuse increased pigmentation on the trunk and extremities with a mottled or freckled distribution and scaling dermatitis of the feet." Also, along with his paresthesias of the feet, the patient experienced "decreased muscle strength in the lower extremities with quadriceps atrophy."

Weeks after his last hospitalization, the patient was readmitted after several days of uncontrollable diarrhea and vomiting. His "glove and sock" paresthesias had rapidly progressed, and he was also experiencing weakness of the upper and lower extremities. After 2 days of neurologic analysis, Guillain-Barré syndrome was suspected. All other symptoms remained undiagnosed and the patient was discharged at the request of his wife, who agreed to continue rehabilitation at home. A urine sample was obtained and sent to a laboratory for heavy metal analysis due to the patient's diverse multi-organ symptoms, gastrointestinal complaints, and polyneuropathy. When the results revealed arsenic levels of 3.66 mg/L, the patient's wife was questioned about possible arsenic exposure at work or home. She denied any exposure, and consequently the physician suspected that an error may have occurred in the laboratory. The physician asked the wife to obtain another urine sample at home in order to repeat the heavy metal test. She returned the sample 2 days later, and the results were approximately 0.05 mg/L, which reflected an arsenic level below what is considered toxic.

Three weeks later, the patient was again readmitted to the hospital with dehydration, hypotension, diarrhea, and vomiting. Laboratory tests revealed hypoproteinemia, leukopenia, thrombocytopenia, abnormal liver function, and metabolic acidosis. His condition continued to worsen despite treatments, and the patient died of multisystem organ failure 3 days later. Before his death, however, a 24-hour urine specimen and portions of hair and fingernails were sent to a laboratory for arsenic analysis. The wife, initially rejecting the physician's recommendation, eventually consented to autopsy. Findings from the autopsy included pulmonary edema, hypoplasia of the bone marrow, partial necrosis of the liver, focal ulceration of the esophagus and stomach with 100 mL of recent blood in the stomach, and scarring of the renal cortices.[1]

From the autopsy findings and the results from the final urine specimen, the cause of death was determined to be arsenic poisoning. The decedent's wife was tried for murder when reports of marital problems surfaced. Evidence against her included a change in the man's will 3 weeks before his death, which left her as the sole heir of his estate. The wife, however, testified that her late husband often complained of depression and had spoken of suicide. It was never determined whether the wife murdered him or he self-administered the arsenic as a suicide attempt.[1]

HISTORY

Arsenic compounds have been used for both therapeutic and malevolent purposes since 3000 BCE.[2] Galen used realgar (As_4S_4) to treat ulcers. Hippocrates, Aristotle, and Pliny the Elder also believed in the medicinal properties of arsenicals.[3] In 1786, Fowler's solution, which contained 1% arsenic trioxide (As_2O_3), was created and then used for over 150 years to treat many illnesses such as syphilis, leukemia, and psoriasis. By the early 1900s, physicians used arsenic to treat a variety of ailments, including pellagra, malaria, amebiasis, trypanosomiasis, anemia, asthma, and dermatitis herpetiformis, among several others.[4] Since then, arsenic has been replaced by nontoxic drugs to treat these illnesses. Recently, arsenical compounds have been used in pesticides, herbicides, fungicides, rodenticides, and chemical warfare.[5]

Arsenic is a metalloid that exists in elemental, gaseous, organic, and inorganic forms. Inorganic arsenicals exist in trivalent (arsenite) and pentavalent (arsenate) states. Elemental arsenic is considered nontoxic, even if eaten in significant quantities, due to its insolubility in bodily fluids.[3] Organic arsenic compounds also exhibit low toxicity and are excreted faster than inorganic compounds.[3] Inorganic pentavalent arsenicals are much less poisonous than trivalent compounds. Trivalent arsenicals include realgar (As_4S_4) and orpiment (As_2S_3). Other examples of trivalent arsenicals include arsenic trioxide (As_2O_3), which has been called "the poison of poisons," and arsine gas (AsH_3). Throughout history, arsenic trioxide has remained a popular poisoning agent because of its availability, inexpensiveness, and lack of taste and odor. Arsenic trioxide is also called "white arsenic" because its appearance resembles that of sugar. After arsine, arsenic trioxide is the most toxic arsenic compound. Arsine's high toxicity can be attributed to the fact that it is inhaled instead of absorbed through the skin or gastrointestinal tract.[3]

For centuries, arsenic has been used for homicidal and very rarely suicidal purposes.[6] One of the earliest documented cases involving homicidal arsenic poisoning was when

Nero poisoned Britannicus to gain his Roman throne in 55 CE.[3] In the Middle Ages, arsenic poisoning rapidly gained popularity in political life. In 1577, Swedish King Erik XIV, the oldest son of Gustav Vasa, was murdered by his brother via arsenic poisoning.[4] In Renaissance Italy, members of the Borgia family, who were alleged masters of the use of poisons in assassinations, used a white powder known as "La Cantarella" to murder political opponents. It is believed that the white powder consisted of arsenic and an unidentified sweetener.[2] After Napoleon Bonaparte was killed, cancer was found in his stomach. Arsenic was found in his nails, and many believed the cancer was related to a slow poisoning by arsenic.[4]

Goeie Mie of the Netherlands was one of the most famous arsenic poisoners of the 19th century. Between 1867 and 1884, she poisoned over 100 friends and relatives. After opening life insurance policies in their names, she administered arsenic trioxide in milk to her victims. Of the 102 victims, 45 became seriously ill and developed neurologic problems, and 27 died. Sixteen of those poisoned were her relatives.[7]

In the 19th century, arsenic became the most popular poison in France, with phosphorus the second most popular. At the end of that century, its use declined due to the development of a highly sensitive assay for arsenic.[3]

In the early 1900s, an arsenic murder ring in Philadelphia was discovered. The members posed as "faith healers" or "witch doctors" and offered medical and spiritual care to vulnerable Italian immigrants. After gaining a target's trust, a ring member would insure that person's spouse or relative, poison the victim, and collect the insurance money. Arsenic is practically undetectable when slipped into someone's food or drink, and because of this, the arsenic ring thought it was a "miracle drug." The ring members, however, did not realize that arsenic is a metallic substance and does not decompose. This feature made it easy for police to find physical evidence against the ring in suspected victims.[8]

Arsenic poisoning has long been present in literature. In Joseph Kesselring's 1941 play *Arsenic and Old Lace*, two old ladies used cyanide and arsenic in wine to poison their gentlemen visitors. People have reported to precondition themselves with sublethal doses of arsenic and consequently become less sensitive to arsenic

poisoning. Novelist Dorothy Sayers used this feature to write narratives involving the use of arsenic as a homicidal agent.[2]

POTENTIAL DELIVERY METHODS

Arsenic is absorbed by the gastrointestinal, respiratory, intravenous, and mucosal routes.[5] Inorganic arsenic is tasteless and odorless. In criminal poisoning cases, arsenic is commonly administered via the victim's food or drink and is subsequently absorbed by the gastrointestinal tract in the small intestine and colon.

TOXICOLOGIC MECHANISMS

Arsenic has multiple mechanisms of toxicity. One mechanism involves the impairment of cellular respiration by inhibition of enzymes containing thiol groups (-SH) and the uncoupling of oxidative phosphorylation.[9,10] Arsenic metabolites typically inactivate enzymes involved in DNA synthesis and repair and the cellular energy pathway.[7] Trivalent arsenicals interact with thiol groups of proteins and enzymes in their reduced state, which inhibits enzyme activity. This leads to reduced energy production in the cell and may cause cell damage and death.[4,7] Arsenic also has the ability to replace phosphate molecules in high-energy compounds such as ATP ("arsenolysis").[7,9,10] Substitution of the less stable pentavalent arsenic anion for the stable phosphorous anion in phosphate causes rapid hydrolysis of high-energy compounds.[7] As a result, ATP is not conserved, leading to cell death.[4]

CLINICAL EFFECTS

The earliest effects of arsenic poisoning are severe gastrointestinal symptoms characteristic of acute or subacute intoxication.[7,11] Toxic effects of inorganic arsenicals vary depending on the quantity and type of arsenic ingested and the chronicity of exposure. Manifestations of acute toxicity occur with large doses of potent arsenicals, such as arsenic trioxide. Clinical effects differ for chronic ingestion of lower amounts, such as drinking contaminated water.

Numerous reports of acute intoxication following criminal poisoning have been published. Severe toxicity has been reported with ingestion of 1 mg of arsenic trioxide; a fatal dose is approximately 200–300 mg.[12] Clinical effects may appear minutes, hours, or days after exposure depending on the dose and type of arsenic consumed.[5]

The earliest manifestations of acute poisoning are severe gastrointestinal symptoms of nausea, vomiting, abdominal pain, and diarrhea.[6,7,13] The diarrhea may resemble that seen with cholera and can appear as "rice water." These symptoms occur 10 minutes to several hours after ingestion. The patient often complains of muscle cramps and thirst.[12] Cardiovascular and respiratory symptoms include hypotension, shock, pulmonary edema, acute respiratory distress syndrome, and heart failure.[7,13] The electrocardiogram may reveal prolongation of the QT interval, particularly of the ST segment, and T-wave inversion.[12] Other symptoms include dehydration, headache, lightheadedness, vertigo, and fever.[5]

In less severe cases, gastroenteritis and mild hypotension may develop in acutely poisoned patients and may persist despite intravenous therapies. The prolonged gastrointestinal symptoms indicate possible arsenic poisoning.

Prolonged or additional symptoms may occur for days to weeks after an acute exposure. Neurologic symptoms such as headache, confusion, personality change, irritability, hallucinations, delirium, and seizures may develop or persist.[7] Peripheral neuropathy commonly occurs 1–3 weeks after an acute poisoning. The peripheral neuropathy may last for several years.[7] Progressive neuropathy may be misdiagnosed as Guillain-Barré syndrome.[7,13] Sensory symptoms may include numbness, tingling, lightheadedness, delirium, encephalopathy, muscle weakness, and severe pain following superficial touching of limbs.[5,7] Anorexia and weight loss have also been reported. Respiratory symptoms such as dry cough, hemoptysis, and chest pain may occur and be misinterpreted as viral or bronchial disease.

While chronic exposure to small amounts of inorganic arsenic usually occurs with environmental or occupational exposure, there are rare reports associated with criminal poisoning.[11] Most chronic exposures result from consumption of arsenic-contaminated water over an extended period of time.[14] Symptoms typically develop within a few weeks or months of exposure.[5]

An accumulation of arsenic in skin, hair, and nails causes clinical symptoms such as hyperpigmentation, keratoses of the palms and soles, melanosis, and hair loss (Figure 6.1).[4,5,9,13,14] A combination of melanosis and keratosis in an adult patient almost certainly indicates chronic arsenic poisoning.[4] Inorganic arsenicals are human carcinogens, and a significant relationship between chronic arsenic exposure and skin cancer has been found.[5] Skin lesions may indicate high exposure and are distinctive clinical manifestations of arsenic poisoning. They are one of the most common features of chronic arsenic poisoning.[15] Neuropathy is also a common complication of the nervous system.[9] Other effects include neuritis, paresthesia, and muscle weakness.[5] A metallic taste and garlic odor of the breath and sweat may indicate chronic arsenic poisoning. Other indicators include excessive salivation and perspiration.[12]

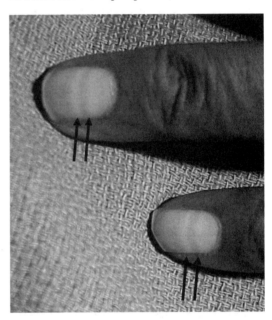

FIGURE 6-1   Mees' lines following arsenic poisoning. Note the white band traversing the width of the nail at the arrows. (See Color Plate 6.)

ANALYTIC DETECTION

The definitive diagnosis of arsenic toxicity can be difficult. Acute arsenic intoxication is commonly diagnosed by an elevated urinary arsenic concentration in association with signs and symptoms consistent with arsenic toxicity. Seafood ingestion itself can markedly increase total urinary arsenic concentrations. When consumption of arsenobetaine in seafood is considered a cause for an elevated total arsenic level, speciation of arsenic can be performed. If urinary arsenic levels are low in a late-presenting case, hair and nail analysis for arsenic can be performed.[4, 5, 14]

CONCLUSION

Arsenic features the key elements of a perfect poisoning agent: It is readily available, inexpensive, tasteless, and odorless. The clinical diagnosis of arsenic toxicity is difficult, as it mimics numerous different disease processes. Analytical techniques are available for detecting arsenic in urine, blood, hair, and nails, but the timing of sample collections and the ingestion of foods that may contain organic arsenic must be taken into consideration when results are reviewed.

REFERENCES

1. Poklis A, Saady JJ. Arsenic poisoning: acute or chronic? *Am J Forensic Med Pathol.* 1990;11(3):226–232.
2. Sambu S, Wilson R. Arsenic in food and water—a brief history. *Toxicol Ind Health.* 2008;24:217–226.
3. Jolliffe DM. A history of the use of arsenicals in man. *J R Soc Med.* May 1993;86:287–289.
4. Saha KC. Review of arsenicosis in West Bengal, India—a clinical perspective. *Environ Sci Technol Rev.* 2003;30(2):127–163.
5. Zelikoff JT, Thomas PT (eds). *Immunotoxicity of Environmental and Occupational Metals.* London: Taylor & Frances; 1998:1–26.
6. Mari F, Polettini A, Lippi D, Bertol E. The mysterious death of Francesco I de' Medici and Bianca Cappello: an arsenic murder? *BMJ.* 2006;333:1299–1301.
7. Vahidnia A, van der Voet GB, de Wolff FA. Arsenic neurotoxicity—a review. *Hum Exp Toxicol.* 2007;26:823–832.
8. Young RJ. Arsenic and no lace: the bizarre tale of a Philadelphia murder ring. *Pa Hist.* 2000;67(3):397–414.
9. Tchounwou PB, Patlolla AK, Centeno JA. Carcinogenic and systemic health effects associated with arsenic exposure—a critical review. *Toxicol Pathol.* 2003;31:575–588.
10. Hall AH. Chronic arsenic poisoning (review article). *Toxicol Lett.* 2002;128:69–72.
11. Franzblau A, Lilis R. Acute arsenic intoxication from environmental arsenic exposure. *Arch Environ Health.* 1989;44(6):385–390.
12. Winship KA. Toxicity of inorganic arsenic salts. *Adv Drug React Ac Pois Rev.* 1984;3:129–160.
13. Scheindlin S. The duplicitous nature of inorganic arsenic. *Mol Interv.* April 2005;5(2):60–64.
14. Kapaj S, Peterson H, Liber K, Bhattacharya P. Human health effects from chronic arsenic poisoning—a review. *J Environ Sci Health A Tox Hazard Subst Environ Eng.* 2006;41(10):2399–2428.
15. Yoshida T, Yamauchi H, Sun G. Chronic health effects in people exposed to arsenic via the drinking water: dose-response relationships in review. *Toxicol Appl Pharmacol.* 2004;198:243–252.

7 | Botulism

William H. Richardson III

CASE STUDY

A 45-year-old woman presented to an emergency department complaining of blurred and double vision, difficulty swallowing, dry mouth, perioral tingling, and difficulty breathing. She had eaten seafood approximately 12 hours prior but denied fever, nausea, vomiting, and diarrhea. Additional history established that no homemade or damaged canned goods were consumed, but a commercial can of tuna and frozen shrimp purchased from a local grocery store were eaten. Her initial vital signs were temperature 97.2°F, blood pressure 130/73 mm Hg, pulse 101 beats per minute, and respiratory rate 24 per minute with 98% oxygen saturations on room air. She had slurred but understandable speech, bilateral sluggish 6-mm pupils, and slight drooping (ptosis) of the left eyelid. Over the next 5 hours, the patient developed ptosis of the right eyelid and was unable to perform extraocular muscle movements but could otherwise follow commands appropriately. The remainder of her initial neurologic examination was normal with strong, symmetric grip and lower extremity strength. Initial laboratory evaluations of serum chemistries, complete blood count, erythrocyte sedimentation rate, urinalysis, and cerebrospinal fluid analysis were normal. A chest radiograph and noncontrast head computed tomography scan were normal. A urine pregnancy test was negative, and a urine drug immunoassay was positive for benzodiazepines as a class.[1]

Approximately 6 hours into the emergency department course, the patient developed short, gasping respirations, and an arterial blood gas yielded the following results: pH 7.11, pCO_2 67 mm Hg, and pO_2 186 mm Hg. She was subsequently intubated and admitted to the intensive care unit. Rapid progression of bulbar muscular weakness, complete bilateral ptosis, and fixed, dilated pupils developed. Weakness progressed in the upper and lower extremities. A working diagnosis of botulism was made, and the state health department was contacted. Stool and serum samples were obtained, and the patient was administered bivalent (A,B) botulinum antitoxin within 18 hours of arrival.[1]

Her condition, however, continued to worsen. Administration of edrophonium 10 mg resulted in no improvement of motor function. Nerve conduction studies and an electromyelogram demonstrated a predominantly motor neuropathy. By day 3 in the hospital, she had developed almost complete motor paralysis except slight movement of the toes on her right foot. On hospital day 5, a stool culture originally sent to the health department was reported to contain type F botulinum toxin. The Centers for Disease Control and Prevention (CDC) was contacted regarding heptavalent (A,B,C1,D,E,F,G) botulinum antitoxin. A single unit vial of the equine heptavalent experimental botulinum antitoxin (H-BAT) was administered on hospital day 7. The following day she was moving digits on both feet, and by the next day, she could weakly shake her head and slightly move her left eyelid. On hospital day 10, the patient could partially open both eyes and weakly move her fingers. Ventilatory support was removed on hospital day 15.

Over the next week, the patient gradually recovered significant motor strength and was discharged to a rehabilitation facility. Subsequent follow-up demonstrated complete neurologic recovery. Although food poisoning was suspected, anaerobic cultures and toxin assays of stool, serum, food samples of tuna and shrimp, and the can containing the tuna from the patient's home could not verify the source of exposure.[1]

HISTORY

Failed attempts at biologic terrorism using botulinum toxin have already occurred. From April 1990 to 1995, the Japanese cult Aum Shinrikyo attempted on several occasions to disperse botulinum toxin at locations in Japan. Cult members initially tried to release the toxin while driving around government buildings in central Tokyo. In June 1993, a spray device was used from a vehicle driven around the imperial palace in Tokyo during the wedding of the crown prince. Just prior to the sarin subway attack in March 1995, a plan to aerosolize botulinum toxin from an improvised briefcase sprayer in the Tokyo subway system was foiled when a cult member did not load the actual toxin in the dispersal device.[2] There were no reported injuries during these attempts to disperse botulinum toxin due to a number of factors: insufficient microbiological facilities, inadequate aerosolization techniques, lack of toxin potency, and internal sabotage. The cult members had obtained *Clostridium botulinum* microbes from soil on a northern Japanese isle.[3]

While modern extremists and terrorists have the capability of acquiring and exploiting botulinum toxin for criminal purposes, the true history begins with state-sponsored development of botulinum toxin during World War II. In 1942, even before the United States began development of botulinum toxin as a bioweapon at Fort Detrick, Maryland, the Japanese had fed deadly *C. botulinum* cultures to prisoners during its Manchuria occupation in the 1930s.[4] Unclassified intelligence from 1947 suggests that Germany also made attempts to develop botulinum toxin as a cross-channel weapon. Although the decision was ultimately made not to implement a vaccination schedule, over a million doses of botulinum toxoid vaccine were made available to the Allied forces in preparation for the Normandy D-Day invasion due to concerns that Germany had weaponized botulinum toxin.[5] There has even been speculation that a high-ranking German officer was assassinated in 1942 by Czech patriots using a bomb containing botulinum toxin, although the preponderance of evidence suggests otherwise.[6]

During the Cold War era, the United States and Soviet Union invested heavily in efforts to develop and weaponize botulinum toxin. Microbiological techniques for culture concentration and purification were optimized to produce maximum amounts of purified toxin until the biologic weapons program in the United States was ended in 1969–1970 by executive order of Richard M. Nixon.[7] Despite the 1972 Biological and Toxin Weapons convention prohibiting bioweapon production and offensive research, evidence exists that proliferation of botulinum toxin offensive programs continued in the former Soviet Union into the 1990s.[8,9] Former Soviet scientists report botulinum toxin testing occurred on Vozrozhdeniye Island in the Aral Sea and describe attempts at splicing the botulinum toxin gene from *C. botulinum* into other bacteria.[8-10]

Following the collapse of the Soviet Union, rogue nations attempted to recruit former Soviet bioweapon scientists, and since the mid-1980s, other countries have produced or are suspected of state-sponsored development of botulinum toxin for biologic weapons.[11] Following the 1991 Persian Gulf War, Iraqi officials admitted to the United Nations inspection team that Iraq had produced over 19,000 L of concentrated botulinum toxin with 10,000 L already weaponized. These included 600-km range missiles and 400-lb bombs containing botulinum toxin.[12]

William C. Patrick III, the former chief of the American offensive biowarfare program at Fort Detrick, Maryland, has suggested that use of botulinum toxin to immobilize an enemy in battle would be difficult due to logistical problems with concentrating and stabilizing the toxin for aerosol dissemination. However, the physical and psychological effects on a civilian population following deliberate release or food contamination with botulinum toxin could be substantial. Intentional release of aerosolized botulinum toxin has been estimated to incapacitate 10% of individuals within 0.5 kilometers downwind of the dispersal site.[8] Therefore the bioterrorist or criminal use of botulinum toxin has significant conceivable public health implications and has been historically recognized as an agent with considerable lethal potential.

POTENTIAL DELIVERY METHODS

Classically, botulism has occurred naturally in humans in three forms: foodborne, intestinal (infant and adult), and wound botulism. Foodborne botulism develops when food contaminated with botulinum toxin is absorbed via the intestinal tract. There is no in vivo colonization of clostridial species with foodborne botulism. Infant and adult intestinal botulism are a direct result of intestinal lumen colonization of *Clostridium* sp. leading to the production of botulinum toxin in vivo. Wound botulism begins as an infectious disease resulting from *C. botulinum* growth in grossly contaminated wounds, often following the subcutaneous injection of black tar heroin.[13]

More recently, an iatrogenic cause of botulism has emerged. The therapeutic use of botulinum toxins type A and B has culminated in inadvertent cases of botulism with systemic manifestations.[14] Criminal exploitation of botulinum toxin is unlikely to involve intestinal or wound botulism, as clostridial growth is required in vivo to produce a slow release of toxin necessary to develop illness.

Aerosolized dissemination is a likely technique to deliver botulinum toxin for reprehensible reasons. Inhalational botulism should be suspected when a large number of cases are geographically and temporally clustered but lack a common dietary exposure.[8] Bioterrorists with large-scale criminal intent would aerosolize particles in a range of 0.3- to 15-μm diameters. Aerosol generators could deliver particles from vehicles, boats, or concealed ground positions typically 1 to 50 kilometers upwind from the intended target population.[15] Many factors including weather conditions, population density, and target environment could significantly impact the timing of symptom onset and extent of casualties from aerosolized botulinum toxin.

Deliberate contamination of food or water is another possible route of botulinum toxin poisoning. In 1977 the largest unintentional outbreak of foodborne botulism in the United States occurred in Michigan and involved 59 patients eating improperly home-canned jalapeño peppers in a restaurant.[16] Following a maleficent act of botulinum toxin poisoning, it would be important to discern the outbreak from a naturally occurring episode of foodborne botulism. It may be difficult to make this distinction because foodborne botulism is now often associated with nonpreserved foods and restaurants, and no longer is it associated with only home-preserved foods.[17]

No cases of waterborne botulism have been reported. Though the potential for water contamination exists, it is an unlikely scenario for several reasons. Botulinum toxin is typically inactivated by standard chlorination water treatments, and the need for large quantities of toxin would make it impractical to contaminate large water reservoirs.[8] Given the large size of most national water reservoirs (3 to 30 million gallons) and the long residence times of water in these reservoirs, intentional contamination is unlikely to cause widespread illness.[18] On a smaller scale, however, untreated water or beverages may contain botulinum toxin for days and should be investigated as a potential source if no other conveyance is identified.[19]

Lastly, malicious injection of an individual with botulinum toxin could present with an appearance similar to cases of therapeutic botulinum toxin injections that resulted in inadvertent systemic symptoms of botulism. The onset and severity of symptoms would depend on the amount and rate of toxin absorption, time to recognition, and treatment. While this potentially lethal delivery method has yet to be described with botulinum toxin, assassination by injecting minute quantities of the biotoxin ricin are described in the death of the Bulgarian dissident Georgi Markov.[20,21]

TOXICOLOGIC MECHANISMS

Botulinum toxin is one of the most potent poisonous substances known. *Clostridium botulinum* is a gram-positive, spore-forming, obligate anaerobic bacillus that produces botulinum toxin. Other strains of *Clostridium baratii* and *Clostridium butyricum* also have this capability.[22] There are eight distinct antigenic types of botulinum toxin that have been identified, and they have been assigned letters A through G with two C subtypes. The toxin types differ slightly in their mechanism of action, but the ultimate pharmacologic effect and clinical symptoms remain the same.[23] Botulinum toxin is a dichain polypeptide in which a 100-kDa heavy chain is linked to a 50-kDa light chain by a single disulfide bond. Following absorption into the bloodstream and transport to the neuromuscular junction in the peripheral nervous system and cranial nerves, the heavy chain binds irreversibly to the presynaptic nerve cell membrane and is taken up via endocytosis.[24] The light chain, a zinc-dependent endopeptidase, then cleaves other peptides inside the neuronal cell that are essential

for release of acetylcholine-containing vesicles. By preventing acetylcholine release at the neuromuscular junction, motor neuron to muscle cholinergic transmission is disrupted and paralysis results.

CLINICAL EFFECTS

As a testament to its potency, the human LD^{50} for intravenous and inhalational exposure with botulinum toxin is estimated at 1 ng/kg and 3 ng/kg, respectively.[7,25,26] The human oral lethal dose is estimated at 1 μg/kg.[27] All forms of human botulism ultimately manifest with the same neurologic clinical picture: a symmetric, descending flaccid paralysis with bulbar musculature and cranial nerve involvement.[8]

Patients exposed to aerosolized botulinum toxin would likely develop botulism in 12–72 hours. The incubation period of inhalational botulism is difficult to predict because so few cases have been reported. Aerosolized exposure in rhesus monkeys has resulted in clinical signs of botulism within 12–80 hours,[28] while the three reported cases of inhalational botulism in humans developed onset of symptoms within 72 hours following a small exposure. These three laboratory workers were exposed from presumed inhalation of contaminated, aerosolized animal fur while performing necropsies on animals exposed to botulinum toxin serotype A. The clinical effects were mild, and all three patients recovered within a week of hospitalization.[29]

Unlike inhalational botulism, patients with foodborne botulism may develop antecedent effects including abdominal cramps or distention, nausea, vomiting, and diarrhea.[30] The speed of onset and severity of clinical symptoms from foodborne botulism depend upon the quantity of toxin absorbed and rate of absorption. Development of clinical symptoms with foodborne botulism ranges from 2 hours to 8 days,[31] but typically the lag time to onset of symptoms and presentation is 12–72 hours. Early stages of the disease are commonly misdiagnosed by physicians because the initial findings are often subtle or similar to other more common ailments. Also, a lag time of up to 24 hours is common before the development of neurologic findings, and this delay can last up to several days as patients vary in the rate of onset of symptoms. Any patient with difficulty swallowing, speaking, or seeing preceded by gastrointestinal symptoms should quickly raise suspicion in healthcare personnel to consider foodborne botulism as an etiology.

Common early neurologic clinical findings of botulism include drooping of the eyelids (ptosis), blurred or double vision (diplopia), enlarged pupils (mydriasis), sluggishly reactive pupils, dysarthria, difficulty articulating, difficulty swallowing, and a nasal quality to the voice. Although the pulse rate is frequently normal, other anticholinergic signs may be present, including dry mouth with pharyngeal injection and constipation. Patients are usually afebrile unless secondary infections are present. As the descending, symmetric motor paralysis initially involves cranial nerves, progression can lead to diaphragmatic weakness and respiratory insufficiency, urinary retention, and complete extremity paralysis. Loss of a protective gag reflex and respiratory hypoventilation may require mechanical ventilation. Deep tendon reflexes may diminish days after initially being normal (Table 7.1). Importantly, sensory loss and mental status changes do not occur as a result of botulinum toxin poisoning. It can be confusing if difficulties with communication occur from fatigue or bulbar palsies, but botulinum toxin does not penetrate the central nervous system.

Botulism is most frequently misdiagnosed as Guillain-Barré syndrome or its Miller–Fisher variant. Other common misdiagnoses include viral syndromes, streptococcal pharyngitis, myasthenia gravis, diseases of the central nervous system (CNS) like stroke, intoxication with CNS depressants, Lambert–Eaton syndrome, and tick paralysis. Less common diagnoses sometimes confused with botulism are CNS infections or tumors, poliomyelitis, psychiatric disease, inflammatory myopathy, and hypothyroidism.[32]

Detecting a malicious outbreak of foodborne botulism may be difficult, as evidenced by an unintentional contamination with a restaurant condiment in Canada in September 1985. Diagnosis of botulism in two sisters who had traveled from Vancouver to Montreal led to the identification of 36 previously unrecognized cases of botulism that had occurred during the preceding 6 weeks. Surveillance in Vancouver then identified other individuals with botulism already hospitalized with other diagnoses. Weeks after the initial cluster was recognized, health department officials discovered more patients hospitalized for disabling neurologic conditions that had begun a month before the first identified cases. All the cases eventually led to identification of a bottle of commercially prepared chopped garlic in soybean oil served at a single, family-style restaurant in Vancouver as the source of type B foodborne botulism. The cases involved thirty patients from four provinces in Canada, five patients from three states in the United States, and one patient from the Netherlands. In these cases, botulism was diagnosed or was being investigated as a possible etiology at a median of 13 days following the onset of illness (range: 2 to 71 days).

Misdiagnoses in these patients included myasthenia gravis, atypical Guillain-Barré

TABLE 7.1 **Signs and Symptoms of Human Botulism**

Gastrointestinal*	Neurologic	General/muscular
Nausea	Double vision	Fatigue
Vomiting	Blurred vision	Dizziness
Abdominal cramps	Dysphagia	Sore throat
Abdominal distention/ileus	Dysarthria	Diaphragmatic weakness
Diarrhea	Dry mouth	Dyspnea
Constipation	Ptosis	Skeletal muscle weakness
	Dilated or fixed pupils	Urinary retention
	Nystagmus	
	Extraocular palsies	
	Facial palsies	
	Decreased gag reflex	
	Paresthesias	
	Extremity weakness	
	Hyporeflexia	
	Ataxia	
	Normal mental status	

*Gastrointestinal symptoms are common with foodborne botulism.

syndrome, cerebrovascular accidents, viral syndromes, psychiatric conditions, inflammatory myopathy, diabetic complications, hyperemesis gravidarum, hypothyroidism, laryngeal trauma, and overexertion. Three of these cases were ultimately recognized in a single neurology practice 500 miles from Vancouver only after a patient's family member inquired about botulism after reading about the Vancouver outbreak.[32] These individuals were discovered to have also eaten sandwiches at the implicated restaurant. Clearly, heightened awareness in medical personnel, local and state health officials, and the lay public would aid in the early recognition of botulism clusters.

Routine testing, such as cerebrospinal fluid analysis, muscle enzymes, and imaging studies, is usually unremarkable in cases of botulism. Tensilon testing with edrophonium chloride may help differentiate myasthenia gravis from botulism. Electromyography (EMG), while not pathognomonic, can identify characteristic patterns associated with botulism. EMG patterns in botulism are characterized by brief, small-amplitude, abundant motor action potentials (BSAP). Another common EMG finding with botulism is an incremental increase in amplitude of small, compound muscle action potentials (CMAP) following high-frequency (50 Hz) repetitive stimulation.[33-35] Electroencephalogram, nerve conduction velocities, and sensory nerve function are normal.

Any afebrile patient with a symmetric, descending paralysis involving bulbar musculature and normal sensorium should be suspected of having botulism.[8] While foodborne botulism produces gastrointestinal symptoms, other routes of exposure likely would not.

ANALYTIC DETECTION

All cases of suspected botulism, regardless of the source, should be reported to hospital epidemiologists, local and state health departments, and the CDC. By law, most states require reporting of botulism to the state health department, thus allowing the appropriate authorities to coordinate the delivery of antitoxin, arrange for definitive laboratory testing, and initiate epidemiologic investigations.[8]

Microbiological testing should not delay treatment when clinical symptoms are highly suggestive of botulism.[17] Antitoxin should be administered to patients once the clinical diagnosis is made because it can prevent but does not reverse paralysis.[28] It can take days to complete the laboratory testing necessary to confirm a case of botulism, therefore early clinical recognition remains the crux of timely treatment of botulism.

In the United States, definitive laboratory testing is available at the CDC and certain state public health laboratories. Samples of serum, stool, gastric contents, and implicated food products should be sent for anaerobic culture and mouse bioassay botulinum toxin studies. Presently, the most sensitive diagnostic test is the mouse bioassay. Mice are injected intraperitoneally with samples suspected of containing botulinum toxin following administration of type-specific antitoxin in order to observe for protective effects. The bioassay can detect extremely small quantities of botulinum toxin, and testing typically is completed in 6 to 24 hours. Delayed deaths are occasionally observed (range: 6 to 96 hours).[36] The results of anaerobic culture specimens are usually available in 7 to 10 days. Polymerase chain reaction testing for *C. botulinum* in human specimens is not yet available.[37]

Following a bioterrorist release of aerosolized botulinum toxin, gastric aspirates and stool samples may be the best sources of detection.[38] Enzyme-linked immunoassays (ELISA) for a botulinum-like neurotoxin have been investigated,[39] but they are not yet available for clinical detection in human specimens. One author has even suggested that ELISA identification of botulinum toxin could likely detect inhalational exposure from swabs of the nasal mucosa in exposed patients within 24 hours.[7]

CONCLUSION

No contemporary cases of human botulinum toxin poisoning with criminal intent have been confirmed. State-supported research and development of botulinum toxin for bioweapons has been reported since the 1940s, and an extremist group has, on at least three occasions, failed in its attempts to disperse aerosolized toxin. The potential harm and intimidation botulinum toxin poisoning poses to the civilian population warrants a heightened clinical suspicion and investigation into suspicious cases. Diagnosis is complicated by the delay of pathognomonic symptoms (resulting in victim dispersal prior to significant illness), difficulty identifying a common source or location of exposure, and confusion with more common diseases that present with similar symptoms. The key to successful diagnosis and treatment is maintaining a heightened awareness in medical personnel and health officials in order to foster early recognition of the disease.

REFERENCES

1. Richardson WH, Frei SS, Williams SR. A case of type F botulism in southern California. *Clin Tox.* 2004;42:383–387.

2. Olson KB. Aum Shinrikyo: once and future threat? *Emerg Infect Dis.* 1999;5:513–516.

3. WuDunn S, Miller J, Broad WJ. How Japan germ terror alerted world. *New York Times.* May 26, 1998:A1, A10.

4. Harris S. Japanese biological warfare research on humans: a case study of microbiology and ethics. *Ann NY Acad Sci.* 1992;666:21–52.

5. Cochrane RC. History of the Chemical Warfare Service in World War II (1 July 1940–15 August 1945). In: *Biological Warfare Research in the United States,* Vol 2. Historical Section, Plans, Training and Intelligence Division, Office of Chief, Chemical Corps, United States Department of the Army; November 1947. Unclassified, archived at the US Army Medical Research Institute of Infectious Disease.

6. Davis RA. The assassination of Reinhard Heydrich. *Surg Gynecol Obstet.* 1971;133:304–318.

7. Middlebrook JL, Franz DR. Botulinum toxins. In: Sidell FR, Takafuji ET, Franz DR, eds. *Medical Aspects of Chemical and Biological Warfare.* Washington, DC: Office of the Surgeon General at TMM Publications; 1997:643–654.

8. Arnon SS, Schechter R, Inglesby TV, et al. Botulinum toxin as a biological weapon- medical and public health management. *JAMA.* 2001;285:1059–1070.

9. Miller J, Engelberg S, Broad WJ. *Germs: Biological Weapons and America's Secret War.* New York: Simon & Schuster; 2002.

10. Alibeck K, Handleman S. *Biohazard.* New York: Random House; 1999.

11. Cole LA. The specter of biological weapons. *Sci Am.* 1996:275:60–65.

12. Zilinskas RA. Iraq's biological weapons: the past as future? *JAMA.* 1997;278:418–424.

13. Werner SB, Passaro D, McGee J, et al. Wound botulism in California, 1951–1998: recent epidemic in heroin injectors. *Clin Infect Dis.* 2000;31:1018–1024.

14. Souayah N, Karim H, Kamin SS, et al. Severe botulism after focal injection of botulinum toxin. *Neurology.* 2006;67:1855–1856.

15. Wiener SL. Strategies for the prevention of a successful biological warfare aerosol attack. *Milit Med.* 1996;161:251–256.

16. Terranova W, Breman JG, Locey RP, Speck S. Botulism type B: epidemiological aspects of an extensive outbreak. *Am J Epidemiol.* 1978;108:150–156.

17. Shapiro RL, Hathaway C, Swerdlow DL. Botulism in the United States: a clinical and epidemiologic review. *Ann Intern Med.* 1998;129:221–228.

18. Nuzzo JB. The biological threat to U.S. water supplies: toward a national water security policy. *Biosecur Bioterror.* 2006;4:147–159.

19. Siegel LS. Destruction of botulinum toxin in food and water. In: Hauschild AH, Dodds KL, eds. *Clostridium Botulinum: Ecology and Control in Foods.* New York: Marcel Dekker Inc; 1993:323–341.

20. Cromptom R, Gall D. Georgi Markov-death in a pellet. *Med Leg J.* 1980;48:51–62.

21. Knight B. Ricin—a potent homicidal poison. *BMJ.* 1979;1:350–351.

22. Harvey SM, Sturgeon J, Dassey DE. Botulism due to *Clostridium baratii* type F toxin. *J Clin Microbiol.* 2002;40:2260–2262.

23. Goldfrank L, Hoffman R, Lewin N, Flomenbaum N, Howland M, Nelson L, eds. *Goldfrank's Toxicologic Emergencies.* 8th ed. New York: McGraw-Hill; 2006.

24. Pellizzari R, Rossetto O, Schiavo G, Montecucco C. Tetanus and botulinum neurotoxins: mechanism of action and therapeutic uses. *Phil Trans R Soc Lond B.* 1999;354:259–268.

25. Burrows WD, Renner SE. Biological warfare agents as threats to potable water. *Environ Health Perspect.* 1999;107:975–984.

26. Gill DM. Bacterial toxins: a table of lethal amounts. *Microbiol Rev.* 1982;46:86–94.

27. Schantz EJ, Johnson EA. Properties and use of botulinum toxin and other microbial neurotoxins in medicine. *Microbiol Rev.* 1992;56:80–99.

28. Franz DR, Pitt LM, Clayton MA, et al. Efficacy of prophylactic and therapeutic administration of antitoxin for inhalational botulism. In: Das Gupta BR, ed. *Botulinum and Tetanus Neurotoxins: Neurotransmission and Biomedical Aspects.* New York: Plenum Press; 1993:473–476.

29. Holzer VE. Botulism from inhalation [in German]. *Med Klin.* 1962;57:1735–1738.

30. Hughes JM, Blumenthal JR, Merson MH, et al. Clinical features of types A and B food-borne botulism. *Ann Intern Med.* 1981;95:442–445.

31. Koenig MG, Drutz D, Mushlin Al, et al. Type B botulism in man. *Am J Med.* 1967;42:208–219.

32. St. Louis ME, Peck SH, Bowering D, et al. Botulim from chopped garlic: delayed recognition of a major outbreak. *Ann Intern Med.* 1988;108:363–368.

33. Valli G, Barbieri S, Scarlato G. Neurophysiological tests in human botulism. *Electromyogr Clin Neurophysiol.* 1983;23:3–11.

34. Masselli RA, Bakshi N. American Association of Electrodiagnostic Medicine case report 16: botulism. *Muscle Nerve.* 2000;23:1137–1144.

35. Cherington M. Clinical spectrum of botulism. *Muscle Nerve.* 1998;21:701–710.

36. Centers for Disease Control and Prevention. *Botulism in the United States 1899–1996: Handbook for Epidemiologists, Clinicians, and Laboratory Workers.* Atlanta, GA: Centers for Disease Control and Prevention; 1998: http://www.cdc.gov/ncidod/dbmd/diseaseinfo/files/botulism.pdf. Accessed September 4, 2009.

37. Szabo EA, Pemberton JM, Gibson AM, et al. Polymerase chain reaction for detection of *Clostridium botulinum* type A, B, E in food, soil and infant faeces. *J Appl Bacteriol.* 1994;76:39–45.

38. Woodruff BA, Griffin PM, McCroskey LM, et al. Clinical and laboratory comparison of botulism from toxin types A, B, and E in the United States, 1975-1988. *J Infect Dis.* 1992;166:1281–1286.

39. Dixit A, Alam SI, Dhaked RK, Singh L. Development of an immunodetection test for a botulinum-like neurotoxin produced by *Clostridium* spp, RKD. *Indian J Med Res.* 2006;124:355–362.

8 | Cyanide

Christopher P. Holstege and Paul M. Maniscalco

CASE STUDY

A 17-year-old boy was at a classmate's house when he complained of "not feeling well," slumped over, and began to have seizures.[1] Prior to this, he was in good health, with no history of medication use or substance abuse. Responding paramedics upon arrival conducted an assessment of the unresponsive patient. Advanced life support interventions were implemented and the patient was intubated to secure his airway and support respiratory effort. Upon arrival at the emergency department, his vitals were as follows: temperature 100°F (37.8°C), blood pressure 98/49 mm Hg, heart rate 79 beats per minute, spontaneous respiratory rate 4. His pulse oximetry was 100% on oxygen. His examination was significant for the following: Glasgow coma score of 3; absent corneal gag and cough reflexes; 5-mm nonreactive pupils; face and neck erythema; weak peripheral pulses; capillary refill time of greater than 6 seconds. His initial laboratory values revealed a serum bicarbonate of 7 mEq/L (anion gap 38), lactic acid 20.3 mmol/L (normal is 0.5–2.2 mmol/L), and an arterial blood gas with a pH of 7.11, pO_2 190 mm Hg, and pCO_2 28 mm Hg.

He became progressively hypotensive and developed a junctional bradycardia, requiring vasopressor therapy and transcutaneous pacing. Repeated simultaneous arterial and venous blood gas analysis revealed an arteriovenous saturation difference of zero, leading to the suspicion of cyanide toxicity. A thiocyanate level (metabolite of cyanide) was markedly elevated at 20.5 mg/L (normal is less than 2 mg/L). Magnetic resonance imaging (MRI) the following day showed cerebellar infarction with tonsillar herniation, diffuse infarcts throughout the frontal and parietal lobes, and edema at the brain stem and upper spinal cord. The victim was subsequently declared brain-dead and life support was removed.

The police investigation led to a confession by the perpetrator of poisoning the patient with 1.5 grams of potassium cyanide that he had purchased at a commercial Internet site and placed in the victim's beverage.

HISTORY

Throughout history, cyanide has been utilized as a poison in warfare and in murder. In ancient Rome, Emperor Nero reportedly used cyanide in the form of cherry laurel water to poison enemies and family members.[2] Louis-Napoléon Bonaparte (Napoleon III) proposed using cyanide on the soldiers' bayonets during the Franco-Prussian War. Hydrogen cyanide and cyanogen chloride were deployed in World War I, but a number of problems (i.e., rapid dissipation) resulted in limited use on the battlefield. During World War II, cyanide (Zyklon B) caused more than 1 million deaths in Nazi gas chambers. In 1978, Jim Jones of the People's Temple in Guyana employed potassium cyanide in a mass suicide, resulting in 913 deaths. In its 1980 campaign, Iraq used chemical weapons including cyanide against the Iranians.[3] In 1982, seven deaths resulted from consumption of cyanide-tainted acetaminophen in Chicago that subsequently led to the requirement of tamper-resistant pharmaceutical packaging in the United States.[4] In 1995, 2 weeks after the sarin subway attacks, the Aum Shinrikyo left potassium cyanide and dilute sulfuric acid in the restrooms of the Japanese subways; the materials were found before they could be employed.[5]

Cyanide has often been used as an agent of murder.[1,6-9] For example, Richard "The Iceman"

Kuklinski claimed to have killed between 100 and 130 individuals as a "hitman" for Italian-American crime families. He reportedly favored the use of cynaide because it killed quickly and was difficult to detect on autopsy. He claimed to have administered it by injection, placement on food, aerosol spray, or simple spillage on the victim's skin.[10] Serial killer Donald Harvey, nicknamed the "Angel of Death," murdered within hospitals where he was employed. He was finally caught after a coroner smelled cyanide during the autopsy of John Powell and subsequently discovered lethal levels of cyanide in his system.[11] Harvey later admitted to the use of cyanide as one means he utilized to kill patients.[12]

In November 2001, a cyanide-laced letter addressed to a New Jersey police department was safely intercepted by a post office. Contents were discovered to be small amounts of copper cyanide mixed with some laundry detergent.[13] In June 2002, Joseph Konopka (also known as "Dr. Chaos") was indicted by a U.S. grand jury on counts of possessing the chemical weapons sodium cyanide and potassium cyanide, which he stored in the Chicago subway system.[14] Also in 2002, nine al-Qaeda-tied Moroccans were arrested in Rome by Italian authorities as they were allegedly planning to poison the water supply of the U.S. embassy with potassium ferrocyanide.[15] The U.S. Department of Homeland Security in November 2003 issued a five page warning to law enforcement and emergency response personnel regarding al-Qaeda's development of a device specifically for dissemination of cyanogen chloride and hydrogen cyanide through building air intakes or ventilation systems and or enclosed spaces like mass transportation vehicles. The blunt warning stated that "Terrorists have designed a crude chemical dispersal device fabricated from commonly available materials, which is designed to asphyxiate its victims."[16]

ROUTES OF EXPOSURE

Cyanide consists of one atom of carbon bound to one atom of nitrogen by three molecular bonds ($C\equiv N$). Inorganic cyanides (also known as cyanide salts) contain cyanide in the anion form (CN^-) (Table 8.1). Cyanide salts react readily with water to form hydrogen cyanide (HCN). Hydrogen cyanide is a colorless gas at standard temperature and pressure with a reported bitter

TABLE 8.1 **Inorganic Cyanide Compounds Examples (*Cyanide Salts*)**

Common name	Chemical formula
Barium cyanide	$Ba(CN)_2$
Beryllium cyanide	$Be(CN)_2$
Cadmium cyanide	$Cd(CN)_2$
Calcium cyanide	$Ca(CN)_2$
Cesium cyanide	CsCN
Cobalt cyanide	$Co(CN)_2$
Copper cyanide	CuCN
Ferric cyanide	$Fe(CN)_3$
Gold cyanide	AuCN
Lithium cyanide	LiCN
Magnesium cyanide	$Mg(CN)_2$
Potassium cyanide	KCN
Potassium gold cyanide	$KAu(CN)_2$
Potassium silver cyanide	$KAg(CN)_2$
Mercuric cyanide	$Hg(CN)_2$
Rubidium cyanide	RbCN
Silver cyanide	AgCN
Sodium cyanide	NaCN
Strontium cyanide	$Sr(CN)_2$

TABLE 8.2 **Examples of Plants That Contain Cyanogenic Glycosides**

Plant (common name)	Plant (Latin name)	Cyanogenic glycoside
Bitter almonds	*Prunus dulcis*	Amygdalin
Apricot	*Prunus armeniaca*	Amygdalin
Black cherry	*Prunus serotina*	Amygdalin
Sorghum	*Sorghum sp.*	Dhurrin
Cassava	*Manihot sp.*	Linamarin
Wild lima beans	*Phaseolus lunatus*	Linamarin
Bamboo shoots	*Bambusa vulgaris*	Taxiphyllin
Bird's-foot trefoil	*Lotus corniculatus*	Linamarin
Oil flax	*Linum usitatissimum*	Linamarin

Note: There are numerous other plants that contain cyanogenic glycosides. Also, the plants listed here may contain more than one type of cyanogenic glycoside.

odor. Cyanogen gas, a dimer of cyanide, reacts with water and breaks down into the cyanide anion. Cyanogen's formula is $(CN)_2$. Cyanogen chloride (CNCL) is a colorless gas that is easily condensed; it is listed as Schedule 3 by the Chemical Weapons Convention.

Organic compounds that have a cyano group bonded to an alkyl residue are known as nitriles. For example, methyl cyanide is also known as acetonitrile (CH_3CN); if ingested, it can be metabolized by the liver to hydrogen cyanide. Many plants contain cyanogenic glycosides (Table 8.2).[17,18] For example, ingested amygdalin is biotransformed by intestinal enzymes to cyanide. A substance marketed by alternative medicine practiioners called Laetrile contains amygdalin and can be purchased on the Internet. Laetrile, when administered by intravenous infusion, bypasses the necessary enzymes in the gastrointestinal tract to liberate cyanide from the amygdalin and does not cause toxicity. If ingested, however, Laetrile can cause cyanide poisoning.[19]

The absorption of cyanide can occur via all routes (inhalation, ingestion, dermal, parenteral), depending on the type of cyanide compound. Rapid diffusion through the lungs followed by direct distribution to target organs accounts for the rapid lethality associated with hydrogen cyanide (HCN) inhalation. The dose of cyanide required to produce toxicity is dependent on the form of cyanide, the duration of exposure, and the route of exposure. For example, the median oral lethal dose of potassium cyanide in an untreated adult is 140–250 mg, and an airborne concentration of 270 ppm (μg/mL) of HCN may be immediately fatal.[1]

TOXICOLOGIC MECHANISMS

Cyanide is an inhibitor of multiple enzymes in the human body.[20] For example, cytochrome oxidase is an enzyme essential for oxidative phosphorylation and thereby aerobic energy production. It functions in the electron transport chain within mitochondria, converting glucose into adenosine triphosphate (ATP). Cyanide induces cellular hypoxia by inhibiting cytochrome oxidase.[20,21] Despite sufficient oxygen supply to the mitochondria, oxygen cannot be utilized, and ATP molecules are no longer formed.[22] Unincorporated hydrogen ions accumulate, and lactate levels rise because of aerobic energy metabolism failure. As a result, laboratory values following cyanide poisoning reveal acidemia, hyperlactemia, and an elevation of venous oxygen concentration.

CLINICAL EFFECTS

No reliable pathognomonic clinical effect is associated with acute cyanide poisoning.[23] The time to onset of clinical effects depends on the dose and route of exposure as well as the type of cyanide-containing compound. Such effects can occur within seconds of inhalation of HCN or several minutes following ingestion of an inorganic cyanide salt. The clinical effects of cyanogenic glycosides and nitriles often are delayed, and the time course varies up to 24 hours depending on their rate of biotransformation.[24] The initial clinical effects of acute cyanide poisoning may be nonspecific, thereby making the correct diagnosis difficult. Clinical manifestations may reflect rapid dysfunction of oxygen-sensitive organs, with central nervous system and cardiovascular findings predominating. The signs and symptoms associated with the cyanide-induced central nervous system toxicity include headache, lightheadedness, anxiety, restlessness, agitation, confusion, lethargy, seizures, and coma.[7] Cardiovascular responses to cyanide are complex. Clinically, an initial period of bradycardia and hypertension may occur, followed by hypotension with reflex tachycardia; the terminal event, however, is commonly reported as bradycardia and hypotension.[1,7]

Gastrointestinal toxicity may occur following ingestion of inorganic cyanide and cyanogens and includes abdominal pain, nausea, and vomiting. These symptoms are caused by hemorrhagic gastritis, which is frequently identified on necropsy, and are thought to be secondary to the corrosive nature of cyanide salts.[23] Reports of cutaneous manifestations vary. A cherry-red skin color has been described as a result of increased venous hemoglobin oxygen saturation, which results from decreased utilization of oxygen at the tissue level.[25] This finding may be evident on funduscopic examination, where veins and arteries may appear similar in color. The occurrence of cyanosis may be seen in some cases likely secondary to cardiovascular collapse.[26]

Survivors of marked acute poisoning may develop delayed neurologic sequelae.[27] Parkinsonian effects (i.e., rigidity, bradykinesia) are most common.[7] These neurologic effects often do not develop immediately and may be delayed over weeks to months.

LABORATORY TESTING

Because of the associated nonspecific signs and symptoms and the delay in laboratory cyanide confirmation, clinicians must rely on routine laboratory studies to raise suspicion of cyanide poisoning. The triad of laboratory findings suggestive of cyanide poisoning include (1) a narrow arterial–venous oxygen difference, (2) an anion gap metabolic acidosis, and (3) an elevated lactate concentration.[1] Blood gas analysis can provide rapid clues to the diagnosis of cyanide toxicity. The arterial pH correlates inversely with cyanide concentration.[28] The finding of an elevated venous oxygen saturation and a narrow arterial–venous oxygen difference also may suggest cyanide toxicity.[29] This finding is not specific for cyanide and could represent cellular poisoning from other agents such as carbon monoxide, hydrogen sulfide, and sodium azide. An anion gap metabolic acidosis with a profound lactic acidosis is found in numerous critical illnesses and is a nonspecific finding. A significant association, however, exists between blood cyanide and plasma lactate concentrations.[28]

There are several electrocardiographic (ECG) findings associated with cyanide poisoning described in published case reports. Sinus tachycardia has been described as an early ECG finding.[7,30] Elevation or depression of the ST segment or a shortened ST segment with fusion of the T wave into the QRS complex has been described.[7] With significant toxicity, ECG findings include bradycardia, atrial fibrillation, ventricular fibrillation, and atrioventricular blocks.[1,29,31,32]

The early onset of diffuse cerebral edema with loss of gray–white differentiation may be a clue to the diagnosis of acute cyanide poisoning.[8] Computerized tomography (CT) and MRI of the head may reveal basal ganglia damage to the globus pallidus, putamen, and hippocampus.[1]

Blood cyanide determination can confirm toxicity.[1] Whole blood or serum usually is analyzed. Whole-blood concentrations are twice serum concentrations as a result of cyanide sequestration in red blood cells. Cyanide may be found in the tissues of healthy subjects. Background whole-blood concentrations in nonsmokers range between 0.02 and 0.5 mg/L.[33,34] Cigarette smokers have been found to have mean whole blood cyanide levels of 0.4 mg/L, more than 2.5 times the mean of nonsmokers.[35] At cyanide concentrations between 0.5 and 1.0 mg/L, victims may be confused, flushed, and tachycardic. At blood levels between 1.0 and 2.5 mg/L, stupor and agitation can appear. Levels greater than 2.5 mg/L are associated with coma and are potentially fatal.[6]

The literature illustrates how difficult the diagnosis of cyanide poisoning is to reliably establish at autopsy. The indicative morphological findings are difficult to unequivocally recognize or may even be completely missing.[6]

CONCLUSION

Cyanide exists in numerous different chemical compounds. Cyanide salts (i.e., potassium cyanide) are the most frequently associated with criminal poisoning in modern society. Cyanide should be considered in the differential diagnosis of rapid-onset coma with associated metabolic acidosis. The finding of elevated venous oxygen saturation and a narrow arteriovenous oxygen difference also suggests the possibility of cyanide toxicity. Blood cyanide determination can confirm toxicity.

As soon as a diagnosis of cyanide poisoning is suspected, law enforcement should be immediately notified by the healthcare team to allow them to expeditiously begin to investigate not only the background and personal history of the victim(s), but determine the context in which the poisoning occurred. For example, law enforcement will need to rapidly determine if this poisoning was an isolated event (e.g., a planned assassination), or whether there other intended victims as might be reflected in similar hospitalizations. Since the onset of clinical effects due to cyanide toxicity is rapid, a complete accounting of the victim's movements is critical as is a determination of people with whom the victim has recently interacted. In the case of victims affiliated with military or political organizations, the investigation should include examination of any confidential meetings the victim may have had and of identifying adversaries who would stand to gain from the victim's demise. Intelligence

sources should be immediately queried to determine the capabilities of suspected adversaries in terms of researching, developing or employing cyanide as a political or military weapon.

REFERENCES

1. Peddy SB, Rigby MR, Shaffner DH. Acute cyanide poisoning. *Pediatr Crit Care Med.* 2006;7(1):79–82.
2. Baskin S, Brewer TG. *Cyanide Poisoning.* Falls Church, Virginia: Office of The Surgeon General—Department of the Army; 1997.
3. Rajaee F. *The Iran-Iraq War—The Politics of Aggression.* Gainesville, FL: University Press of Florida; 1993.
4. Wolnik KA, Fricke FL, Bonnin E, et al. The Tylenol tampering incident—tracing the source. *Anal Chem.* 1984;56(3):466A–470A, 474A.
5. Oshita M, Sato N, Yoshihara H, et al. Ethanol-induced focal cell necrosis via microcirculatory disturbance in the perfused rat liver. *Alcohol Alcohol (Suppl).* 1991;1:317–320.
6. Musshoff F, Schmidt P, Daldrup T, Madea B. Cyanide fatalities: case studies of four suicides and one homicide. *Am J Forensic Med Pathol.* 2002;23(4):315–320.
7. Chin RG, Calderon Y. Acute cyanide poisoning: a case report. *J Emerg Med.* 2000;18(4):441–445.
8. Varnell RM, Stimac GK, Fligner CL. CT diagnosis of toxic brain injury in cyanide poisoning: considerations for forensic medicine. *Am J Neuroradiol.* 1987;8(6):1063–1066.
9. Padwell A. Cyanide poisoning. Case studies of one homicide and two suicides. *Am J Forensic Med Pathol.* 1997;18(2):185–188.
10. Carlo P. *Ice Man: Confessions of a Mafia Contract Killer.* New York: St. Martin's Press; 2006.
11. Anonymous. Lethal doses. *Time;* August 24,1987.
12. Whalen W, Martin B. *Defending Donald Harvey: The Case of America's Most Notorious Angel-of-Death Serial Killer.* Cincinnati: Clerisy Press; 2005.
13. Parry W. Cyanide traces found in N.J. letter. *Associated Press.* November 11, 2001.
14. Warmbir S, Herguth RC, Main F, et al. "Dr. Chaos" held in cyanide case. *Chicago Sun-Times.* March 12, 2002.
15. Hundley T. 4 Moroccans held in suspected plot against U.S. embassy in Rome. *Chicago Tribune.* Feburary 20, 2002.
16. Anonymous. *Terrorist Chemical Device.* U.S. Department of Homeland Security Information Bulletin, September 16, 2003.
17. Sousa AB, Soto-Blanco B, Guerra JL, Kimura ET, Gorniak SL. Does prolonged oral exposure to cyanide promote hepatotoxicity and nephrotoxicity? *Toxicology.* 2002;174(2):87–95.
18. Frehner M, Scalet M, Conn EE. Pattern of the cyanide-potential in developing fruits: implications for plants accumulating cyanogenic monoglucosides *(Phaseolus lunatus)* or cyanogenic diglucosides in their seeds *(Linum usitatissimum, Prunus amygdalus). Plant Physiol.* 1990;94(1):28–34.

19. Hall AH, Linden CH, Kulig KW, Rumack BH. Cyanide poisoning from laetrile ingestion: role of nitrite therapy. *Pediatrics.* 1986;78(2):269–272.

20. Way JL, Leung P, Cannon E, et al. The mechanism of cyanide intoxication and its antagonism. *Ciba Found Symp.* 1988;140:232–243.

21. Pettersen JC, Cohen SD. Antagonism of cyanide poisoning by chlorpromazine and sodium thiosulfate. *Toxicol Appl Pharmacol.* 1985;81(2):265–273.

22. Maduh EU, Borowitz JL, Isom GE. Cyanide-induced alteration of the adenylate energy pool in a rat neurosecretory cell line. *J Appl Toxicol.* 1991;11(2):97–101.

23. Gill JR, Marker E, Stajic M. Suicide by cyanide: 17 deaths. *J Forensic Sci.* 2004;49(4):826–828.

24. Thier R, Lewalter J, Selinski S, Bolt HM. Possible impact of human CYP2E1 polymorphisms on the metabolism of acrylonitrile. *Toxicol Lett.* 2002;128(1–3):249–255.

25. Singh BM, Coles N, Lewis P, Braithwaite RA, Nattrass M, FitzGerald MG. The metabolic effects of fatal cyanide poisoning. *Postgrad Med J.* 1989;65(770):923–925.

26. van Heijst AN, Douze JM, van Kesteren RG, et al. Therapeutic problems in cyanide poisoning. *J Toxicol Clin Toxicol.* 1987;25(5):383–398.

27. Messing B, Storch B. Computer tomography and magnetic resonance imaging in cyanide poisoning. *Eur Arch Psychiatry Neurol Sci.* 1988;237(3):139–143.

28. Baud FJ, Borron SW, Megarbane B, et al. Value of lactic acidosis in the assessment of the severity of acute cyanide poisoning. *Crit Care Med.* 2002;30(9):2044–2050.

29. Johnson RP, Mellors JW. Arteriolization of venous blood gases: a clue to the diagnosis of cyanide poisoning. *J Emerg Med.* 1988;6(5):401–404.

30. Lam KK, Lau FL. An incident of hydrogen cyanide poisoning. *Am J Emerg Med.* 2000;18(2):172–175.

31. Cooper M, Powers K, Rusnack R et al. Cyanide ingestion: preventing the cascade. *Dimens Crit Care Nurs.* 1998;17(2):83–90.

32. Geller RJ, Barthold C, Saiers JA, Hall AH. Pediatric cyanide poisoning: causes, manifestations, management, and unmet needs. *Pediatrics.* 2006;118(5):2146–2158.

33. Hall AH, Rumack BH. Clinical toxicology of cyanide. *Ann Emerg Med.* 1986;15(9):1067–1074.

34. Hernandez T, Lundquist P, Oliveira L et al. Fate in humans of dietary intake of cyanogenic glycosides from roots of sweet cassava consumed in Cuba. *Nat Toxins.* 1995;3(2):114–117.

35. Ballantyne B. Artifacts in the definition of toxicity by cyanides and cyanogens. *Fundam Appl Toxicol.* 1983;3(5):400–408.

9 | Dioxin

Christopher P. Holstege

CASE STUDY

n October of 1997, a 30-year-old woman developed follicular pustules on her face that gradually increased in size and number.[1] Six months later, she presented to the Department of Dermatology at the University of Vienna Medical School in Austria for a second opinion.[2] She was diagnosed with acne fulminans and treated with high-dose steroids and antibiotics. Her inflammation had subsided, but hundreds of cysts developed on her face, auricular areas, eyelids, genital region, limbs, and trunk. Chloracne was suspected, and a subsequent level of 2,3,7,8-tetrachlorodibenzo-*p*-dioxin (TCDD) was found to be 144,000 pg TCDD per gram of blood fat, which was the highest level ever recorded in a human. The calculated body burden was 1.6 mg (or 25 µg/kg).[2] Her disease progressed and her face became densely covered with cysts. She was reported to have numerous other clinical effects, including nausea, vomiting, epigastric pain, anorexia, weight loss, and amenorrhea. Her laboratory values were significant for elevation of her triglycerides, cholesterol, amylase, lipase, transaminases, C-reactive protein, and alkaline phosphatase. She had a transient thrombocytopenia, normocytic/normochromic anemia, and leukocytosis, with decreased natural killer cells.

Four other individuals working at the same institute also were found to be poisoned with TCDD. A criminal investigation was initiated, but the cause of the outbreak has to date not been solved.

HISTORY

The term *dioxin* represents a family of compounds called the polychlorinated dibenzo-*p*-dioxins (PCDDs). The PCDDs are associated with a larger class of compounds called the polyhalogenated aromatic hydrocarbons. This class includes such agents as the PCDDs, polyhalogenated napthalenes, polyhalogenated biphenyls (i.e., PCB), polyhalogenated dibenzofurans, tetrachloroazobenzene, and tetrachloroazo-oxybenzene.[3] The basic structure of a PCDD is two benzene rings joined via two oxygen bridges at adjacent carbons on each of the benzene rings. There are 75 distinct types of PCDDs. The most thoroughly studied is TCDD, which is also the only PCDD reportedly used in criminal poisonings.

Numerous past industrial accidents have exposed human populations to the polyhalogenated aromatic hydrocarbons. The most notorious instances include the 1953 BASF accident in Germany, the 1963 Philips-Duphar facility explosion in the Netherlands, the 1968 Yusho disease in Japan, the 1973 Coalite explosion in England, the 1976 Seveso disaster in Italy, and the 1979 Yu-Cheng disease in Taiwan. In addition, Operation Ranch Hand during the Vietnam War exposed U.S. troops to dioxin and led to numerous long-term investigative studies of that population of soldiers.

There are only two reported criminal poisoning incidents associated with dioxins, and both incidents involved the use of TCDD. The first incident was depicted in the introductory Case Study above. The second case involves President Viktor Yushchenko of Ukraine (see Chapter 1).[4,5] Both of these incidents remain unsolved.

ROUTES OF EXPOSURE

Dioxins are well absorbed by inhalation, ingestion, and dermal contact. The formation of a noncovalent complex between TCDD and the human transport protein, α-fetoprotein (AFP), has resulted in a stable complex that increases the water solubility of TCDD significantly.[6] This complex manifests higher toxicity against specific cell lines; AFP may facilitate TCDD transport into cells and enhance toxic effects.

McConnell et al. in 1978 described the effects of TCDD on primates.[7] They administered TCDD by gavage. The earliest notable effects occurred 3 days later when a puffiness of the eyelids occurred and caused a narrowing of the openings. The first primate died 14 days after a 70-μg/kg dose. By 30 days, all had lost some or all of their nails, and their skin had developed a dry crusty texture. Laboratory tests revealed the development of leukocytosis, elevated erythrocyte sedimentation rate, thrombocytopenia, and elevated triglycerides.

The median toxic dose in humans is reported as 0.1 μg/kg.[8,9] Following absorption, dioxins are widely distributed throughout the body with the highest concentrations found in the fat, pancreas, liver, and skin; the lowest concentrations are in the nervous tissue, lungs, and kidneys. Elimination is primarily via the feces with enterohepatic recirculation. The reported elimination half-life varies but is approximately 7 years at lower concentrations in humans.[10]

TOXICOLOGIC MECHANISMS

Chloracne (also known as *halogen acne*) was reportedly coined by Herxheimer in 1899 and is the most consistent reported finding in humans exposed to TCDD.[11-13] Chloracne is a symmetrical dermatologic condition involving the change of undifferentiated sebaceous gland cells to keratinocytes, resulting in a disappearance of sebaceous glands and the substitution of closed comedones (blackheads) and keratin cysts.[14] Levels above 650 pg of TCDD per gram of fat are necessary to develop these lesions of chloracne that may persist for over 30 years.[15]

TCDD may induce d-aminolevulinic acid synthetase (ALA) in genetically susceptible individuals.[16] This subsequently induces porphyria cutanea tarda, characterized by uroporphyrinuria, photosensitivity, and mechanical fragility of the skin.[3]

TCDD also induces a sustained increase in triglycerides by increasing triglyceride synthesis in the liver, decreasing lipoprotein lipase activity, and enhancing lipolysis.[17-19] Dioxin stimulates the aryl hydrocarbon receptor, which in turn depresses adipogenesis and leads to a wasting syndrome. It induces CYP1A-1 and -2 activity as well as a fibrosis and steatosis of the liver.[20,21]

CLINICAL EFFECTS

Dioxins have been associated with many human health problems.[22] Reports describing dioxin's clinical effects vary widely in the literature. Several factors complicate the interpretation of the data regarding the effects of exposure in humans, including the route of the exposure, the presence of other chemicals, the total dioxin body burden, the duration of dioxin exposure, the age of the person exposed, the preexisting health of the exposed person, the use of surrogate markers (i.e., chloracne) rather than a dioxin level itself in studies, and the limits in the statistical power of studies to detect adverse health effects. Animal models have been utilized to further elucidate potential health effects.

The dermatologic effects following dioxin exposure may be pronounced and have been well described.[2,23-26] Chloracne is a symmetrical dermatologic eruption of comedones, cysts, and pustules.[11] Comedones are delayed in their development (weeks to months) following exposure.[27] The malar crescent of the face and retroauricular folds are the areas of the skin most commonly involved. The cheeks, forehead, neck, forearms, trunk, back, legs, and genitalia are also commonly afflicted.[28] The nose, eyelids, and the auricular region are typically spared, except in patients with markedly elevated levels.[27] The hands, forearms, feet, and legs are involved less. Other dermatologic effects that have been reported include:

- Hyperproduction of melanin by a normal number of melanocytes[14]
- Cystic lesions containing straw-colored fluid, especially on the face in the "crow's feet" area, giving a "plucked chicken skin" appearance[13,28]
- Lesions in the axilla that may mimic hidradenitis suppurativa
- Xerosis, alopecia, and granuloma annulare
- Hypertrichosis, primarily involving the temporal area of the face and the eyebrows, occurring primarily in association with TCDD-induced porphyria cutanea tarda[13,20]
- Punctate keratoderma, primarily involving the palms and soles[1]

- Palpebral edema and meibomian gland cysts
- Hyperhidrosis of the palms and the soles
- Increased nail growth and nail plate thickening[27]

TCDD causes peripheral neuropathies.[29] Sensory neuropathies tend to be delayed in onset, persistent, and most commonly affect the legs. Polyneuropathic electromyogram abnormalities are frequently observed. The neuritis may cause limb pain of disabling severity. The motor nerves are rarely affected. Severe myalgias of the extremities, shoulders, and thorax have been reported.

Anorexia, irritability, weight loss, fatigue, headache, and insomnia have all been associated with TCDD toxicity.[23] Gastrointestinal symptoms, including nausea, vomiting, abdominal pain, and gastritis may occur. Hepatitis and pancreatitis have been reported. Studies have suggested a link between TCDD exposure and ischemic vascular disease.

ANALYTIC DETECTION

The early diagnosis of acute TCDD toxicity following a criminal poisoning would be difficult. Depending on the time after exposure that the tests are drawn, routine laboratory tests may reveal a pattern consistent for TCDD exposure. When reviewed separately, such laboratory abnormalities might not raise suspicion. However, a persistent rash along with such a pattern of laboratory abnormalities should raise suspicion for TCDD toxicity.[2]

Numerous abnormalities in laboratory values have been reported following TCDD exposure, including transient anemia, leukocytosis, thrombocytopenia, and decreased numbers of natural killer cells. Publications of human TCDD toxicity have also reported an elevation of the erythrocyte sedimentation rate, C-reactive protein, fibrinogen, and uroporphyrins.[27] Prolonged elevation of gamma-glutamyltransferase has been documented in numerous reports of TCDD toxicity.[30,31] TCDD may also induce a transient increase in other transaminases, lipase, and amylase. TCDD-induced alternations in serum lipid levels have been demonstrated with elevated triglycerides, characterized in the medical literature.[17,31,32] Elevated total cholesterol and lowered HDL may also occur.[31]

In testing specifically for TCDD, a number of different methods may be utilized. The primary method of determining TCDD in biologic samples is gas chromatography with mass spectrometry (GC-MS). Sample preparation is critical, and extensive extraction and sample clean-up are required to separate TCDD from organic contaminants.[33] Extreme care must also be used to ensure that all reagents and equipment used in the analysis are free of TCDD contamination.

Another test recently developed is called DR CALUX bioassay (dioxin responsive chemically activated luciferase expression).[34,35] This bioassay uses a cell line, which contains the luciferase reporter gene under control of a murine dioxin-responsive enhancer. In response to exposure to dioxins and dioxin-like chemicals, DR CALUX rat hepatoma cell line synthesizes luciferase in a dose-dependant way that can reportedly be quantified by an enzymatic light-producing reaction.

CONCLUSION

The diagnosis of acute dioxin toxicity following a criminal poisoning is difficult, especially early in the clinical course. Human toxicity with many of the different polyhalogenated aromatic hydrocarbons would give rise to a similar clinical pattern. There is a common clinical triad of findings associated with acute TCDD toxicity: the development of a progressive rash that slowly progresses to classic chloracne, peripheral neuropathy, and new-onset but persistent hyperlipidemia. Testing samples for TCDD must be performed meticulously both to avoid the loss of TCDD from the sample being tested and to avoid TCDD contamination from material and equipment used to perform the analysis.

REFERENCES

1. Geusau A, Jurecka W, Nahavandi H, et al. Punctate keratoderma-like lesions on the palms and soles in a patient with chloracne: a new clinical manifestation of dioxin intoxication? *Br J Dermatol.* 2000;143(5):1067–1071.
2. Geusau A, Abraham K, Geissler K, et al. Severe 2,3,7,8-tetrachlorodibenzo-p-dioxin (TCDD) intoxication: clinical and laboratory effects. *Environ Health Perspect.* 2001;109(8):865–869.
3. Kimbrough RD. The toxicity of polychlorinated polycyclic compounds and related chemicals. *CRC Crit Rev Toxicol.* 1974;2(4):445–448.
4. Walker NJ, Crockett PW, Nyska A, et al. Dose-additive carcinogenicity of a defined mixture of "dioxin-like Compounds." *Environ Health Perspect.* 2005;113(1):43–48.
5. Holt E. Doctor sues clinic over Yushchenko poisoning claims. *Lancet.* 2005;365(9468):1375.
6. Sotnichenko AI, Severin SE, Posypanova GA, et al. Water-soluble 2,3,7,8-tetrachlorodibenzo-p-dioxin complex with human alpha-fetoprotein: properties, toxicity in vivo and antitumor activity in vitro. *FEBS Lett.* 30 1999;450(1–2):49–51.
7. McConnell EE, Moore JA, Dalgard DW. Toxicity of 2,3,7,8-tetrachlorodibenzo-p-dioxin in rhesus monkeys *(Macaca mulatta)* following a single oral dose. *Toxicol Appl Pharmacol.* 1978;43(1):175–187.
8. Kociba RJ, Keeler PA, Park CN, et al. 2,3,7,8-tetrachlorodibenzo-p-dioxin (TCDD): results of a 13-week oral toxicity study in rats. *Toxicol Appl Pharmacol.* 1976;35(3):553–574.
9. Stevens KM. Agent Orange toxicity: a quantitative perspective. *Hum Toxicol.* 1981;1(1):31–39.
10. Needham LL, Gerthoux PM, Patterson DG, et al. Serum dioxin levels in Seveso, Italy, population in 1976. *Teratog Carcinog Mutagen.* 1997;17(4-5):225–240.
11. Poland AP, Smith D, Metter G, et al. A health survey of workers in a 2,4-D and 2,4,5-T plan with special attention to chloracne, porphyria cutanea tarda, and psychologic parameters. *Arch Environ Health.* 1971;22(3):316–327.
12. Rosas Vazquez E, Campos Macias P, Ochoa Tirado JG, et al. Chloracne in the 1990s. *Int J Dermatol.* 1996;35(9):643–645.
13. Brodkin RH, Schwartz RA. Cutaneous signs of dioxin exposure. *Am Fam Physician.* 1984;30(3):189–194.
14. Pastor MA, Carrasco L, Izquierdo MJ, et al. Chloracne: histopathologic findings in one case. *J Cutan Pathol.* 2002;29(4):193–199.
15. Coenraads PJ, Olie K, Tang NJ. Blood lipid concentrations of dioxins and dibenzofurans causing chloracne. *Br J Dermatol.* 1999;141(4):694–697.
16. Poland A, Glover E. 2,3,7,8-Tetrachlorodibenzo-p-dioxin: a potent inducer of aminolevulinic acid synthetase. *Science.* 1973;179(72):476–477.
17. Gorski JR, Weber LW, Rozman K. Reduced gluconeogenesis in 2,3,7,8-tetrachlorodibenzo-p-dioxin (TCDD)-treated rats. *Arch Toxicol.* 1990;64(1):66–71.
18. Olsen H, Enan E, Matsumura F. 2,3,7,8-Tetrachlorodibenzo-p-dioxin mechanism of action to reduce lipoprotein lipase activity in the 3T3-L1 preadipocyte cell line. *J Biochem Mol Toxicol.* 1998;12(1):29–39.
19. Roth WL, Weber LW, Stahl BU, et al. A pharmacodynamic model of triglyceride transport and deposition during feed deprivation or following treatment with 2,3,7,8-tetrachlorodibenzo-p-dioxin (TCDD) in the rat. *Toxicol Appl Pharmacol.* 1993;120(1):126–137.
20. Caramaschi F, del Corno G, Favaretti C, et al. Chloracne following environmental contamination by TCDD in Seveso, Italy. *Int J Epidemiol.* 1981;10(2):135–143.
21. Poland A, Clover E, Kende AS, et al. 3,4,3',4'-Tetrachloro azoxybenzene and azobenzene: potent inducers of aryl hydrocarbon hydroxylase. *Science.* 1976;194(4265):627–630.

22. Holstege C. Effects of dioxins on human health. *J Toxicol Clin Toxicol.* 2005;43(5):407–408.

23. Van Miller JP, Marlar RJ, Allen JR. Tissue distribution and excretion of tritiated tetrachlorodibenzo-p-dioxin in non-human primates and rats. *Food Cosmet Toxicol.* 1976;14(1):31–34.

24. Geusau A, Schmaldienst S, Derfler K, et al. Severe 2,3,7,8-tetrachlorodibenzo-p-dioxin (TCDD) intoxication: kinetics and trials to enhance elimination in two patients. *Arch Toxicol.* 2002;76(5–6):316–325.

25. Geusau A, Tschachler E, Meixner M, et al. Cutaneous elimination of 2,3,7,8-tetrachlorodibenzo-p-dioxin. *Br J Dermatol.* 2001;145(6):938–943.

26. Geusau A, Tschachler E, Meixner M, et al. Olestra increases faecal excretion of 2,3,7,8-tetrachloro-di-benzo-p-dioxin. *Lancet.* 1999;354(9186):1266–1267.

27. Poskitt LB, Duffill MB, Rademaker M. Chloracne, palmoplantar keratoderma and localized scleroderma in a weed sprayer. *Clin Exp Dermatol.* 1994;19(3):264–267.

28. McDonagh AJ, Gawkrodger DJ, Walker AE. Chloracne—study of an outbreak with new clinical observations. *Clin Exp Dermatol.* 1993;18(6):523–525.

29. Oliver RM. Toxic effects of 2,3,7,8 tetrachlorodi-benzo 1,4 dioxin in laboratory workers. *Br J Ind Med.* 1975;32(1):49–53.

30. Sweeney MH, Calvert GM, Egeland GA, et al. Review and update of the results of the NIOSH medical study of workers exposed to chemicals contaminated with 2,3,7,8-tetrachlorodibenzodioxin. *Teratog Carcinog Mutagen.* 1997;17(4-5):241–247.

31. Martin JV. Lipid abnormalities in workers exposed to dioxin. *Br J Ind Med.* 1984;41(2):254–256.

32. Pelclova D, Fenclova Z, Preiss J, et al. Lipid metabolism and neuropsychological follow-up study of workers exposed to 2,3,7,8-tetrachlordibenzo-p-dioxin. Int Arch *Occup Environ Health.* 2002;75:S60–S66.

33. Chlorianted dibenzo-p-dioxins (update). In: *Registry AfTSaD.* U.S. Department of Health and Human Services; 1998:507–508.

34. Aarts JM, Denison MS, Cox MA, et al. Species-specific antagonism of Ah receptor action by 2,2′,5,5′-tetrachloro- and 2,2′,3,3′4,4′-hexa-chlorobiphenyl. *Eur J Pharmacol.* 1995;293(4):463–474.

35. Sanderson JT, Aarts JM, Brouwer A, et al. Comparison of Ah receptor-mediated luciferase and ethoxyresorufin-O-deethylase induction in H4IIE cells: implications for their use as bioanalytic tools for the detection of polyhalogenated aromatic hydrocarbons. *Toxicol Appl Pharmacol.* 1996;137(2):316–325.

10 | Drugs of Abuse

Rachel Haroz and Susan Ney

CASE STUDY

On November 28, 1953, Frank Olson fell 170 feet to his death from a 10th floor room in the Statler Hotel in Manhattan, New York. He was a biochemist, an expert in aerobiology with the United States Army, and an employee of the Central Intelligence Agency (CIA). At the time, the death was deemed a suicide.[1] Twenty-two years later the Rockefeller commission and congressional hearings revealed that Olson's death had been preceded 9 days prior by the surreptitious administration of 70 µg of lysergic acid diethylamide (LSD) in a glass of Cointreau during a military retreat at Deep Creek Lodge in Maryland.[2] Olson developed hallucinations shortly after ingesting the LSD. Those hallucinations were followed by depression, paranoia, and ultimately his death.[3]

Despite congressional hearings, a repeat autopsy 40 years later, and a subsequent intriguing homicide investigation, the actual course of Frank Olson's death is still controversial.[1,3] This administration of LSD was part of an extensive program, Project MK ULTRA, that was launched on April 13, 1953, by the CIA and was headed by Dr. Sidney Gottlieb.[1] The aim was "research and development of chemical, biological, and radiological materials capable of employment in clandestine operations to control human behavior."[2] Although the project focused largely on LSD, other drugs such as barbiturates, amphetamines (including 3,4-methylenedioxymethampheamine), sodium pentothal, alcohol, scopolamine, marijuana, psilocybin, heroin, and mescaline were included. These drugs were administered to civilian and military personnel as well as thousands of other unwitting participants, generally without any informed consent or medical prescreening. For instance, in Operation Midnight Climax, prostitutes would lure subjects, generally businessmen, to safe houses disguised as bordellos. The men were then administered LSD and observed behind two-way mirrors.[2, 4]

HISTORY

The term "drugs of abuse" is broad and encompasses numerous categories of pharmacologic agents. Several drugs of abuse are discussed in other chapters within this book. This chapter will focus on four drugs: benzoylmethylecgonine (cocaine), methamphetamine, LSD, and 3,4-methylenedioxymethamphetamine (MDMA or ecstasy).

Cocaine, derived from leaves of the *Erythroxylum coca* plant, has been used by humans as a stimulant for over 5000 years.[5] Until the late 19th century, cocaine was generally consumed in small amounts by chewing leaves and drinking cocaine-laced wines such as Vin Mariani; thus harmful side effects were rare. In 1884, Sigmund Freud declared that cocaine was a miracle drug. At the same time, Merck increased production from less than a pound in 1883 to 158,352 pounds in 1886. Concurrently, chemical advances allowed for more purified cocaine to be available, and abuse increased exponentially.[6] Despite government efforts, cocaine use continued to increase and peaked dramatically in the United States in the 1980s with the spread of crack, a freebase and cheaper form than the powder.[7] Currently, cocaine is a Schedule II drug under the Controlled Substances Act (CSA) of 1970.

Although cocaine is often associated with violent crime, intentional criminal poisoning is not frequently reported. There are, however, cases of prenatal, infant, and child deaths determined to be homicides. In *State* v. *McKnight*, the South Carolina Supreme Court upheld a ruling that intrauterine fetal demise was caused by the known ingestion of cocaine by the pregnant McKnight. Cocaine metabolites were found in the fetus's system. The verdict was homicide by child abuse, with a subsequent 20-year prison term.[8] In September of 2000, rescue personnel found a 10-month-old female infant experiencing ventricular fibrillation and apnea. Despite initial resuscitation, the infant died. The parents initially claimed the child had eaten rat poison, but later admitted that 2 hours before calling for assistance, the infant's 2-year-old brother was found eating crack cocaine and also feeding it to the infant. Investigators found crack cocaine throughout the house and in the infant's crib. At autopsy, the infant was found to have two "crack rocks," 0.3 cm in diameter, in her duodenum. The cause of death was determined to be cocaine poisoning by homicide.[9] In another case in West Branch, Michigan, a woman pled guilty to attempted manslaughter after her infant died from cocaine intoxication caused by ingestion of the mother's breast milk.[10] In a different case, syringes with cocaine were found in a supermarket. One syringe was found piercing a pear. The pear flesh tested positive for cocaine, indicating injection. Product tampering was suspected, but it did not appear that there were any casualties.[11]

Methamphetamine (MA) is a derivative of amphetamine. First synthesized by the Germans and Japanese in the late 19th century, it became popular during World War II. At that time, Japan, Germany, and the United States supplied their military personnel with MA to increase performance and reduce flight fatigue. Postwar spread of MA from surplus army supplies led to the "first epidemic" in Japan, and subsequently MA popularity grew in the western United States in the 1960s. Production and distribution at that time were largely controlled by San Francisco Bay-area motorcycle gangs but were eventually taken over by Mexican traffickers and spread east.[12] MA abuse today is rampant both in the United States and globally. With 25 million users, amphetamine ranks second after cannabis in prevalence of abuse. Currently, MA is a Schedule II drug under the CSA. Deaths related to MA intoxication and violence are common, but like cocaine, criminal poisoning is rare and intentional poisonings have not been reported. The Supreme Court of Hawaii recently overturned a manslaughter conviction for a woman who smoked MA during the late stages of pregnancy, causing the death of her newborn child.[13]

LSD was first synthesized in 1938 by the Swiss biochemist Albert Hofmann. He accidentally exposed himself to the drug in 1943, leading to the first LSD "trip."[14] A potent hallucinogen and psychedelic, LSD quickly became popular. Within medical communities, LSD was believed to induce a model for psychosis and was used to further investigate schizophrenia and potential medications for its treatment.[4] Other research focused on LSD as a possible adjunct in psychotherapy. At the same time, Timothy Leary, a Harvard psychology professor, advocated LSD use and encouraged people to "Tune in. Turn on. Drop out."[7] Despite being outlawed in 1965 and a subsequent decrease in use, LSD is still widely available. Naturally occurring lysergic acid can be found in the fungus *Claviceps purpurea*, and in the morning glory plants *Rivea corymbosa* and *Ipomoea violacea*.[15] LSD is currently a Schedule I drug under the CSA.

MDMA was first synthesized in 1912 by Anton Köllisch for Merck as an intermediate precursor for another chemical. It remained relatively obscure for several decades. In the 1970s, it gained popularity in psychotherapy, and its use among youth continued to grow into the 1980s and 1990s with the rise of the rave culture.[16,17] MDMA is currently a Schedule I drug under the CSA. Criminal poisoning with MDMA is rare. Recently two teenagers were charged with homicide after providing a 16-year-old girl with MDMA and then failing to call emergency services when she had an adverse reaction.[18]

POTENTIAL DELIVERY METHODS

Cocaine comes in several forms. Coca leaves are generally chewed but can be steeped into teas and beverages. Cocaine hydrochloride is a water-soluble powder and can be injected intravenously (Figure 10.1), injected subcutaneously ("skin popping"; Figure 10.2), as well as absorbed through mucous membranes by nasal insufflation and vaginal or rectal administration.[19] Two alkaloid forms, crack and freebase, have lower melting points and can therefore be smoked and thus inhaled. In addition, coca paste, or "bazooka," a form of coca leaves, water, sulfuric acid, and kerosene, is smoked in South America.[20] Cocaine hydrochloride is available medically in the form of a powder and topical solution in various concentrations as an anesthetic for medical procedures. It is also mixed into a topical anesthetic solution with tetracaine and adrenaline (TAC). Toxicity from mucosal exposure to the solution has been reported, and toxicity from dermal exposure is certainly possible.[21]

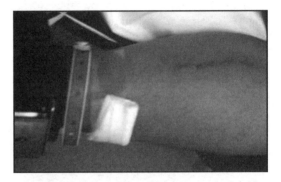

FIGURE 10-1   **Track marks in an intravenous drug abuser** (See Color Plate 7.)

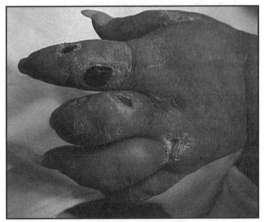

FIGURE 10-2   **Skin popping on a hand of a subcutaneous injecting drug abuser** (See Color Plate 8.)

Methamphetamine hydrochloride is usually a powder that can be injected intravenously, smoked, nasally insufflated, or ingested. It may also come in capsule or tablet form. The crystal form, or "ice," is generally smoked. Other, more novel methods of administration include transrectal administration and "parachuting." Parachuting involves placing the MA in a wrapper prior to ingestion, thus allowing it to unravel in the gastrointestinal tract in an attempt to prolong the duration of action.[22,23]

LSD can be found in liquid, powder, gelatin sheet, or tablet form. It is usually ingested, although reports exist of nasal insufflation, subcutaneous and intravenous injection, smoking, and conjunctival instillation. The liquid form is often ingested on sugar cubes or blotter paper that has been soaked in LSD.[15]

MDMA is generally found in tablet form (Figure 10.3), but it may appear as a powder or in capsules. It is usually ingested, but it can be injected, smoked, or nasally insufflated.[24]

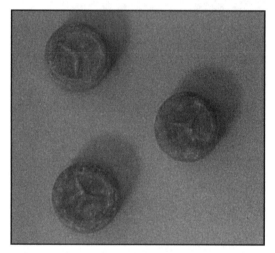

FIGURE 10-3 **MDMA tablets** (See Color Plate 9.)

TOXICOLOGIC MECHANISMS

Cocaine exhibits its effects through several different mechanisms. Peripherally, it blocks reuptake of catecholamines such as norepinephrine, causing stimulation of α and β adrenergic and dopamine receptors, which then leads to an increase in sympathomimetic symptoms. In the central nervous system (CNS), cocaine mainly acts by blocking dopamine reuptake, leading to euphoria and CNS stimulation. Cocaine also blocks sodium channels. In low doses, it acts as an anesthetic at sensory neurons, and at higher doses, it may block cardiac conduction, leading to dysrhythmias.[19,25,26]

Methamphetamine exhibits similar action to cocaine centrally and peripherally, albeit by a slightly different mechanism. Methamphetamine increases production and release of dopamine, blocks reuptake of catecholamines, inhibits catecholamine breakdown by monoamine oxidase, and leads to depletion of dopamine and serotonin.[27,28]

The exact mechanism of action of LSD has not been elucidated. It appears that LSD may act as a partial agonist and antagonist of serotonin (5-hydroxytryptamine, or 5-HT).[29] LSD may also act as an agonist and antagonist on postsynaptic dopamine receptors.[15]

MDMA is structurally and pharmacologically similar to methamphetamine. In addition, it acts as a hallucinogen. It increases release of dopamine and serotonin, blocks serotonin reuptake, and inhibits monoamine oxidase. It also has activity at α_2-adrenergic, M_1-muscarinic, and H_1 receptors and may exhibit less activity at M_2-, α_1-, and β-adrenergic receptors.[17,30,31]

CLINICAL EFFECTS

Cocaine and methamphetamine are potent stimulants, and exposure to them leads to a wide variety of mostly sympathomimetic symptoms. Patients may present complaining of agitation, confusion, chest pain, dyspnea, palpitations, headache, abdominal pain, weakness, hallucinations, and seizures.[32] Clinical findings may reveal hyperthermia, tachycardia, tachypnea, hypertension, change in behavior, focal neurologic findings, seizures, mydriasis, diaphoresis, hyperthermia, and hyperactive bowel sounds.[33] Patients may also present with choreiform movements and, after methamphetamine use, bruxism.[33]

Chest pain and dyspnea are common complaints after cocaine exposure but may also be seen with methamphetamine use.[32,34] These symptoms may be due to cardiac ischemia or infarction, aortic dissection, pneumothorax, asthma exacerbation, "crack lung," and pulmonary edema (cardiac and noncardiac).[32-35] Dysrhythmias are more common with cocaine use due to cocaine's sodium-channel-blocking properties; dysrhythmias may manifest as atrial fibrillation, ventricular fibrillation, ventricular tachycardia, and torsade de pointes.[35]

While the cardiovascular effects of cocaine and methamphetamine are similar, the duration is different. Symptoms from cocaine use subside more rapidly, with heart rate and blood pressure returning to baseline within 30 minutes. Symptoms from methamphetamine use may continue for several hours.[26] Abdominal pain secondary to gastrointestinal ischemia may result in ulceration, bowel perforation, or ischemic colitis.[26,36] Other findings may include rhabdomyolysis, renal failure, and multi-organ failure.[33]

Neurologically, patients may have intracranial hemorrhages, strokes, and seizures as well as psychosis.[26,32] These conditions are largely due to significant hypertension and vasospasm,[26,32] but in both methamphetamine and cocaine use, some cases may be the result of a vasculitis.[37] With methamphetamine, the vasculitis has a typical beaded pattern on angiography.[37] In addition, patients with repeated cocaine and methamphetamine use over several days may present with hypotension, bradycardia, and a depressed mental status secondary to catecholamine depletion.[38] Cocaethylene is an active metabolite of coingestion of alcohol and cocaine, and while less potent than cocaine, it has a longer duration of action, which may account for some cocaine-related symptoms (e.g., coronary vasospasm, hepatotoxicity) seen long after the last use of cocaine.

A unique presentation of methamphetamine is "meth mouth" (Figure 10.4). Vasoconstriction decreases saliva production and flow. In combination with the overall poor hygiene and bruxism, the teeth become decayed on the buccal and anterior surfaces, and periodontal disease ensues.[39]

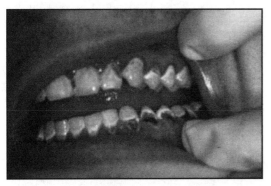

FIGURE 10-4   **Meth mouth of a chronic methamphetamine abuser**
(See Color Plate 10.)
Used with permission from Dr. John A. Svirksy

Laboratory values may vary based on the presentation. Basic chemistry panels may demonstrate acidosis, hyperglycemia, hypokalemia (early in toxicity) or hyperkalemia (late in toxicity), and elevation of renal function tests (i.e., creatinine). Creatine phosphokinase and cardiac enzymes may be elevated, indicating rhabdomyolysis and myocardial infarction.[26] Electrocardiograms may show a dysrhythmia,

prolonged intervals, or ST-elevation myocardial infarctions.[35] Chest x-rays may demonstrate widening of the mediastinum in aortic dissection, pneumothorax, vasocongestion, or free air below the diaphragm. Abdominal x-rays may show body-stuffed packets (of drugs). Cerebral CT scans may demonstrate a stroke, either ischemic or hemorrhagic.[26] Lumbar puncture may show red blood cells or xanthochromia consistent with intracranial bleeding.[26] Cardiac catheterization may result in normal coronaries or may show diseased vessels.

Signs and symptoms of LSD exposure are initially sympathomimetic: nausea, flushing, chills, tachycardia, hypertension, tremors, mydriasis, hyperthermia, hyperreflexia, and piloerection.[15] Some will also experience dizziness, weakness, sleepiness, paresthesias, and blurry vision. The hallmark hallucinations usually start within 20 to 60 minutes and last 6 to 12 hours.[40] These hallucinations are described as largely visual but can be auditory. Rarely synesthesia, the mixing of senses, occurs. Time may become distorted and mood labile. People on LSD may discuss "oneness with the universe," but they may also experience feelings of extreme anxiety, paranoia, or fear. Trauma may be self-inflicted or unintentional.[15] "Flashbacks" may occur and are generally similar to prior LSD experiences but usually less intense. Rarely, people will have prolonged or permanent pyschosis; this is more common in patients with underlying mental illness.[15]

Although largely seen as a benign exposure, LSD use has led to significant morbidity and mortality. In 1972, eight individuals mistakenly snorted LSD. They presented to the emergency department with varying degrees of respiratory failure, tachycardia, hyperthermia, hypertension, and a universal coagulopathy. With supportive care, including mechanical ventilation, all eight survived.[41] In another case, an 18-year-old man presented with confusion, agitation, hypertension, and hyperthermia with an axillary temperature of 106.4°F (41.3°C). He recovered within 18 hours with supportive care that included aggressive cooling.[42] LSD exposure, however, can also prove fatal. In 1975, a 34-year-old man died of unknown causes; autopsy revealed unusually high tissue levels of LSD. Death was determined to be secondary to LSD toxicity.[43] In another case in 1985, a 25-year-old man died after hospital admission; based on medical and toxicologic analysis, the cause of death was determined to be LSD toxicity. An antemortem serum LSD level of 14.4 ng/mL was significantly higher than the previously highest recorded level of 9.5 ng/mL in patients who survived.[44]

The clinical presentation of LSD is such that routine tests are not necessary and generally normal if performed. However, as in the previous example, lab abnormalities may exist in extreme cases including leukocytosis, neutrophilia, elevations in LDH, liver transaminases, uric acid, and blood glucose as well as a coagulopathy.[45]

MDMA users may present with both sympathomimetic and hallucinogenic symptoms. They may initially experience palpitations, blurry vision, dry mouth, sweating, and bruxism. They may feel extra energy, euphoria, extroversion, increased empathy, increased sociability, mild perceptual disturbances, and changed perception of colors and sounds.[17] Some patients also experience ataxia and confusion.[24] Initial exam findings may reveal a change in mental status, agitation, tachycardia, hypertension, hyperthermia, and mydriasis. The hyperthermia, in combination with sweating and increased physical activity, may lead to dehydration, compensated by consumption of water.[46] Cases of subsequent rhabdomyolysis, liver failure, and multi-organ failure have been reported.[46] Profound hyponatremia has been reported with sodium levels ranging from 107 to 128 mmol/L.[47] The cause may be multifactorial. MDMA appears to cause an inappropriate secretion of the antidiuretic hormone (SIADH).[47] In addition to the dehydration and water consumption, SIADH leads to hyponatremia, which subsequently contributes to a change in mental status, seizures, cerebral edema, brain herniation, and death.[47] Case reports have also illustrated that fatalities may occur with ingestion of only one tablet, usually in young females.[48]

Routine laboratory testing in cases of MDMA abuse may reveal hyponatremia. In the setting of liver failure, raised serum transaminases, hypoglycemia, and elevated prothrombin time may be observed. Creatinine phosphokinase and creatinine may be elevated, indicative of rhabdomyolysis and renal failure. Head CT scans may show cerebral edema or brain herniation.

In addition, MDMA tablets may contain various other substances such as 3,4-methylenedioxyethylamphetamine (MDEA), 3,4-methylenedioxyamphetamine (MDA), as well as nonamphetamines, including but not limited to caffeine, dextromethorphan, paramethoxyamphetamine (PMA), ketamine, ephedrine, or acetaminophen.[49]

ANALYTIC DETECTION

The initial screening for cocaine is usually an immunoassay of the urine, which usually detects a metabolite of cocaine, benzoylecgonine. It may remain positive for up to 72 hours after cocaine use.[50] Gas chromatography-mass spectrometry (GC-MS) can detect cocaine in the urine up to 14 days.[51] Postmortem redistribution may not be significant for cocaine, evidenced by a strong correlation between femoral and heart blood concentrations. Cocaine and its metabolites (benzoylecgonine, ecgonine methyl ester, and ecgonine) can also be found in vitreous humor and correlate with heart and peripheral blood concentrations.[52] Actual cocaine and metabolite levels, however, have a wide distribution and do not correlate with the clinical picture or severity of findings.[51] There is no known toxic level of cocaethylene. GC-MS is the most specific test for cocaethylene.[53]

Although methamphetamine has been reported to have a "toxic level" of 5 µg/mL, a retrospective review of deaths in Japan revealed that half of the methamphetamine poisoning cases had a serum less than this level.[54] Testing specifically for methamphetamine and its metabolites, including amphetamine, can be done on blood, urine, saliva, or hair. Urine and saliva can be tested using GC-MS, with urine resulting in positive tests 3 days after drug use and saliva for only 24 hours.[55] Hair can be tested using cation-selective exhaustive injection and sweeping micellar electrokinetic chromatography; these methods have been reported to give positive results months after exposure.[56] Elevated magnesium, calcium, and creatinine postmortem may point to methamphetamine overdose.

LSD use can be detected by immunoassay of the urine but has many false positives. Therefore, confirmation testing by high-performance liquid chromatography or gas chromatography is often necessary and can be done on the blood or urine.[57] At autopsy, edema throughout the abdominal organs, brain, and lungs may be found.[43] The postmortem levels of LSD in the blood may be lower than the antemortem levels, likely due to redistribution.[44]

MDMA is often not detected on routine drug-of-abuse tests. While GC-MS has the widest application, there are many alternative methods (e.g., immunoassay, electrophoresis, and high-performance liquid chromatography) for determining if MDMA is present in blood or urine.[58-60] However, MDMA has nonlinear kinetics, which make blood concentrations difficult to interpret and correlation of concentrations with clinical effects even more difficult.[61] Extremely divergent MDMA levels have produced fatalities.[62]

It should be noted that urine drug tests are an indication of exposure but cannot be used to determine impairment. Any test that is to be used for legal purposes should be obtained and processes observing a strict chain of custody. Results of positive tests should be confirmed by a second, more specific method, such as GC-MS.

CONCLUSION

Although actual cases of criminal poisoning by cocaine, methamphetamine, LSD, and MDMA are rare, some have been reported. Positive tests for cocaine and methamphetamine on routine drug testing are usually deemed secondary to recreational use, not intentional poisoning. Meanwhile, LSD and MDMA are usually not detected on any routine tests. In addition, no specific "toxic levels" exist for any of these drugs. Therefore a suspicious history and clinical symptoms in the right setting should lead investigators to further testing.

REFERENCES

1. Shane S. Son probes strange death of WMD worker. *San Francisco Chronicle.* September 12, 2004:A5.
2. Joint Hearing before the Select Committee on Intelligence and the Subcommittee on Health and Scientific Research of the Committee on Human Resources United States Senate First ed. Washington: US Government Printing Office; 1977.
3. Starrs J. *A Voice for the Dead: A Forensic Investigator's Pursuit of the Truth in the Grave.* New York: G.P. Putnam's Sons; 2005.
4. Ulrich RF, Patten BM. The rise, decline, and fall of LSD. *Perspect Biol Med.* 1991;34(4):561–578.
5. Calatayud J, Gonzalez A. History of the development and evolution of local anesthesia since the coca leaf. *Anesthesiology.* 2003;98(6):1503–1508.
6. Karch SB. Cocaine: history, use, abuse. *J R Soc Med.* 1999;92(8):393–397.
7. Bailey BJ. Looking back at a century of cocaine—use and abuse. *Laryngoscope.* 1996;106(6):681–683.
8. Smith M. Child safety: homicide by child abuse: South Carolina upholds conviction under "Crack Mom" law. *J Law Med Ethics.* 2003;31(3):457–458.
9. Havlik DM, Nolte KB. Fatal "crack" cocaine ingestion in an infant. *Am J Forensic Med Pathol.* 2000;21(3):245–248.
10. English E. Woman pleads guilty in case of infant who was killed by cocaine. *The Bay City Times.* January 11, 2007.
11. Tomlinson JA, Crowe JB, Ranieri N, Kindig JP, Platek SF. Supermarket tampering: cocaine detected in syringes and in fruit. *J Forensic Sci.* 2001;46(1):144–146.
12. Anglin MD, Burke C, Perrochet B, Stamper E, Dawud-Noursi S. History of the methamphetamine problem. *J Psychoactive Drugs.* 2000;32(2):137–141.
13. Kobayashi K. Meth mother's conviction overturned. *The Honolulu Advertiser.* November 30, 2005.
14. Montagne M. LSD at 50: Albert Hofmann and his discovery. *Pharm Hist.* 1993;35(2):70–73.
15. Kulig K. LSD. *Emerg Med Clin North Am.* 1990;8(3):551–558.
16. Freudenmann RW, Oxler F, Bernschneider-Reif S. The origin of MDMA (ecstasy) revisited: the true story reconstructed from the original documents. *Addiction.* 2006;101(9):1241–1245.
17. Milroy CM. Ten years of "ecstasy." *J R Soc Med.* 1999; 92(2):68–72.
18. Brown I. Charges will make people less likely to call for help. *The News Tribune.* June 13, 2007.
19. Brownlow HA, Pappachan J. Pathophysiology of cocaine abuse. *Eur J Anaesthesiol.* 2002;19(6):395–414.
20. Warner EA. Cocaine abuse. *Ann Intern Med.* 1993;119(3):226–235.
21. Vinci RJ, Fish S, Mirochnick M. Cocaine absorption after application of a viscous cocaine-containing TAC solution. *Ann Emerg Med.* 1999;34(4, pt 1): 498–502.
22. Harris DS, Boxenbaum H, Everhart ET, et al. The bioavailability of intranasal and smoked methamphetamine. *Clin Pharmacol Ther.* 2003;74(5):475–486.
23. Cantrell FL, Breckenridge HM, Jost P. Transrectal methamphetamine use: a novel route of exposure. *Ann Intern Med.* 2006;145(1):78–79.
24. Topp L, Hando J, Dillon P, et al. Ecstasy use in Australia: patterns of use and associated harm. *Drug Alcohol Depend.* 1999;55(1-2):105–115.
25. Benowitz NL. Clinical pharmacology and toxicology of cocaine. *Pharmacol Toxicol.* 1993;72(1):3–12.
26. Boghdadi MS, Henning RJ. Cocaine: pathophysiology and clinical toxicology. *Heart Lung.* 1997;26(6):466–483, 484–465 (quiz).
27. Logan BK. Amphetamines: an update on forensic issues. *J Anal Toxicol.* 2001;25(5):400–404.
28. Newton TF, De La Garza R, Kalechstein AD, et al. Cocaine and methamphetamine produce different patterns of subjective and cardiovascular effects. *Pharmacol Biochem Behav.* 2005;82(1):90–97.

29. Glennon RA. Do classical hallucinogens act as 5-HT2 agonists or antagonists? *Neuropsychopharmacology.* 1990;3(5-6):509–517.

30. Morton J. Ecstasy: pharmacology and neurotoxicity. *Curr Opin Pharmacol.* 2005;5(1):79–86.

31. Schifano F. A bitter pill. Overview of ecstasy (MDMA, MDA) related fatalities. *Psychopharmacology* (Berl). 2004;173(3-4):242–248.

32. Albertson TE, Derlet RW, Van Hoozen BE. Methamphetamine and the expanding complications of amphetamines. *West J Med.* 1999;170(4):214–219.

33. Romanelli F, Smith KM. Clinical effects and management of methamphetamine abuse. *Pharmacotherapy.* 2006;26(8):1148–1156.

34. Jones JH, Weir WB. Cocaine-induced chest pain. *Clin Lab Med.* 2006;26(1):127–146, viii.

35. Chakko S. Arrhythmias associated with cocaine abuse. *Card Electrophysiol Rev.* 2002;6(1-2):168–169.

36. Herr RD, Caravati EM. Acute transient ischemic colitis after oral methamphetamine ingestion. *Am J Emerg Med.* 1991;9(4):406–409.

37. Stoessl AJ, Young GB, Feasby TE. Intracerebral haemorrhage and angiographic beading following ingestion of catecholaminergics. *Stroke.* 1985;16(4):734–736.

38. Glauser J, Queen JR. An overview of non-cardiac cocaine toxicity. *J Emerg Med.* 2007;32(2):181–186.

39. Curtis EK. Meth mouth: a review of methamphetamine abuse and its oral manifestations. *Gen Dent.* 2006;54(2):125–129, 130 (quiz).

40. Nichols DE. Hallucinogens. *Pharmacol Ther.* 2004; 101(2):131–181.

41. Eveloff HH. The LSD syndrome. A review. *Calif Med.* 1968;109(5):368–373.

42. Klock JC, Boerner U, Becker CE. Coma, hyperthermia, and bleeding associated with massive LSD overdose, a report of eight cases. *Clin Toxicol.* 1975;8(2):191–203.

43. Griggs EA, Ward M. LSD toxicity: a suspected cause of death. *J Ky Med Assoc.* 1977;75(4):172–173.

44. Fysh RR, Oon MC, Robinson KN, et al. A fatal poisoning with LSD. *Forensic Sci Int.* 1985;28(2):109–113.

45. Friedman SA, Hirsch SE. Extreme hyperthermia after LSD ingestion. *JAMA.* 1971;217(11):1549–1550.

46. Hartung TK, Schofield E, Short AI, Parr MJE, Henry JA. Hyponatraemic states following 3,4-methylenedioxymethamphetamine (MDMA, "ecstasy") ingestion. *Q J Med.* 2002;95(7):431–437.

47. Budisavljevic MN, Stewart L, Sahn SA, et al. Hyponatremia associated with 3,4-methylenedioxymethamphetamine ("Ecstasy") abuse. *Am J Med Sci.* 2003;326(2):89–93.

48. Parrott AC. Is ecstasy MDMA? A review of the proportion of ecstasy tablets containing MDMA, their dosage levels, and the changing perceptions of purity. *Psychopharmacology (Berl).* 2004;173(3-4):234–241.

49. Tanner-Smith EE. Pharmacological content of tablets sold as "ecstasy": results from an online testing service. *Drug Alcohol Depend.* 2006;83(3):247–254.

50. Ambre JJ, Connelly TJ, Ruo TI. A kinetic model of benzoylecgonine disposition after cocaine administration in humans. *J Anal Toxicol.* 1991;15(1):17–20.

51. Weiss RD, Gawin FH. Protracted elimination of cocaine metabolites in long-term high-dose cocaine abusers. *Am J Med.* 1988;85(6):879–880.

52. Duer WC, Spitz DJ, McFarland S. Relationships between concentrations of cocaine and its hydrolysates in peripheral blood, heart blood, vitreous humor and urine. *J Forensic Sci.* 2006;51(2):421–425.

53. Rose JS. Cocaethylene: a current understanding of the active metabolite of cocaine and ethanol. *Am J Emerg Med.* 1994;12(4):489–490.

54. Inoue H, Ikeda N, Kudo K, et al. Methamphetamine-related sudden death with a concentration which was of a "toxic level." *Leg Med.* 2006;8(3):150–155.

55. Huestis MA, Cone EJ. Methamphetamine disposition in oral fluid, plasma, and urine. *Ann N Y Acad Sci.* 2007;1098:104–121.

56. Lin YH, Lee MR, Lee RJ, et al. Hair analysis for methamphetamine, ketamine, morphine and codeine by cation-selective exhaustive injection and sweeping micellar electrokinetic chromatography. *J Chromatogr A.* 2007;1145(1-2):234–240.

57. Johansen SS, Jensen JL. Liquid chromatography-tandem mass spectrometry determination of LSD, ISO-LSD, and the main metabolite 2-oxo-3-hydroxy-LSD in forensic samples and application in a forensic case. *J Chromatogr B Analyt Technol Biomed Life Sci.* 2005;825(1):21–28.

58. Skrinska VA, Gock SB. Measurement of 3,4-MDMA and related amines in diagnostic and forensic laboratories. *Clin Lab Sci.* 2005;18(2):119–123.

59. Peters FT, Samyn N, Lamers CT, et al. Drug testing in blood: validated negative-ion chemical ionization gas chromatographic-mass spectrometric assay for enantioselective measurement of the designer drugs MDEA, MDMA, and MDA and its application to samples from a controlled study with MDMA. *Clin Chem.* 2005;51(10):1811–1822.

60. Pirnay SO, Abraham TT, Huestis MA. Sensitive gas chromatography-mass spectrometry method for simultaneous measurement of MDEA, MDMA, and metabolites HMA, MDA, and HMMA in human urine. *Clin Chem.* 2006;52(9):1728–1734.

61. Garcia-Repetto R, Moreno E, Soriano T, et al. Tissue concentrations of MDMA and its metabolite MDA in three fatal cases of overdose. *Forensic Sci Int.* 2003; 135(2):110–114.

62. De Letter EA, Bouche MP, Van Bocxlaer JF, et al. Interpretation of a 3,4-methylenedioxymethamphetamine (MDMA) blood level: discussion by means of a distribution study in two fatalities. *Forensic Sci Int.* 2004;141(2-3):85–90.

11 | Gamma-Hydroxybutyrate

Jenny J. Lu and Timothy B. Erickson

CASE STUDY

In January 1999, 15-year-old Samantha Reid became fatally ill after consuming a Mountain Dew beverage, which was laced with gamma-hydroxybutyrate (GHB). She and two female friends had been given drinks at a party in Grosse Isle, Michigan. Reid told a friend that her drink tasted "gross," but continued consuming it. Within minutes she was vomiting and subsequently lost consciousness. Evidence during the court trial suggested that it was hours before the girls were taken to the hospital, where Reid was intubated and later died.[1] One of the other two girls also lost consciousness but survived. The third girl developed drowsiness but did not become seriously ill as a result of ingesting her drink. There was no evidence of sexual misconduct. Tests indicated high levels of GHB in Reid's body. There were four men, ranging from 18 to 25 years of age, with whom the victims were visiting at the time of the incident and who had offered the victims the tainted drinks. These men were charged in what is considered to be the first prosecution of a GHB-poisoning death in the United States. Three were convicted of involuntary manslaughter and two counts of "mixing a harmful substance in a drink."[1] The fourth defendant, in whose apartment the crime occurred, was convicted of accessory to manslaughter after the fact, poisoning, delivery of marijuana, and possession of GHB.[1,2] Prosecuting attorney Doug Baker stated that "the weapon in this case— that which brought about the death and near death of the complainants—was not a knife, not a gun, but a drug, just as fatal as any other weapon."[3] Their convictions were overturned in March 2003 by the Michigan Court of Appeals but reinstated by the Michigan Supreme Court in August 2003.

HISTORY

GHB was isolated in 1960 and investigated initially as a potential analog of the inhibitory neurotransmitter gamma-aminobutyric acid (GABA), with the ability to traverse the blood–brain barrier. Shortly after, it was found to be naturally occurring in the mammalian brain.[4,5] Its initial use as an anesthetic never gained widespread acceptance in the United States due to adverse effects, including seizure-like activity, inadequate analgesia, and unpredictable anesthetic duration.[6-8]

Beginning in the 1970s, GHB showed promise as a treatment for narcolepsy by increasing rapid eye movement sleep. GHB became popular with bodybuilders during the 1980s as an anabolic steroid alternative. It was readily available at health food stores and at gymnasiums until nonprescription sales of GHB were banned by the FDA after reports of at least 57 cases of toxicity from GHB ingestion.[9]

Despite the FDA's ban, GHB was popularized in the 1990s as an illicit recreational drug among adolescents and young adults. Unsubstantiated rumors linking GHB to actor River Phoenix's death contributed to its high profile. Recreational use of GHB also became problematic in Europe, particularly during music festivals and "rave" parties.[10] In 2000, GHB was classified by the United States National Institute on Drug Abuse as an illicit "club drug," and it became a Schedule I drug under the Controlled Substance Act with the passage of the Hillory J. Farias and Samantha Reid Date-Rape Drug Prohibition Act of 2000.

More recently, GHB has gained notoriety as a drug to facilitate sexual assault, owing to its colorless and purportedly odorless qualities, as well as its rapidly intoxicating and amnestic effects. It often goes unnoticed in the beverages of victims who become sedated or comatose within minutes after consuming the drug.

Between 1990 and 2000, the Drug Enforcement Administration (DEA) documented over 9600 overdoses and law enforcement encounters involving GHB in 45 states.[11] Between 1995 and 2000, there were 65 DEA-documented deaths related to GHB.[11] In a study of selected emergency departments, the Drug Abuse Warning Network (DAWN) found an alarming increase in GHB-associated visits to emergency departments, from 55 in 1994 to a peak of 4969 visits in 2000. By 2002, the number of GHB-associated visits had declined to 3330.[12]

Today, GHB's main clinical use in the United States is in the treatment of cataplexy associated with narcolepsy (under the product name Xyrem).[13,14] It became a dually scheduled drug in 2002 (I and III) with the FDA approval of this medically formulated GHB product, which is available only through a restricted distribution program.[13]

POTENTIAL DELIVERY METHODS

GHB is available as a clear liquid (free acid, 4-hydroxybutyric acid), white powder (sodium salt, sodium oxybate), tablet, or capsule. Its taste has been described as "salty" or "rubbery." It is sold illicitly under various street names (Table 11.1). GHB can be synthesized from recipes and ingredients obtainable through the Internet. Synonyms for the chemical names of GHB and its precursors are significant for concealing the identity of illicit GHB products.

GHB is most commonly ingested in the liquid form and is often coingested with alcohol or other recreational drugs. Typical GHB abuse/misuse occurs in males with a history of drug abuse, young adults at "raves," or victims of poisoning for the purposes of sexual assault. The concentration of a capful or a teaspoon of a "street dose" has been reported to vary from 500 mg to 5 g per dose,[15] costing from $5 to $25 per capful.[11]

Absorption is dose-dependent and elimination kinetics are nonlinear, as indicated by increases in half-life with dose. Plasma peaks occur between 20 and 45 minutes.[6] The half-life of an oral dose of 12.5 mg/kg is 15 to 20

TABLE 11.1 Common Street and Chemical
Names for GHB

Common street names	
Liquid X	Blue nitro
Liquid ecstasy	Everclear
Grievous bodily harm	Gamma G
Scoop	Oxy-sleep
Cherry meth	Poor man's heroin
Soap	Vita-G
Salty water	Zonked
Organic quaalude	Insom-X
Growth hormone booster	Invigorate
Easy lay	Longetivity
Georgia homeboy	Liquid E
Somatomax	Bioski
Goop	Nature's quaalude

Chemical Names
4-Hydroxy butyrate
Gamma hydrate
Gamma-hydroxybutyrate sodium
Gamma-hydroxybutyric acid
Gamma-OH
Sodium oxybate
Sodium oxybutyrate

minutes.[15] GHB levels have been reported to clear from serum approximately 8 hours after an oral dose of 75 to 100 mg/kg.[15,16] Serial urine levels of GHB appear to decline rapidly and become undetectable after 12 hours. Only small percentages of GHB ranging from 1–5% are eliminated in the urine.[6,15,16] Oral fluid from healthy volunteers after a single oral dose of GHB at 25 mg/kg was found to have a detection window of 150 minutes.[6]

Analogues of GHB, including gamma-butyrolactone (GBL) and 1,4-butanediol (BD) (found in industrial solvents often used in paint thinner and floor strippers as well as in consumer nail care products), are converted to GHB following oral administration. Poisonings and deaths after consumption of these chemicals, which have similar but delayed effects to that of GHB, have been documented.[17] Sales of "chemistry kits" containing GHB precursors have attempted to circumvent laws restricting GHB.[18] GHB precursors might account for a significant percentage of GHB-related overdoses.[17,19] Currently, both GBL and 1,4-BD are listed as controlled substance analogues.[14] Numerous other GHB analogs exist, including gamma-valerolactone (GVL), gamma-hydroxyvaleric acid (GHV), and tetrahydrofuran (THF).

TOXICOLOGIC MECHANISMS

GHB has at least two distinct binding sites: It is an agonist at the GHB receptor, and it is a weak agonist at the $GABA_B$ receptor. GHB is found naturally in the mammalian brain. GHB within the normal brain is synthesized from GABA in GABAergic neurons.

CLINICAL EFFECTS

GHB rapidly crosses the blood–brain barrier to enter the central nervous system. It possesses a steep dose-response curve; overdose and coma can easily occur with illicit use. Doses of 10 mg/kg typically cause anxiolysis and myorelaxation, although amnesia is also reported at this dose; sleep can be induced with 20–30 mg/kg; and doses of 50 mg/kg or higher produce anesthesia/coma.[20] Illicit use of GHB typically involves doses between 20 and 35 mg/kg, although this is a gross estimation.[7,21]

While a history of GHB ingestion is often obtainable from witnesses or first responders, the healthcare provider should consider the possibility of coingestants such as drugs (commonly MDMA) or alcohol. GHB in combination with another depressant agent could result in greater central nervous system (CNS) effects than either alone.[18] GHB and ethanol coingestion may produce other adverse effects, including gastrointestinal disturbances, hypotension, and decreased oxygen saturation.[22]

Additional effects of GHB intoxication may include vomiting, sedation and somnolence, respiratory depression with loss of gag reflexes, and coma. The alteration in consciousness is frequently expressed using the Glasgow coma scale (GCS), and a significant number of patients will present with GCS scores of less than eight, prompting the clinician to protect the patient's airway through endotracheal intubation. It is important to note that the original purpose of the GCS was to monitor mental status in head trauma patients. A lower initial GCS score on presentation in GHB intoxication may portend a longer period of time of recovery. A retrospective study of 88 patients reported that the mean time to consciousness in nonintubated patients presenting with an initial GCS of 13 or less was 146 minutes (range: 16–389 minutes).[23] Spontaneous awakening from the "GHB coma" has been described as unpredictable and surprisingly sudden, commonly occurring just prior to placement of the endotracheal tube.

Although CNS depression is classically described, agitation, excitement, and combativeness have paradoxically been reported with GHB use; in some cases, agitation was noted to alternate with somnolent periods.[10,13,14,24] Animal studies and human anesthesia studies support these nonsedative or stimulant effects.[24] In a prospective observational study of 66 patients with GHB toxicity (in which 40 manifested agitation as described in the medical record), 21 were negative for other stimulants by screen or history.[24] An emergence phenomenon including myoclonic jerking motions, transient confusion, and combativeness has been witnessed. Bradycardia, hypothermia, and hypotension have also been noted (Table 11.2).[23]

TABLE 11.2 GHB Clinical Effects (Reported)

System	Signs and symptoms
Vital signs	Hypo-/hypertension, hypo-thermia, bradycardia
Respiratory	Respiratory depression, apnea, Cheyne–Stokes respirations
Gastrointestinal	Vomiting, diarrhea
Neurologic	Sedation, coma, confusion, hallucinations, vertigo, ataxia, weakness, amnesia, seizure-like activity, dizziness, vertigo, nystagmus, miosis/mydriasis
Endocrine	Hyperglycemia
Psychiatric	Agitation, aggression, impaired judgment
Metabolic	Respiratory acidosis

GHB and precursors GBL and 1,4-BD are physically and psychologically addictive. With regular, prolonged use, GHB tolerance and dependency may occur, although there have been relatively few controlled studies in either humans or animals to examine this ability.[18] Regular use can involve dosing every few hours on a daily basis for weeks to months to years, with doses reaching greater than 25 g daily.[15,18,25] Withdrawal syndromes may set in within a few hours following an abrupt cessation or reduction in GHB intake. Symptoms and signs, which may be similar to withdrawal from sedative-hypnotics, include anxiety, insomnia and tremor, muscular cramping, and possibly deterioration into frank delirium.[26,27] Withdrawal followed by death

in one patient has been reported.[13] Symptoms may last from 3 to 15 days.[13] Treatment includes benzodiazepines, with very high doses for severe withdrawal. Adding barbiturates, mood stabilizers (e.g., gabapentin), and low-dose antipsychotics in severe cases has been suggested.[13,26]

ANALYTIC DETECTION

Most routine hospital toxicology screens do not test for GHB or its precursors. Methods employing gas chromatography-mass spectrometry (GC-MS) to measure blood and urine concentrations of GHB are not routinely available in hospital laboratories. Blood and urine specimens must be sent to one of a few national reference laboratories,[17] although results are unlikely to be returned in a timely enough manner to be clinically useful. Serum and urine can be tested for the presence of GHB, quantitatively and qualitatively, depending on the analytic technique. Appropriate cutoff levels must be selected, and careful interpretation of results is required in order to distinguish between endogenous and exogenous GHB serum concentrations.[28,29]

Legally defensible cutoff values for endogenous GHB concentrations are not clearly defined, in part due to the wide distribution of endogenous concentrations. Due to its rapid metabolism and elimination, the window for detection of GHB is very short, and GHB concentrations may return to endogenous levels by the time a specimen is sampled. This brief window makes proof of GHB poisoning problematic in most cases of sexual assault. A "negative" GHB test result could potentially be detrimental to the alleged victim's case by misleading a jury into believing that there is no evidence of GHB poisoning.

As discussed earlier, serum and urine GHB levels are reported to be undetectable by 8 and 12 hours after ingestion, respectively. The probability of obtaining a positive result may increase if specimens are collected during the period when the patient is symptomatic.[16] In a case series of 16 patients with suspected GHB poisoning and GCS of eight or lower, confirmatory testing demonstrated significant GHB levels in the serum (range: 45–295 mg/L; median 180 mg/L) and in the urine (range: 432–2407 mg/L). Quantitative GHB levels did not correlate with the degree of coma or time to awakening (range: 30–190 minutes; median: 120

minutes). More than half of the patients were found to have coingestants, most commonly alcohol. Ecstasy, ketamine, and dextromethorphan were not tested in any of the subjects.[16]

Hair testing for GHB was first described in 1994. GHB is detectable in hair and has been documented in a case of sexual assault 1 month after a single GHB exposure.[30] Because GHB is endogenous and present in hair under physiological conditions, cautious interpretation of GHB presence in hair should be made. There is a wide distribution of endogenous concentrations, from 0.5 to 12 ng/mg.[21] Segmented hair analysis allows the patient's own hair to be used as his or her own control to compare endogenous GHB concentrations with concentrations resulting from exposure.[21,31] Ideally, hair testing should complement hair and urine testing, rather than substituting for either.

Other potential tests, including urine organic acid analysis, have been studied to provide more accessible and timely diagnostic testing for suspected acute overdoses with GHB or its precursor 1,4-BD.[17] Studies investigating potential surrogate markers of GHB administration may expand the window of detection to 48 hours.[32] An ultra-rapid procedure to detect gamma-hydroxybutyric acid in blood and urine using GC-MS has been developed but is currently not available.[33]

Quick-test kits (Drink Detective and Drink Guard), which detect various drug-facilitated sexual assault drugs in beverages, are commercially available but need further investigation due to rater, drug, and drink variability. In one study, the overall sensitivity for Drink Detective and Drink Guard was 69% and 37.5%, respectively. Overall specificity was 87.9% for Drink Detective and 76.6% for Drink Guard.[34]

Laboratory testing to be considered by the healthcare provider includes a metabolic panel, arterial blood gas measurement, ethanol concentration, electrocardiogram (ECG), chest radiograph, and computed tomography of the brain. U waves without significant hypokalemia have been reported to represent GHB intoxication on cardiac electrophysiology, hypothesized to result from ventricular repolarization.[35] Electroencephalogram (EEG) patterns induced by GHB intoxication have been reversed with ethosuximide, clonazepam, and phenobarbital. L-Dopa had no effect on GHB-induced EEG patterns, and phenytoin worsened EEG patterns.[35]

POSTMORTEM TOXICOLOGY

It should be emphasized that interpretation of GHB levels is complicated by its natural presence in the body and its rapid elimination after ingestion. In fatalities where GHB intoxication is suspected, samples of urine, blood, and vitreous fluids should be analyzed as part of the comprehensive toxicology testing. Urine and vitreous fluids may be particularly important in death investigations due to forensically significant postmortem production of GHB in blood specimens.[36] Urine appears to be less susceptible to postmortem GHB production than blood. Tissue levels between endogenous and fatal overdose situations appear to be at least at an order-of-magnitude difference.[37]

In a retrospective case series of 10 fatalities associated with GHB, the average postmortem GHB level in cases considered to be directly attributable to GHB (n = 8) was 231 mg/L (range: 77–370 mg/L).[37] In a review of seven adult fatalities attributed to GHB, concentrations of GHB ranged from 27 to 1030 mg/L.[35] These findings are in contrast to one case series where GHB was not suspected to be a cause of death and measured concentrations of GHB were between 0 and 18 mg/L.[37] Another analysis of 40 fatalities unrelated to GHB demonstrated blood concentrations of GHB less than 30 mg/L and urine concentrations of GHB less than 20 mg/L, reflecting endogenous levels.[29] Interpretation of postmortem GHB concentrations should be based on comparative data obtained using the same technique.

CONCLUSION

Although a history of GHB ingestion may be provided by the patient or witnesses, it is critical to consider other contributory causes for altered mental status, including head trauma, coingestants, metabolic, and medical causes. Other toxicologic causes include, but are not limited to, sedative-hypnotics, alcohol ingestion, carbon monoxide poisoning, antipsychotics, and opioids. The environment in which the patient was found, as well as the patient's medical and social history, may aid in the diagnosis. Initial clinical clues are often nonspecific, and maintaining a high index of suspicion for

GHB intoxication will help guide the approach to treatment of the patient (Table 11.3). Finally, GHB testing and interpretation of results can prove to be a challenge given the brief window for obtaining specimens and the difficulties in interpreting low or negative GHB concentrations.

TABLE 11.3 **Pitfalls in Detecting GHB Poisoning**

- Failure to consider GHB intoxication/poisoning as a diagnosis
- Failure to provide adequate supportive treatment
- Failure to consider coingestions
- Failure to exclude other causes for altered mental status
- Failure to understand complexity of GHB testing and interpretation of results
- Failure to associate GHB with alleged cases of sexual assault

REFERENCES

1. *State of Michigan v Nicolas E. Holtschlag, et al,* No. 226715 Wayne Circuit Court, LC No. 99-473103 (State of Michigan Court of Appeals, October 19, 2004).
2. GHB [transcript]. CBS News. CBS. February 10, 2000.
3. Anonymous. GHB death trial begins in Detroit. The Michigan Daily. February 10, 2000. Page 3A.
4. Wong CG, Gibson KM, Snead OC. From the street to the brain: neurobiology of the recreational drug γ-hydroxybutyric acid. *Trends Pharmacol Sci.* 2004;25(1):29–34.
5. Crunelli V, Emri Z, Leresche N. Unraveling the brain targets of γ-hydroxybutyric acid. *Curr Opin Pharmacol.* 2006;6(1):44–52.
6. Brenneisen R, Elsohly MA, Murphy TP, et al. Pharmacokinetics and excretion of gamma-hydroxybutyrate (GHB) in Healthy Subjects. *J Anal Toxicol.* 2004;28(8):625–630.
7. Gonzalez A, Nutt DJ. Gamma hydroxy butyrate abuse and dependency. *J Psychopharmacol.* 2005;19(2):195–204.
8. Kam PC, Yoong FF. Gamma-hydroxybutyric acid: an emerging recreational drug. *Anaesthesia.* 1998;53(12):1195–1198.
9. Centers for Disease Control (CDC). Multistate outbreak of poisonings associated with illicit use of gamma hydroxy butyrate. *MMWR.* 1990;39(47):861–863.
10. Drasbek KR, Christensen J, Jensen K. Gamma-hydroxybutyrate—a drug of abuse. *Acta Neurol Scand.* 2006;114(3):145–156.
11. GHB. *Drug Facts.* Drug Enforcement Agency (DEA). September; 2001.
12. Club Drugs, 2001 Update. The Dawn Report. Drug Abuse Warning Network. Substance Abuse and Mental Health Services Administration; Oct, 2002.
13. Britt GC, McCance-Katz EF. A brief overview of the clinical pharmacology of "club drugs." *Subst Use Misuse.* 2005;40(9-10):1189–1201.
14. Couper FJ, Thatcher JE, Logan BK. Suspected GHB overdoses in the emergency department. *J Anal Toxicol.* 2004;28(6)481–484.
15. Miotto K, Darakjian J, Basch J, et al. Gamma-hydroxybutyric acid: patterns of use, effects and withdrawal. *Am J Addict,* 2001;10(3):232–241.
16. Sporer KA, Chin RL, Dyer JE, et al. γ-Hydroxybutyrate serum levels and clinical syndrome after severe overdose. *Ann Emerg Med.* 2003;42(1):3–8.
17. Quang, LS, Levy HL, Law T, et al. Laboratory diagnosis of 1,4-BD and GHB overdose by routine urine organic acid analysis. *Clin Toxicol.* 2005;43(4):321–323.
18. Nicholson KL, Balster RL. GHB: a new and novel drug of abuse. *Drug Alcohol Depend.* 2001;63(1):1–22.
19. Thai D, Dyer JE, Jacob P, Haller CA. Clinical pharmacology of 1,4-butanediol and gamma-hydroxybutyrate after oral 1,4-butanediol administration to healthy volunteers. *Clin Pharmcol Ther.* 2007;81(2):178–184.
20. Kintz P, Villain M, Pélissier AL, Cirimele V, Leonetti G. Unusually high concentrations in a fatal GHB case. *J Anal Toxicol.* 2005;29(6):582–585.
21. Kintz P, Villain M, Cirimele V, Ludes B. GHB in postmortem toxicology. Discrimination between endogenous production from exposure using multiple specimens. *Forensic Sci Int.* 2004;143(2-3):177–181.
22. Thai D, Dyer JE, Benowitz NL, Haller CA. Gamma-hydroxybutyrate and ethanol effects and interactions in humans. *J Clin Psychopharmcol.* 2006;26(5):524–529.
23. Chin RL, Sporer KA, Cullison B, Dyer JE, Wu TD. Clinical course of γ-hydroxybutyrate overdose. *Ann Emerg Med.* 1998;31(6):716–722.
24. Zvosec DL, Smith SW. Agitation is common in γ-hydroxybutyrate toxicity. *Am J Emerg Med.* 2005;23(3):316–320.
25. McDaniel CH, Miotto, KA. Gamma-hydroxybutyrate (GHB) and gamma butyrolactone (GBL) withdrawal: five case studies. *J Psychoactive Drugs.* 2001;33(2):143–149.
26. McDonough M, Kennedy N, Glasper A, Bearn J. Clinical features and management of gamma-hydroxybutyrate (GHB) withdrawal: a review. *Drug Alcohol Depend.* 2004;75(1):3–9.
27. Dyer JE, Roth B, Hyma BA. Gamma-hydroxybutyrate withdrawal syndrome. *Ann Emerg Med.* 2001;37(2):147–153.
28. Crookes CE, Faulds MC, Forrest AR, Galloway JH. A reference range for endogenous gamma-hydroxybutyrate in urine by gas chromatography-mass spectrometry. *J Anal Toxicol.* 2004;28(8):644–649.

29. Eliott SP. Further evidence for the presence of GHB in postmortem biological fluid: implications for the interpretation of findings. *J Anal Toxicol.* 2004;28(1):20–26.

30. Kintz P, Cirimele V, Jamey C, Ludes B. Testing for GHB in hair by GC/MS/MS after a single exposure. Application to document sexual assault. *J Forensic Sci.* 2003;48(1):195–200.

31. Goulle JP, Cheze M, Pepin G. Determination of endogenous levels of GHB in human hair. Are there possibilities for the identification of GHB administration through hair analysis in cases of drug-facilitated sexual assault? *J Anal Toxicol.* 2003;27(8):574–580.

32. Larson SJ, Putnam EA, Schwanke CM, Pershouse MA. Potential surrogate markers for gamma-hydroxybutyrate administration may extend the detection window from 12 to 48 hours. *J Anal Toxicol.* 2007;31(1):15–22.

33. Villain M, Cirimele V, Ludes B, Kintz P. Ultra-rapid procedure to test of γ-hydroxybutyrate acid in blood and urine by gas chromatography-mass spectrometry. *J Chromatogr B Analyt Technol Biomed Life Sci.* 2003;792(1):83–87.

34. Beynon CM, Sumnall HR, McVeigh J, Cole JC, Bellis MA. The ability of two commercially available quick test kits to detect drug-facilitated sexual assault drugs in beverages. *Addiction.* 2006;101:1413–1420.

35. Li J, Stokes SA, Woeckener A. A tale of novel intoxication: seven cases of γ- hydroxybutyric acid overdose. *Ann Emerg Med.* 1988;31(6):723–728.

36. Mazarr-Proo S, Kerrigan S. Distribution of GHB in tissues and fluids following a fatal overdose. *J Anal Toxicol.* 2005;29(5):398–400.

37. Caldicott DG, Chow FY, Burns BJ, et al. Fatalities associated with the use of γ-hydroxybutyrate and its analogues in Australasia. *Med J Aust.* 2004;181(6):310–313.

12 | Hypoglycemics

Adam K. Rowden and Kelli D. O'Donnell

CASE STUDY

A 48-year-old man presented to the emergency department with a decreased level of consciousness. He was previously in good health and used no medications. His wife reported that he had just completed 2 days of extensive diving prior to his loss of consciousness. Despite this history, the medical team recognized that his clinical presentation was not consistent for decompression sickness, especially when he was found to be hypoglycemic with a glucose of 5.4 mg/dL (normal levels are 70–150 mg/dL). The victim remained in a persistent vegetative state for more than 2 months before expiring from multisystem organ failure.

Subsequent laboratory studies revealed an elevated insulin level at 75 mU/L (normal level in the fasting state is below 20 mU/L) when he first presented that continued to climb over the ensuing few hours to 240 mU/L. A low C-peptide (below detection limits of 0.1 nmol/L) drawn from his presenting blood work confirmed the diagnosis of exogenous insulin administration. This finding raised suspicions for a possible criminal poisoning, and the local police were contacted.

The victim's wife, a nurse, produced a farewell letter allegedly written by her husband. She, however, was later found to have forged this letter. In addition, she was shown to have misled the attending paramedics transporting the victim to the hospital by overstating the extent of the diving exercises done by the victim. She was later convicted of her husband's murder.[1]

HISTORY

Diabetic agents are a diverse group of medications all having the goal of controlling the level of glucose in the blood. To better understand these drugs as agents of criminal poisonings, it is useful to separate them into two classes: those that frequently produce hypoglycemia (dangerously low blood glucose) and those that do not cause hypoglycemia. The agents that are routinely capable of inducing hypoglycemia include insulin, the sulfonylureas, and the meglitinides. There are three other classes of diabetes medications that do not cause hypoglycemia—the biguanides, the glitizones, and the alpha-glucosidase inhibitors. Of these, only the biguanides are thought to be clinically significant in terms of poisonous exposures and will therefore be discussed in more detail.[2-6] Phenformin is a biguanide that was removed from the U.S. market in the 1970s but is still available in some countries.[5]

POTENTIAL DELIVERY METHODS

Insulin is a regulatory hormone that is usually supplied as a white crystal dissolved in solution. This preparation must be administered via a hypodermic needle. It is typically administered therapeutically by injection into the subcutaneous tissue, but it is also effective when injected intramuscularly or intravenously. Orally administered insulin is not absorbed.[7] Recently, an inhaled form of insulin was approved for marketing by the U.S. Food and Drug Administration. The preparation is a white powder that is inhaled and absorbed by the lungs.[8] Experience with poisoning is limited, but this may represent a new delivery method for insulin's use as an agent of criminal poisoning.

The sulfonylureas, meglitinides, and metformin are all oral medications that are not available commercially in an injectable form. There are multiple cases of self-ingestion or attempted homicide with these agents described in the literature.[4,6,9-15] Unintentional poisoning, however, has also been described with the sulfonylureas due to pharmacy dispensing errors[16,17] and contaminated herbal products.[18]

TOXICOLOGIC MECHANISMS

Insulin is a naturally occurring hormone secreted by the pancreas. Its main purpose is to act as a regulatory hormone to control blood glucose levels. In response to high blood glucose, the pancreas secretes insulin. Insulin then signals muscle tissue and the liver to take up glucose. When blood glucose levels fall, insulin secretion stops and the liver and muscle tissues stop taking up glucose. Diabetics either produce inadequate amounts of insulin or are resistant to insulin. In diabetic patients, insulin is used to either replace the body's lack of insulin or to provide more insulin in those who are resistant to it. The sulfonylurea and the meglitinide classes of medications act on the pancreas to secrete more insulin,[2-4,19] thereby lowering blood glucose levels.

Overdose of insulin, in both diabetic and nondiabetic patients, results in low blood sugar.[5] Excess insulin stimulates muscle tissue and liver to absorb glucose from the blood. The typical counter regulatory response that prevents low blood sugar is overrun, and the tissues continue to absorb glucose despite dangerously low levels of blood glucose. This reaction can also occur in diabetics who are not poisoned but who either miss a meal or have coexistent illness that can result in labile blood sugar. Those poisoned by sulfonylureas or meglitinides have reactions that are similar to those described with insulin because toxic amounts of these medications stimulate the pancreas to oversecrete insulin.[3-5]

Metformin's mechanism of action is not completely understood. It is thought to decrease the liver's ability to secrete stored glucose and to increase muscle tissue's ability to absorb glucose.[3,4,6,14,20] The toxic effect of metformin is not fully understood either but appears to result from an increase in lactate production and a decrease in the hepatic metabolism of lactate.[21-23]

CLINICAL EFFECTS

Insulin, the sulfonylureas, and the meglitinides cause toxicity by inducing hypoglycemia. The clinical effects of hypoglycemia are well documented in the literature but vary considerably from case to case.[5,24] Symptoms of hypoglycemia typically involve the central nervous system (CNS) because the brain, unlike other organs, is nearly exclusively dependent on glucose as a fuel source.[7] Other organ systems, primarily the cardiovascular system, also manifest symptoms either in direct response to hypoglycemia or as a result of the catecholamine surge associated with CNS dysfunction from hypoglycemia.[5,7]

A patient with hypoglycemia typically presents with altered mental status. Rapid assessment of blood glucose is considered routine care in all mentally impaired patients. The alterations of consciousness can range from simple confusion and agitation to frank coma with respiratory depression.[5,24] Fixed pupils are also described.[5] Focal neurologic findings, such as muscular weakness on one side, which resemble a cerebral vascular accident (CVA) or stroke have often been described.[25-27] Isolated seizures, status epilepticus,[5,7,28] and cerebral edema[29] have been reported with hypoglycemia.

Other organ systems can be affected by hypoglycemia. Frequently, the cardiovascular system is involved. Common cardiac manifestations include tachycardia and rhythm disturbances.[24,30,31] Hypokalemia is also reported after an episode of hypoglycemia.[5,28] Other symptoms frequently encountered with hypoglycemia include diaphoresis, anxiety, nausea, and vomiting.[5,24]

If recognized and treated rapidly, the clinical effects of hypoglycemia, including coma and seizures, will resolve with the correction of blood glucose.[4,5] This is accomplished with oral glucose if the patient is cooperative or with intravenous dextrose solution. The neurologic findings, however, may be permanent if hypoglycemia persists for too long despite adequate treatment.[5,7,24,26,28] If hypoglycemia persists even longer, death occurs from cardiopulmonary collapse.[5]

The time from exposure to onset of hypoglycemia can vary widely because of the many products and preparations available. Insulin is available in short-, intermediate-, and long-acting preparations. Depending on which preparation is used, the delay to peak effect can range from 30 minutes to 24 hours.[2,5] Delay from insulin exposure to symptomatic hypoglycemia has been reported to be as long as 18 hours.[7] The duration of action can be 36 hours at therapeutic dosages[2,5] and longer still in massive overdoses that allow for recurrent episodes of hypoglycemia. In a case

of long-acting insulin overdose, recurrent hypoglycemia lasted 6 days.[32]

Insulin must be given via a hypodermic needle, which may leave evidence of injection, including bruising or an area that is raised and red. Typically, insulin is injected into the skin and may leave a deposit of insulin,[5] which may be noticed on physical exam.

Likewise, hypoglycemia from sulfonylurea ingestion can be delayed and persistent.[4] The entire class of sulfonylureas has delayed onset of action and persistent therapeutic effect. The time from exposure with sulfonylurea to hypoglycemia can range from as little as 4 hours to as many as 21 hours.[33-36] Recurrent hypoglycemia can occur for at least 24 hours, and, after massive overdoes, it has been reported to last as long as 27 days.[37]

The meglitinides are a newer class of diabetes drugs that are capable of producing hypoglycemia.[4,9,10,38,39] They have much shorter onset and duration of action than the sulfonylureas and are therefore capable of having delayed or persistent hypoglycemia. There is limited experience with these medications in poisonings.

Unlike insulin, the sulfonylureas, and meglitinides, metformin is very unlikely to produce hypoglycemia when taken in overdose. Reports exist of hypoglycemia associated with metformin poisoning, but most of these involve polypharmacy ingestions and/or unclear histories.[4,5,14,15,22] Based on the bulk of evidence and the pharmacologic mechanism, hypoglycemia after exclusive metformin exposure would not be expected unless other agents or diseases are present.

Acute metformin exposure is frequently a benign event, rarely resulting in serious morbidity and mortality.[4,5,14,15] In a large case series of adults and children that included accidental and intentional poisonings, the mortality rate was 0.2%.[14]

The initial clinical effects in those poisoned with metformin are frequently vague. Nausea, vomiting, diarrhea, and abdominal pain are reported as early symptoms.[5,14,40-42] These symptoms along with tachycardia, agitation, and lethargy were among the most commonly encountered complaints of exposed patients.[5,14,40-42]

Metformin is believed to cause death by a process known as lactic acidosis.[5,14,40-42] This process usually results in severe metabolic derangements that lead to multisystem organ failure and death. High serum lactates are encountered along with low serum pH. A large anion gap acidosis is also present in those severely poisoned by metformin. Cardiopulmonary collapse, decreased cardiac output, shock, and cardiac dysrhythmias lead to death.[3-7,40,42-44]

Those seriously poisoned with metformin are frequently treated with intravenous bicarbonate therapy. They may receive some form of dialysis in an attempt both to correct the metabolic derangements and to remove metformin.[4,13,40,42-47]

ANALYTIC DETECTION

Insulin levels can be detected by high-performance liquid chromatography (HPLC) that can also distinguish human insulin from cow- and pig-derived insulin.[48] Postmortem and antemortem samples of blood should be obtained for analysis of glucose and insulin levels. Postmortem vitreous humor samples are invalid, as the glucose level is abnormally low.[48] Rare disease states, such as insulinomas, can result in hypoglycemia and a high insulin level. Laboratory testing in suspected cases of poisonings by diabetic agents is fairly well established. Insulin secreted from the pancreas is accompanied by the protein C-peptide. Exogenous insulin does not contain the C-peptide. In cases of poisoning with exogenous insulin, the C-peptide levels would be low and insulin levels would be high.[11]

In poisonings with sulfonylureas and meglitinides, both the C-peptide and insulin levels would be high because these medications stimulate the pancreas to secrete the body's own insulin. In these cases, screening tests for these medications are available. The technique usually used in these screenings is HPLC.[11,49] Due to the large number of available medications, false negative screens have been reported, and further testing may be needed if suspicion is high.[50,51]

Metformin generally does not affect insulin or glucose levels. Assays to detect blood and tissue levels are available and generally use HPLC.[52]

CONCLUSION

Diabetic agents represent a diverse group of medications all aimed at controlling blood sugar. Most potential criminal poisoning agents alter the body's ability to maintain proper control of blood glucose, usually resulting in hypoglycemia. Deaths resulting from diabetic agent poisoning can mimic natural death, resembling seizures, strokes, and other disease states. In situations where suspicion exists, blood samples from early in the hospital stay should be stored for forensic testing. In addition, efforts should be made to identify those having access to the victim as well as to determine the nature and extent of their knowledge regarding diabetic agents.

REFERENCES

1. Koskinen PJ, Nuutinen HM, Laaksonen H, et al. Importance of storing emergency serum samples for uncovering murder with insulin. *Forensic Sci Int.* 1999;105(1):61–66.
2. Carlton FB Jr. Recent advances in the pharmacologic management of diabetes mellitus. *Emerg Med Clin North Am.* 2000;18(4):745–753.
3. Harrigan RA, Nathan MS, Beattie P. Oral agents for the treatment of type 2 diabetes mellitus: pharmacology, toxicity, and treatment. *Ann Emerg Med.* 2001;38(1):68–78.
4. Rowden AK, Fasano CJ. Emergency management of oral hypoglycemic drug toxicity. *North Am.* 2007;25(2):347–356.
5. Spiller HA. Management of antidiabetic medications in overdose. *Drug Safety.* 1998;19(5):411–424.
6. Spiller HA, Sawyer TS. Toxicology of oral antidiabetic medications. *Am J Health Syst Pharm.* 2006;63(10):929–938.
7. Bosse GM. Antidiabetic and hypoglycemic agents. In: Goldfrank Lea, ed. *Goldfrank's Toxicologic Emergencies.* 7th ed. New York: McGraw-Hill; 2002.
8. Exubera [package insert]. New York: Pfizer Pharmaceuticals; 2007.
9. Hirshberg B, Skarulis MC, Pucino F, et al. Repaglinide-induced factitious hypoglycemia. *J Clin Endocrinol Metab.* 2001;86:475–477.
10. Nakayama S, Hirose T, Watada H, et al. Hypoglycemia following a nateglinide overdose in a suicide attempt. *Diabetes Care.* 2005;28:227–228.
11. Waickus CM, de Bustros A, Shakil A. Recognizing factitious hypoglycemia in the family practice setting. *J Am Board Fam Pract.* 1999;12(2):133–136.
12. Brady WJ, Carter CT. Metformin overdose. *Am J Emerg Med.* 1997;15(1):1078.
13. Gjedde S, Christiansen A, Pedersen SB, et al. Survival following a metformin overdose of 63 g: a case report. *Pharmacol Toxicol.* 2003;93(2):98–99.
14. Spiller HA, Quadrani DA. Toxic effects from metformin exposure. *Ann Pharmacother.* 2004;38(5):776–780.
15. Spiller HA, Weber JA, Winter ML, et al. Multicenter case series of pediatric metformin ingestion. *Ann Pharmacother.* 2000;34(12):1385–1388.
16. Shumak SL, Corenblum B, Steiner G. Recurrent hypoglycemia secondary to drug-dispensing error. *Arch Intern Med.* 1991;151(9):1877–1878.

17. Sledge ED, Broadstone VL. Hypoglycemia due to a pharmacy dispensing error. *South Med J.* 1993;86(11):1272–1273.

18. Goudie AM, Kaye JM. Contaminated medication precipitating hypoglycaemia. *Med J Aust.* 2001;175(5):256–257.

19. Eliasson L, Renstrom E, Ammala C, et al. PKC-dependent stimulation of exocytosis by sulfonylureas in pancreatic beta cells. *Science.* 1996;271(5250):813–815.

20. Stumvoll M, Nurjhan N, Perriello G, Dailey G, Gerich JE. Metabolic effects of metformin in non-insulin-dependent diabetes mellitus. *N Engl J Med.* 1995;333(9):550–554.

21. Bailey CJ. Biguanides and NIDDM. *Diabetes Care.* 1992;15(6):755–772.

22. Bailey CJ, Turner RC. Metformin. *N Engl J Med.* 1996;334(9):574–579.

23. Jurovich MR, Wooldridge JD, Force RW. Metformin-associated nonketotic metabolic acidosis. *Ann Pharmacother.* 1997;31(1):53–55.

24. Hoffman JR, Schriger DL, Votey SR, et al. The empiric use of hypertonic dextrose in patients with altered mental status: a reappraisal. *Ann Emerg Med.* 1992;21(1):20–24.

25. Andrade R, Mathew V, Morgenstern MJ, et al. Hypoglycemic hemiplegic syndrome. *Ann Emerg Med.* 1984;13(7):529–531.

26. Malouf R, Brust JC. Hypoglycemia: causes, neurological manifestations, and outcome. *Ann Neurol.* 1985;17(5):421–430.

27. Spiller HA, Schroeder SL, Ching DS. Hemiparesis and altered mental status in a child after glyburide ingestion. *J Emerg Med.* 1998;16(3):433–435.

28. Arem R, Zoghbi W. Insulin overdose in eight patients: insulin pharmacokinetics and review of the literature. *Medicine (Baltimore).* 1985;64(5):323–332.

29. Bourgeois M, Dufourg J. Suicide by insulin. *Ann Med Psychol (Paris).* 1967;125(1):133–140.

30. Leak D, Starr P. The mechanism of arrhythmias during insulin-induced hypoglycemia. *Am Heart J.* 1962;63:688–691.

31. Odeh M, Oliven A, Bassan H. Transient atrial fibrillation precipitated by hypoglycemia. *Ann Emerg Med.* 1990;19(5):565–567.

32. Martin FI, Hansen N, Warne GL. Attempted suicide by insulin overdose in insulin-requiring diabetics. *Med J Aust.* 1977;1(3):58–60.

33. Quadrani DA, Spiller HA, Widder P. Five year retrospective evaluation of sulfonylurea ingestion in children. *J Toxicol Clin Toxicol.* 1996;34(3):267–270.

34. Seltzer HS. Drug-induced hypoglycemia. A review of 1418 cases. *Endocrinol Metab Clin North Am.* 1989;18(1):163–183.

35. Spiller HA, Villalobos D, Krenzelok EP, et al. Prospective multicenter study of sulfonylurea ingestion in children. *J Pediatr.* 1997;131(1, pt 1):141–146.

36. Szlatenyi CS, Capes KF, Wang RY. Delayed hypoglycemia in a child after ingestion of a single glipizide tablet. *Ann Emerg Med.* 1998;31(6):773–776.

37. Ciechanowski K, Borowiak KS, Potocka BA, et al. Chlorpropamide toxicity with survival despite 27-day hypoglycemia. *J Toxicol Clin Toxicol.* 1999;37(7):869–871.

38. Fonseca VA, Kelley DE, Cefalu W, et al. Hypoglycemic potential of nateglinide versus glyburide in patients with type 2 diabetes mellitus. *Metabolism.* 2004;53(10):1331–1335.

39. Nagai T, Imamura M, Iizuka K, et al. Hypoglycemia due to nateglinide administration in diabetic patient with chronic renal failure. *Diabetes Res Clin Pract.* 2003;59(3):191–94.

40. Harvey B, Hickman C, Hinson G, et al. Severe lactic acidosis complicating metformin overdose successfully treated with high-volume venovenous hemofiltration and aggressive alkalinization. *Pediatr Crit Care Med.* 2005;6(5):598–601.

41. Panzer U, Kluge S, Kreymann G, et al. Combination of intermittent haemodialysis and high-volume continuous haemofiltration for the treatment of severe metformin-induced lactic acidosis. *Nephrol Dial Transplant.* 2004;19(8):2157–2158.

42. Teale KF, Devine A, Stewart H, et al. The management of metformin overdose. *Anaesthesia.* 1998; 53(7):698–701.

43. Guo PY, Storsley LJ, Finkle SN. Severe lactic acidosis treated with prolonged hemodialysis: recovery after massive overdoses of metformin. *Semin Dial.* 2006;19(1):80–83.

44. Heaney D, Majid A, Junor B. Bicarbonate haemodialysis as a treatment of metformin overdose. *Nephrol Dial Transplant.* 1997;12(5):1046–1047.

45. Barrueto F, Meggs WJ, Barchman MJ. Clearance of metformin by hemofiltration in overdose. *J Toxicol Clin Toxicol.* 2002;40(2):177–180.

46. Kutoh E. Possible metformin-induced hepatotoxicity. *Am J Geriatr Pharmacother.* 2005;3(4):270–273.

47. Lalau JD, Andrejak M, Moriniere P, et al. Hemodialysis in the treatment of lactic acidosis in diabetics treated by metformin: a study of metformin elimination. *Int J Clin Pharmacol Ther Toxicol.* 1989;27(6):285–288.

48. Rao NG, Menezes RG, Nagesh KR, et al. Suicide by combined insulin and glipizide overdose in a non-insulin dependent diabetes mellitus physician: a case report. *Med Sci Law.* 2006;46(3):263–269.

49. Hoizey G, Lamiable D, Trenque T, et al. Identification and quantification of 8 sulfonylureas with clinical toxicology interest by liquid chromatography-ion-trap tandem mass spectrometry and library searching. 2005;51:1666–1672.

50. Earle KE, Rushakoff RJ, Goldfine ID. Inadvertent sulfonylurea overdosage and hypoglycemia in an elderly woman: failure of serum hypoglycemia screening. *Diabetes Technol Ther.* 2003;5(3):449–451.

51. Klonoff DC. A flaw in the use of sulfonylurea screening to diagnose sulfonylurea overdosages. *Diabetes Technol Ther.* 2003;5(3):453–454.

52. Moore KA, Levine B, Titus JM, et al. Analysis of metformin in antemortem serum and postmortem specimens by a novel HPLC method and application to an intoxication case. *J Anal Toxicol.* 2003;27(8):592–594.

13 | Neuromuscular Blocking Agents

R. Brent Furbee

CASE STUDY

At the Veterans Administration Hospital (VAH) in Ann Arbor, Michigan, the rate of sudden unexpected deaths began to climb in July of 1975. The change was noted to be occurring in the intensive care unit. During the previous year, there had been about six cardiopulmonary arrests per month. In 1975, however, there were 24 such deaths and another 27 in the first 2 weeks of August alone. Initially, the increasing rate appeared only to represent a normal fluctuation in the mortality rate. It was not until August 15, when 3 cardiac arrests occurred in a 20-minute period that criminal activity was suspected. On that day, teams of physicians and nurses moved from patient to patient performing intubations and placing the patients on ventilators. In attendance was the chief of anesthesia, who noted that the patients appeared to have an unexpected lack of muscle tone. When a nerve stimulator from the surgery department indicated paralysis, neostigmine was administered, and the patients dramatically improved. This reinforced the suspicion that a curare-like agent had been used. No such agent had been ordered for any of the patients.

Because the VAHs are federal hospitals, the Federal Bureau of Investigation (FBI) was notified. Working with the FBI, an investigative team consisting of physicians from the Veterans Administration, the Epidemic Intelligence Service of the Centers for Disease Control and Prevention (CDC), and the University of Michigan Medical School was assembled. They began a review of deaths occurring from June 1, 1975, through August 15, 1975. Those were compared with deaths from time periods before and after those months. The rate of suspicious deaths was decidedly higher for the months in question. Particularly unusual were the number of primary respiratory arrests occurring between 4 PM and 12 AM that had a significantly higher than expected rate of successful resuscitations.

The hospital began to accept only emergent admissions. All patients receiving intravenous (IV) drugs were placed on two wards. Nurses were to administer IV medications in the presence of a second nurse. The nursing staff was increased, and identification cards were required. Pancuronium, the suspected agent, was put under strict control.[1,2]

Two nurses were charged with the crime due to several witnesses placing them in close proximity to the patients at the time of their respiratory arrests. However, no one witnessed either nurse injecting a patient, and the murder charges were dropped. They were eventually convicted of conspiracy and poisoning, but those convictions were reversed.[3]

HISTORY

Curare was first used by South American Indians for hunting, but its date of discovery is not recorded. They used it to coat the tips of arrows and darts. It was derived from the plants *Chondrodendron tomentosum* and *Strychnos toxifera*.[4] In the mid-1500s, it was introduced to Europe. Sir Walter Raleigh is often credited with its introduction, although some argue that others were responsible for its appearance in Europe.[5] Humboldt and Bonpland were the first trained scientists to view the preparation of the poison.

Claude Bernard observed that when frogs received subcutaneous injects of curare, they appeared to die, though their hearts continued to beat. Bernard incorrectly concluded that this was due to curare's action on motor nerves.

However, Bernard's pupil, Alfred Vulpian, attributed paralysis to action at the then recently described motor end-plate.[5,6] Since that time, several agents have been developed with fewer side effects and greater efficacy.[7]

The first reported use of neuromuscular blockers (NMBs) for murder occurred in 1961 when physician Carl Coppolino was tried for the murder of his wife and his neighbor. He was accused of injecting both with succinylcholine and was found guilty of second-degree murder.[8] Since then, several healthcare workers have been accused of homicide with NMBs.[2,3,9-14] Rarer, but still reported, are cases involving nonmedical suspects.[15]

As an aside, there are a number of compounds capable of causing paralysis that are not classically considered in this class of drugs. For example, organophosphates and carbamates can cause fasciculations and paralysis by inhibiting acetylcholinesterase. The most common mode of exposure is ingestion of a concentrated solution or high-dose inhalation. Nicotine can be absorbed from the gastrointestinal tract, lung, or skin. It stimulates nicotinic acetylcholine (ACh) receptors causing fasciculations and paralysis in high doses. It is usually accompanied by nausea, vomiting, and weakness. Potassium salts, discussed in Chapter 17, can cause paralysis without fasciculation. Finally, familial hyper- or hypokalemic paralysis, a condition that often presents with severe weakness or paralysis, may be confused with a criminal event.

POTENTIAL DELIVERY METHODS

Onset of intravenously injected NMBs is rapid (Table 13.1). Intramuscular administration is also relatively rapid. Ingestion of a typical intravenous dose is unlikely to be life-threatening. There is little information concerning the oral route, but the fact that hunters and their families eat meat killed with curare suggests it is not well absorbed orally. While material safety data sheets for pancuronium, vecuronium, and succinylcholine warn against oral exposure, rat and mouse data for ingestion suggest very large doses are required for lethality.[16-18]

TOXICOLOGIC MECHANISMS

For muscles to contract, ACh is released from the nerve ending as a result of depolarization (Figure 13.1). As the inner aspect of the nerve

TABLE 13.1 Pharmacokinetics of Intravenous Neuromuscular Blockers

Agent	Onset of Action (Minutes)	Duration of Action (Minutes)
Atracurium	2–4	30–60
Doxacurium	4–6	90–120
Mivacurium	2–4	12–18
Pancuronium	4–6	120–180
Pipecuronium	2–4	80–100
Rocuronium	1–2	30–60
Succinylcholine	1–1.5	5–8
Tubocurarine	4–6	80–120
Vecuronium	2–4	60–90

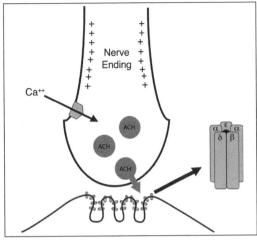

FIGURE 13-1 Depolarization of the nerve ending causes release of acetylcholine (ACh)

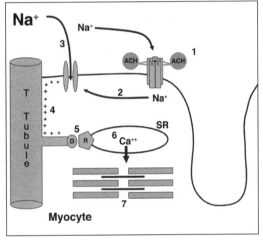

FIGURE 13-2 Acetylcholine (ACh) triggers a cascade of events resulting in muscle contraction

ending becomes more positive, calcium enters. This causes vesicles containing ACh to fuse with the cell membranes releasing that neurotransmitter into the synaptic cleft. ACh crosses the synaptic cleft and attaches to nicotinic receptors on the motor end-plates located on the muscle. This site of attachment is constructed of five protein subunits that form a channel on the muscle cell membrane. There are two α subunits and a single β, δ, and ε subunit (Figure 13.1). Two ACh molecules attach to two subunits each. They engage an α unit and either a δ or ε subunit (Figure 13.2, step 1). These attachments open the sodium channel of the receptor, and as sodium ions enter, the interior of the cell membrane starts to become more positive, causing the voltage-dependent sodium channels to open (Figure 13.2, step 2). With a larger influx of sodium (Figure 13.2, step 3), the cell membrane starts to depolarize, engaging the T tubules (Figure 13.2, step 4). The dihydropyridine and ryanodine receptors are activated in turn (Figure 13.2, step 5), and calcium is released from the sarcoplasmic reticulum (Figure 13.2, step 6). Calcium then binds with troponin C to cause muscle contraction (Figure 13.2, step 7).

Nondepolarizing Neuromuscular Blockers

Most nondepolarizing neuromuscular blockers (NDNMBs) cause paralysis by attaching to the α subunit of the nicotinic receptors, thereby blocking the attachment of ACh and preventing the sequence of events necessary for muscle contraction.

Depolarizing Neuromuscular Blockers

Succinylcholine is the only commonly used member of the depolarizing neuromuscular blockers (DNMBs). Nicotine is also capable of producing depolarizing neuromuscular blockade and has been used as a paralytic agent for animals. To cause paralysis, two molecules of the DNMB must bind to the two α subunits of the nicotinic receptors on the motor end-plate. This binding briefly causes the entry of sodium ions and activates muscle contraction. Thus, at the onset of DNMBs action, fasciculation (muscle twitching) is seen for a few seconds. Fasciculations do not occur with nondepolarizing agents. Succinylcholine remains attached to the receptor subunits and essentially allows the myocyte to "fire" but will not let it recover. Muscle cells remain in the depolarized state and do not respond to further ACh release, thus leaving the muscle paralyzed until succinylcholine is metabolized.

CLINICAL EFFECTS

The onset of symptoms occurs within 1 to 6 minutes of injection, depending on the rate and dose. DNMB, such as succinylcholine, causes fasciculations just prior to the onset of paralysis. Muscles of the eyes, jaw, and larynx tend to relax first. Recovery occurs in reverse order. Fasciculations are frequently noted in the pectoralis and abdominal muscles. They subside in a few minutes as paralysis ensues. NDNMBs do not cause fasciculations and tend to be slower in onset. Succinylcholine administration has been associated with hyperkalemia in patients with rhabdomyolysis, head injury, or spinal injury, as well as crush injury, burns, sepsis, and a number of other conditions.

D-tubocurarine and, to a lesser extent, mivacurium, doxacurium, and atracurium, can cause histamine release. This reaction can manifest as bronchospasm, salivation, increased bronchiolar secretion, and hypotension and occasionally death. Pancuronium, vecuronium, pipecuronium, and rocuronium may do so to a lesser degree.

Cardiovascular effects vary with different agents, but tachycardia is relatively common. The cardiac muscle is protected from paralysis because contraction is not produced via a motor end-plate.[19]

Neuromuscular paralytic agents are available in the hospital setting and are not controlled substances. They have rapid onset and appear to induce coma. The NMBs, however, whether depolarizing or nondepolarizing, have minimal central nervous system effect. Even though they are not always believed, patients who survive exposure can frequently identify their assailant. Interestingly, many healthcare workers are unaware that paralysis does not alter consciousness. In a survey by Loper et al., approximately 50% of medical/surgical staff and 70% of critical care nurses believed that pancuronium had anxiolytic properties.[20]

ANALYTIC DETECTION

Laboratory detection is possible but is not rapidly available in most hospitals. Kerskes et al. described the use of high-performance liquid chromatography-electrospray ionization-mass spectrometry (LC-ESI-MS) for the detection of quaternary nitrogen muscle relaxants such as pancuronium and rocuronium.[21]

Because of its use in homicidal poisoning, the detection of succinylcholine has been the subject of much study. Gao and coworkers were able to detect succinylcholine to a concentration of 0.250 µg/mL in human plasma, but concentrations may be well below that in postmortem specimens.[22] They applied their method in a patient receiving 1 mg/kg as an IV bolus. The initial plasma concentration of 33 µg/mL declined to 0.11 µg/mL in 3 minutes. By 4 minutes, it was undetectable. In postmortem specimens, such attempts at obtaining levels would be of little use.

LeBeau and Quenzer of the FBI Laboratory in Quantico, Virginia, released results of a small study of succinylmonocholine in patients who had *not* been injected with succinylcholine prior to death.[23] They were able to identify small concentrations of the compound in autopsy tissue from the six patients they studied. They concluded that "succinylmonocholine is not an exclusive indicator of exposure to the parent drug, succinylcholine."

Pitts et al. addressed the succinylmonocholine issue by measuring choline instead.[24] They suggested that choline is produced from succinylcholine and not succinylmonocholine, which may be an endogenous compound, because the choline they recovered never exceeded that expected for succinylcholine. Subsequently, choline would reflect the administration of the paralytic agent.[25]

Reversal agents may also be useful in determining the presence of NDNMBs. As in the cases reported by Stross and Kroll, the administration of neostigmine suggested the presence of NMB.[1,2] Edrophonium, neostigmine, or physostigmine in conjunction with atropine can reverse the effects of the nondepolarizing agents.

CONCLUSION

Use of NMBs have been used by both medical and nonmedical personnel for attempted murder have been reported. Victims who survive can often recall the events, as the NMBs have no amnestic properties. Cases where the criminal administration of NMBs may have occurred may be clinically suspected through the use of nerve stimulation studies or when clinical effects can be reversed. Analytic detection is possible for the NDNMBs. Studies have suggested other markers may be useful for the detection of the DNMB succinylcholine.

REFERENCES

1. Kroll P, Silk K, Chamberlain K, Ging R. Denying the incredible: unexplained deaths in a Veterans Administration hospital. *Am J Psychiatry.* 1977;134(12):1376–1380.

2. Stross JK, Shasby M, Harlan WR. An epidemic of mysterious cardiopulmonary arrests. *N Eng J Med.* 1976;295(20):1107–1110.

3. Yorker BC, Kizer KW, Lampe P, et. al . Serial murder by healthcare professionals. *J Forensic Sci.* 2006;51(6):1362–1371.

4. Bowman WC. Neuromuscular block. *Br J Pharmacol.* 2006;147:S277–S286.

5. Black J. Claude Bernard on the action of curare. *BMJ.* 1999;319(7210):622.

6. Cousin MT. Vulpian and not Claude Bernard first proposed the hypothesis of the motor end-plate as the site of action of curare. *Anesthesiology.* 2002;97(2):527–528.

7. Gyermek L. Development of ultra short-acting muscle relaxant agents: history, research strategies, and challenges. *Med Res Rev.* 2005;25(6):610–654.

8. Maltby JR. Criminal poisoning with anaesthetic drugs: murder, manslaughter, or not guilty. *Forensic Sci.* 1975;6(1-2):91–108.

9. Alpers A. Criminal act or palliative care? Prosecutions involving the care of the dying. *J Law Med Ethics.* 1998;26(4):308–331.

10. McGraw S. Notorious murders/not guilty? The Bill Sybers case. In: Bardsley M, ed. *Crime Library.* Court TV. 2005.

11. Park GR, Khan SN. Murder and the ICU. *Eur J Anaesthesiol.* 2002;19(9):621–623.

12. Ramsland K. All about Efren Saldivar. In: Bardsley M, ed. *Crime Library.* Court TV. 2005.

13. Siegel H, Rieders F, Holmstedt B. The medical and scientific evidence in alleged tubocurarine poisonings. A review of the so-called Dr. X case. *Forensic Sci Int.* 1985;29(1-2):29–76.

14. Stewart J. *Blind Eye: How the Medical Establishment Let a Doctor Get Away with Murder.* New York: Simon & Schuster; 1999.

15. Maeda H, Fujita MQ, Zhu BL, et al. A case of serial homicide by injection of succinylcholine. *Med Sci Law.* 2000;40(2):169–174.

16. ANON. *Material Safety Data Sheet—Pancuronium Bromide.* Irvine, CA: Teva Sicor Pharmaceuticals; 2005:1–6.

17. ANON. *Material Safety Data Sheet—Succinylcholine chloride.* Houston, TX: Science Lab; 2005:1–5.

18. Chemical Safety Associates. *Material Safety Data Sheet—Vecuronium.* San Diego, CA: Sicor Pharmaceuticals; 2004:1–6.

19. Mohrman D, Heller L. *Cardiovascular Physiology—Lange Physiology Series.* 6th ed. New York: McGraw-Hill; 2006;19–46.

20. Loper KA, Butler S, Nessly M, Wild L. Paralyzed with pain: the need for education. *Pain.* 1989; 37(3):315–316.

21. Kerskes CH, Lusthof KJ, Zweipfenning PG, Franke JP. The detection and identification of quaternary nitrogen muscle relaxants in biological fluids and tissues by ion-trap LC-ESI-MS. *J Anal Toxicol.* 2002;26(1):29–34.

22. Gao H, Roy S, Donati F, Varin F. Determination of succinylcholine in human plasma by high-performance liquid chromatography with electrochemical detection. *J Chromatogr Biomed Sci Appl.* 1998;718(1):129–134.

23. LeBeau M, Quenzer C. Succinylmonocholine identified in negative control tissues. *J Anal Toxicol.* 2003;27(8):600–601.

24. Pitts NI, Deftereos D, Mitchell G. Determination of succinylcholine in plasma by high-pressure liquid chromatography with electrochemical detection. *Br J Anaesth.* 2000;85(4):592–598.

25. Pitts NI, Deftereos D, Mitchell G. Determination of succinylcholine in plasma by high-pressure liquid chromatography with electrochemical detection. *Br J Anaesthesia.* 2000;85(4):592–598.

14 | Opioids

Ziad N. Kazzi and Kevin S. Barlotta

CASE STUDY

On October 23, 2002, over 40 Chechen terrorists took 914 people hostage in the Dubrovka Theater Center in Moscow, Russia, during the musical *Nord-Ost*. The terrorists repeatedly threatened to detonate explosive and destroy the theater if their political demands were not met by the Russians. After several days of captivity, Russian special forces, known as spetsnaz, stormed the theater 15 minutes after introducing a mysterious aerosolized gas into its ventilation system. This gas, believed to be a mixture of carfentanyl (a fentanyl derivative) and halothane (an anesthetic), resulted in a massive inhalation exposure, leaving 127 hostages and the Chechen terrorists dead. Victims initially treated by the health-care teams were reported to exhibit classic signs of opioid toxicity consisting of miosis and depressed consciousness and respiratory function. This incident captured the world's attention and generated controversy over the use of aerosolized opiates.[1-3]

HISTORY

Opiates are the naturally derived narcotics, such as morphine and codeine, found in opium. Opium is isolated from the poppy plant *Papaver somniferum*. Opioids include opiates and other substances that bind to opioid receptors. Opioids include semisynthetic compounds such as hydrocodone, hydromorphone, oxycodone, and fentanyl. Heroin is the only opioid currently listed as a Schedule I drug by the U.S. Drug Enforcement Administration, primarily due to its rapid onset, clinical effects (euphoria and sedation), and high abuse potential. These drugs all have potent analgesic and sedative properties but different pharmacokinetic properties.

Long before its categorization by Linnaeus as *Papaver somniferum*, opium was recognized for its medicinal uses as a remedy to a variety of ailments. As early as the third century BCE, Egyptian and Sumerian civilizations began extracting the sap from the immature seeds of the opium poppy for use as an analgesic. Morphine, named after the Greek god of dreams Morpheus, was isolated from opium in 1804 by German chemist Friedrich Sertürner. The isolation of codeine followed in 1832. With the invention of the hypodermic needle in 1853, morphine's use became widespread. Decades later, heroin was synthesized by Dresser by diacetylating morphine. Opioids are frequently associated with addiction. Their abuse remains a worldwide threat to public health and a continued, potentially lethal, vehicle for misuse and criminal poisoning.[4]

Opioids are often utilized in palliative care and can be administered in excess, thereby leading to an accusation of euthanasia.[5] Even for medical experts, it is difficult to distinguish between relieving suffering and intentionally hastening death.[6] Because of this, it is often difficult to prosecute such cases for murder. For example, in one small study, five U.S. physicians were indicted for murder related to opioid overdose deaths, with none found guilty.[7] In 2003, a 53-year-old German physician was investigated for possible murder after her use of morphine to treat multiple hospital patients led to several deaths at the private Paracelsus Hospital Silbersee in Langenhagen, Germany. Suspicions were raised when health insurance companies monitoring patients' files for the preceding 2 years found extremely high costs and dosages of morphine without evidence of severe pain and suffering among the patients.[8] Controversy even encompassed the death of Sigmund Freud, which is thought by some to have been hastened by the administration of morphine.[9]

There are notorious cases in which opioids were utilized in criminal poisoning. One of the most notable involved Dr. Harold Frederick Shipman of Great Britain who was convicted of murdering 15 of his patients. He is actually thought to have killed hundreds of his patients using morphine and diamorphine (heroin) in a murderous career that spanned more than two decades, earning him the notoriety of the most prolific British serial killer (see Chapter 26).[10,11]

POTENTIAL DELIVERY METHODS

Opioids can be administered through a variety of routes including oral consumption, intravenous injection, topical application, rectal deposition, and intranasal as well as pulmonary inhalation (smoking). Historically, opioids have been abused through intravenous administration, but subcutaneous administration ("skin popping") has become another common avenue of abuse (Figure 14.1). Currently, oral administration has regained popularity due to the availability of oral opioid preparations and the risks associated with intravenous abuse, including viral hepatitis and HIV infections.[12,13]

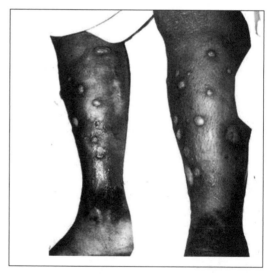

FIGURE 14-1 **Subcutaneous injection of opioids (skin popping) resulting in multiple ulcers of the legs.** (See Color Plate 11.)

Transdermal delivery is a route used by patients who are chronically dependent on opioid analgesia. These patches usually contain a large amount of the drug and can lead to significant central nervous system (CNS) depression or death if they are ingested, licked, chewed, or smoked, or if they are inadvertently or intentionally placed on the skin in a manner inconsistent with the instructions given with the prescription.[14]

Occasionally, "body packers" (i.e., individuals who ingest opioid-laden packets to smuggle them through border inspections) are poisoned when the packet contents spill into their gastrointestinal tract, leading to significant morbidity and mortality (Figure 14.2).[15]

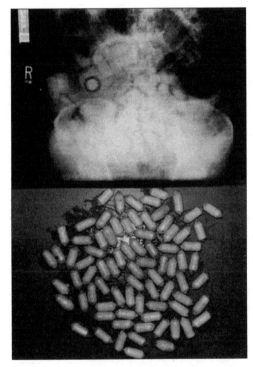

FIGURE 14-2   Body packer carrying multiple condoms filled heroin.
Reprinted with permission from Dr. CV Wetli.

As noted previously, a novel method of delivery was used in Moscow when Chechen terrorists were subdued with a potent aerosolized fentanyl derivative (carfentanyl).[1]

TOXICOLOGIC MECHANISMS

Opioids exert their clinical effects by binding to specific CNS receptors. These receptors consist of three major classes (mu, kappa, and delta; or OP3, OP2, and OP1). Various opioids have different affinity profiles with respect to the opioid receptors; hence the differences in the clinical effects. For example, mu receptors are primarily responsible for the sensation of euphoria, and specific opioids are preferred for abuse due to their potent mu receptor agonism.[16]

CLINICAL EFFECTS

Opioid poisoning can have widespread clinical manifestations depending on the agent used, dose, method of delivery, and the presence of a coingestant(s). The classic toxidrome consists of miosis (pupillary constriction) and respiratory and CNS depression. Although pinpoint pupils are often associated with opioid poisoning, one should not rely on them exclusively in making the diagnosis. Gastrointestinal motility is decreased. CNS and respiratory depression can lead to a number of potentially serious secondary effects including anoxic brain injury, aspiration pneumonia, and muscle breakdown (rhabdomyolysis). The onset of clinical effects for oral ingestion of opioids varies, but most are within 30 to 60 minutes; the effects of inhalation or injection are more rapid (within 5 minutes). Duration of clinical effects depends upon the specific opioid drug and a person's preexisting health and physical status.

Acute lung injury has been associated with opioid poisoning. It manifests as bilateral, noncardiogenic pulmonary edema leading to shortness of breath and cough after toxic patients resume breathing. Such individuals often produce pink-frothy sputum and develop hypoxemia. Rales are often heard on clinical examination.[17] The cause and mechanism of this injury is not well understood.[18]

Several opioids cause additional nonclassic signs and symptoms that confound clinical diagnosis. For example, tramadol, propoxyphene, and meperidine may cause seizures.[19-21] Propoxyphene and methadone can directly cause cardiac conduction abnormalities (prolonged QRS and QTc intervals) and dysrhythmias.[22,23] Movement disorders may also be seen with drugs such as fentanyl, including life-threatening chest wall rigidity.[24]

Certain opioids, like meperidine, fentanyl, propoxyphene, dextromethorphan, and tramadol, have serotonergic properties and may lead to a serotonin syndrome when combined with other serotonin agonists.[25-27] Serotonin syndrome manifests as a triad of neuro-excitatory features including neuromuscular hyperactivity (tremor, clonus, myoclonus), autonomic hyperactivity (diaphoresis, fever, tachycardia), and altered mental status.[27]

Adulterants or contaminants may confound the clinical presentation of a patient presenting with opioid toxicity. For example, clenbuterol-contaminated heroin produced an outbreak of an atypical clinical illness consisting of tachycardia, palpitations, hypokalemia, and hyperglycemia.[28] Heroin adulterated with quinine has been reported to produce cardiotoxicity due to the quinine-induced sodium channel blockade and QRS interval prolongation.[29,30]

The opioid toxidrome may be mimicked by nonopioid agents such as clonidine, barbiturates, valproic acid, oxymetazoline, and antipsychotics. Pontine strokes may occasionally manifest with miosis and CNS and respiratory depression.[31,32]

Diagnostic chest radiographs may reveal findings of noncardiogenic pulmonary edema while arterial blood gases may reveal low arterial oxygen pressure. Other laboratory abnormalities such as leukocytosis are neither consistent nor clinically useful.[17]

In summary, patients who are poisoned with opioids typically present with a triad of miosis along with CNS and respiratory depression. Although these signs should lead healthcare and law enforcement personnel to suspect exposure to opioids, other substances and diseases can mimic opioid toxicity (e.g., clonidine toxicity and tetrahydrozoline toxicity). The possibility of atypical presentations stemming from coingestants, drug-to-drug interactions, and drug-specific effects must also be considered.

ANALYTIC DETECTION

Commercial immunoassays (e.g., EMIT, by Dade-Behring; TDx, by Abbott) are designed to detect naturally occurring opiates (morphine and codeine). Specific gas chromatography-mass spectrometry (GC-MS) analysis protocols are available for confirming natural, synthetic, and semisynthetic opioid compounds from urine specimens. In addition, specific immunoassays and GC-MS protocols are available for detection of methadone and propoxyphene.

Poppy seeds that are used in culinary settings, such as in poppy seed bagels, contain codeine and morphine and can produce a positive result in morphine and codeine assays. These levels rise in urine rapidly and may be detectable up to 3 days in urine and 1 day in serum.[33] Detection of 6-monoacetylmorphine in urine differentiates poppy seed ingestion from heroin (diacetylmorphine) abuse.[34]

CONCLUSION

Criminal opioid poisoning poses several diagnostic and forensic challenges. Criminal investigators and medical personnel need to pay special attention to the clinical findings, keeping in mind the specific characteristics of each opioid. Diagnostic testing is available for all substances, but immunoassays have specific limitations. The habits, lifestyle, and associations of opioid victims may reveal information that may guide the police in their investigation of suspicious deaths.

REFERENCES

1. Wax PM, Becker CE, Curry SC. Unexpected "gas" casualties in Moscow: a medical toxicology perspective. *Ann Emerg Med.* 2003;41(5):700–705.
2. Coupland RM. Incapacitating chemical weapons: a year after the Moscow theatre siege. *Lancet.* 2003;362(9393):1346.
3. Stanley T. Human immobilization: is the experience in Moscow just the beginning? *Eur J Anaesthesiol.* 2003;20(6):427–428.
4. Baraka A. Historical aspects of opium. *Middle East J Anaesthesiol.* 1982;6(5):289–302.
5. Reuzel RP, Hasselaar GJ, Vissers KC, et al. Inappropriateness of using opioids for end-stage palliative sedation: a Dutch study. *Palliat Med.* 2008;22(5):641–646.
6. Sprung CL, Ledoux D, Bulow HH, et al. Relieving suffering or intentionally hastening death: where do you draw the line? *Crit Care Med.* 2008;36(1):8–13.
7. Reidenberg MM, Willis O. Prosecution of physicians for prescribing opioids to patients. *Clin Pharmacol Ther.* 2007;81(6):903–906.
8. Tuffs A. German doctor is investigated for killing 76 patients with morphine. *BMJ.* 2003;327(7419):830
9. Burchell HB, Pierach CA. Freud's death. *Arch Intern Med.* 2000;160(1):118.
10. Pounder DJ. The case of Dr. Shipman. *Am J Forensic Med Pathol.* 2003;24(3):219–226.
11. Knox EG. An epidemic pattern of murder. *J Public Health Med.* 2002;24(1):34–37.
12. Thiblin I, Eksborg S, Petersson A, et al. Fatal intoxication as a consequence of intranasal administration (snorting) or pulmonary inhalation (smoking) of heroin. *Forensic Sci Int.* 2004;139(2-3):241—247.

13. Hughes AA, Bogdan GM, Dart RC. Active surveillance of abused and misused prescription opioids using poison center data: a pilot study and descriptive comparison. *Clin Toxicol.* 2007;45(2):144–151.

14. Teske J, Weller JP, Larsch K, et al. Fatal outcome in a child after ingestion of a transdermal fentanyl patch. *Int J Legal Med.* 2007;121(2):147–151.

15. Utecht MJ, Stone AF, McCarron MM. Heroin body packers. *J Emerg Med.* 1993;11(1):33–40.

16. Hosztafi S. The pharmacology of heroin. *Acta Pharm Hung.* 2003;73(3):197–205.

17. Duberstein JL, Kaufman DM. A clinical study of an epidemic of heroin intoxication and heroin-induced pulmonary edema. *Am J Med.* 1971;51:704–714.

18. Helpern M, Rho YM. Deaths from narcotism in New York City. Incidence, circumstances, and postmortem findings. *N Y State J Med.* 1966;66:2391–2408.

19. Spiller HA, Gorman SE, Villalobos D, et al. Prospective multicenter evaluation of tramadol exposure. *J Toxicol Clin Toxicol.* 1997;35(4):361–364.

20. Sloth Madsen P, Strøm J, Reiz S, et al. Acute propoxyphene self-poisoning in 222 consecutive patients. *Acta Anaesthesiol Scand.* 1984;28(6):661–665.

21. Beaule PE, Smith MI, Nguyen VN. Meperidine-induced seizure after revision hip arthroplasty. *J Arthroplasty.* 2004;19(4):516–519.

22. Stork CM, Redd JT, Fine K, et al. Propoxyphene-induced wide QRS complex dysrhythmia responsive to sodium bicarbonate—a case report. *J Toxicol Clin Toxicol.* 1995;33(2):179–183.

23. Staikowsky F, Candella S, Raphael M. Dextropropoxyphene and the cardiovascular system: about two cases of acute poisoning with cardiac conduction abnormalities. *J Opioid Manag.* 2005;1(5):240–243.

24. Fahnenstich H, Steffan J, Kau N, Bartmann P. Fentanyl-induced chest wall rigidity and laryngospasm in preterm and term infants. *Crit Care Med.* 2000;28(3):836–839.

25. Ailawadhi S, Sung KW, Carlson LA, Baer MR. Serotonin syndrome caused by interaction between citalopram and fentanyl. *J Clin Pharm Ther.* 2007;32(2):199–202.

26. Bush E, Miller C, Friedman I. A case of serotonin syndrome and mutism associated with methadone. *J Palliat Med.* 2006;9(6):1257–1259.

27. Gillman PK. Monoamine oxidase inhibitors, opioid analgesics and serotonin toxicity. *Br J Anaesth.* 2005;95(4):434–441.

28. Centers for Disease Control and Prevention. Atypical reactions associated with heroin use—five states, January-April 2005. *MMWR.* 2005;54(32):793–796.

29. Ruttenber AJ, Luke JL. Heroin-related deaths: new epidemiologic insights. *Science.* 1984;226(4670):14–20.

30. Christie DJ, Walker RH, Kolins MD, et al. Quinine-induced thrombocytopenia following intravenous use of heroin. *Arch Intern Med.* 1983;143(6):1174–1175.

31. Bamshad MJ, Wasserman GS. Pediatric clonidine intoxications. *Vet Hum Toxicol.* 1990;32(3):220–223.

32. Mitchell AA, Lovejoy FH, Goldman P. Drug ingestions associated with miosis in comatose children. *J Pediatr.* 1976;89(2):303–305.

33. Struempler RE. Excretion of codeine and morphine following ingestion of poppy seeds. *J Anal Toxicol.* 1987;11:97–99.

34. Mule SJ, Casella GA. Rendering the poppy-seed defense defenseless: identification of 6-monoacetylmorphine in urine by gas chromatography/mass spectroscopy. *Clin Chem.* 1988;34:1427–1430.

15 | Organophosphates (Nerve Agents)

Christopher P. Holstege and Kahoko Taki

CASE STUDY

On March 20, 1995, five two-man teams of the Aum Shinri-kyo cult carried out a nerve agent attack in Tokyo, Japan.[1-3] At 7:55 AM, during peak commuting time, the assailants placed sarin-filled bags on the subway train floor and pierced them with sharpened umbrella tips. The first emergency call was received by the Tokyo fire department at 8:09 AM, and in the ensuing hour, emergency medical authorities were inundated with calls for aid from multiple subway stations. A total of 131 ambulances and 1364 emergency medical technicians were dispatched, with 688 people transported to hospitals by emergency rescue vehicles. More than 4000 people found their own way to medical facilities in taxis, private cars, or on foot. The lack of emergency decontamination facilities and protective equipment resulted in a secondary exposure of medical staff (135 ambulance staff and 110 staff in the main receiving hospital reported symptoms). Having initially been misinformed that a gas explosion had caused burns and carbon monoxide poisoning, medical centers nevertheless began treating for organophosphate exposure based on the clinical effects they encountered. An official announcement by the police that sarin had been identified came to the hospitals via television news, reportedly 3 hours after the release. Overall, 12 people died, 54 were severely injured, and approximately 980 were mildly to moderately affected. The majority of the 5000 seeking help were worried that they might have been exposed, many with psychogenic symptoms.

HISTORY

Organophosphates were developed as pesticides and are utilized throughout the world. These pesticides include agents such as malathion, parathion, and chlorpyrifos. There are a number of organophosphates that have been manufactured as chemical warfare agents ("nerve agents"), including tabun, soman, sarin, cyclosarin, VX, and the Russia V-type agent designated VR.[4] These agents are among the most potent toxins known to humankind. Tabun, sarin, soman, and cyclosarin are more volatile than the V-agents and evaporate from the skin more rapidly, therefore failing to penetrate skin unless occluded. Sarin is the most volatile of the nerve agents, possessing a volatility similar to that of water. The less volatile an agent is, the more persistent it is on terrain and material. The vapor densities of all these agents are heavier than air, and subsequently, they sink to the ground.

The discovery of nerve agents occurred in the 1930s when German scientists were attempting to improve upon existing organophosphate pesticides.[4] The German military manufactured the nerve agents tabun, sarin, and soman, but for unclear reasons, their use in combat never occurred during World War II. The Iraqi military used nerve agents against the Iranian military in the mid-1980s; this was the first known use of these agents on a battlefield.[5] In 1988, Iraq used sarin against the Kurds.[6] In 1994, a terrorist sarin gas attack occurred in Matsumoto, Japan, resulting in the deaths of seven people, with more than 200 exposed civilians seeking medical attention.[7] In 1995, another terrorist sarin gas attack occurred in Japan, resulting in 12 deaths, with more than 5000 civilians presenting to medical facilities believing they had been exposed.[1-3] In 1996, the U.S. government acknowledged that troops operating during the Gulf War in 1991 were potentially exposed to sarin after an Iraqi chemical weapons dump was destroyed at Khamisiyah.[8] On May 17, 2004, a roadside bomb containing sarin detonated near a U.S. military convoy in Iraq, requiring two military personnel to be treated for exposure.

POTENTIAL DELIVERY METHODS

Organophosphates can be delivered by numerous routes. Absorption can occur via ingestion, inhalation, dermal exposure, or parenteral exposure. Nerve agents were designed for warfare, and each agent's volatility is different. Sarin is the most volatile, with most reported exposures occurring via inhalation, whereas VX is less volatile and more persistent in the environment.

TOXICOLOGIC MECHANISMS

Acetylcholine (ACh) is a neurotransmitter found throughout the nervous system, including the central nervous system (CNS), the autonomic nervous system, and at the skeletal muscle motor end-plate.[9] ACh acts in both the CNS and peripheral nervous system by binding to and activating muscarinic and nicotinic cholinergic receptors.

The enzyme acetylcholinesterase (AChE) terminates the activity of ACh within the synaptic cleft. ACh binds to AChE's active site where the enzyme hydrolyzes ACh to choline and acetic acid. These hydrolyzed products rapidly dissociate from AChE so that the enzyme is free to act on another molecule. Organophosphates act by binding to the AChE active site, rendering that enzyme incapable of inactivating ACh. As a result, ACh accumulates in the synapse and excessive stimulation occurs.

Over time, a portion of the bound organophosphate is cleaved, producing a stable covalent bond between the nerve agent and AChE. This process is called *aging*. The time it takes for aging to occur depends upon the nerve agent. Aging occurs within 2 minutes for soman but takes hours for the other organophosphates. Before aging occurs, AChE reactivaters, such as pralidoxime chloride, can remove the nerve agent and restore enzyme function. Once this aged covalent bond forms, however, AChE cannot be reactivated, and activity is not restored until a new enzyme is synthesized.

CLINICAL EFFECTS

The reported clinical effects of organophosphate poisoning have been well described in the literature. The majority of reported cases have been due to either exposure in the occupational setting or suicidal ingestion.[10] Numerous reports of the clinical effects of nerve agent poisoning have been published, either following accidental exposure in the laboratory or following the terrorist attacks in Japan.[11-14] There are reports of organophosphates being utilized in isolated cases of homicide.[15]

The onset, severity, and clinical effects of organophosphate poisoning vary widely (Table 15.1). Both the dose and the route of exposure are factors in determining the clinical effects. The two most prevalent routes of exposure are via dermal droplet contact and via gas inhalation or absorption. The progression of the signs and symptoms can range from a mild and gradual intoxication to cardiopulmonary collapse, seizures, and death within minutes.

TABLE 15.1 **Acute Clinical Effects of Organophosphate Poisoning**

Muscarinic manifestations	
Ophthalmic	Conjunctival injection, lacrimation, miosis, blurred vision, diminished visual acuity, ocular pain
Respiratory	Rhinorrhea, stridor, wheezing, cough, excessive sputum, chest tightness, dyspnea, apnea
Cardiovascular	Bradydysrhythmias, hypotension
Dermal	Flushing, diaphoresis, cyanosis
Gastrointestinal	Nausea, vomiting, salivation, diarrhea, abdominal cramping, tenesmus, fecal incontinence
Genitourinary	Frequency, urgency, incontinence
Nicotinic manifestations	
Cardiovascular	Tachydysrhythmias, hypertension
Striated muscle	Fasciculations, twitching, cramping, weakness, paralysis
CNS manifestations	
Anxiety, restlessness, depression, confusion, ataxia, tremors, seizures, coma, areflexia	

The respiratory system effects of organophosphates tend to be dramatic and are considered to be the major factor leading to death. The development of respiratory failure results from the triad of increased airway resistance, neuromuscular failure, and depression of the central respiratory centers.[11] Intoxication can present with profuse watery nasal discharge, nasal hyperemia, marked salivation, and bronchorrhea. Animal studies have reported weakness of the tongue and pharyngeal muscles leading to airway obstruction.[16] Laryngeal muscle paralysis can result in vocal cord dysfunction and subsequent stridor. A prolonged expiratory phase, cough, and wheezing may manifest as a consequence of lower respiratory tract bronchorrhea and bronchoconstriction. As systemic absorption occurs, respiratory muscle weakness ensues. Organophosphate-induced central apnea may contribute to the patient's demise if supportive therapy is not initiated.

AChE receptors are found throughout the CNS. Due to the ubiquity of these receptors, organophosphate poisoning can produce a large variation in neurologic signs and symptoms. Headache, vertigo, paresthesias, anxiety, insomnia, depression, excessive dreaming, and emotional lability have all been reported following AChE inhibitor exposures.[13] A rapidly progressive decrease in the level of consciousness resulting in coma is seen, with the time from exposure to coma reported as fast as a few seconds.[11] Organophosphate poisoning is associated with seizure initiation, status epilepticus, seizure-related brain damage, and subsequent death.[7,17]

The cardiovascular effects from organophosphate poisoning are variable and can be caused by either direct cholinergic effects at the heart or nicotinic effects at the autonomic ganglia.[7] Experiments in rats indicate that soman-induced hypertension depends entirely on central muscarinic stimulation.[18] Cardiotoxicity resulting from AChE inhibitors has been divided into three phases. Initially, a period of intense sympathetic activity results in sinus tachydysrhythmias with or without hypertension. Victims may subsequently develop bradydysrhythmias, prolongation of the PR interval, atrioventricular blocks, and hypotension as parasympathetic tone predominates. The third phase occurs with QT prolongation and progression to polymorphous ventricular tachycardia (torsade de pointes). The etiology of the QT prolongation has not been elucidated. These phases can occur at any time while the patient is manifesting clinical signs of toxicity and do not necessarily follow sequentially.

Skeletal muscle activity is initiated at nicotinic receptors at motor end-plates. With early or minimal exposure to AChE inhibitors, symptoms may be vague and consist of muscular weakness and difficulty with ambulation. With increasing exposure, these agents resemble succinylcholine in that they cause muscular fasciculations and subsequent paralysis. Paralysis is especially problematic, as it may mask seizure activity.

Vapors from some organophosphates can rapidly penetrate the conjunctiva and stimulate muscarinic receptors. This causes constriction of both the ciliary and sphincter muscles as well as stimulation of the lacrimal gland. As a result, victims of poisoning experience lacrimation, blurred vision, and miosis. Miosis can develop immediately after vapor exposure or after direct ocular contact with liquid and is the most consistent clinical finding associated with nerve agent vapor exposure. In the Japan sarin attacks, miosis was reported in 89–99% of the victims.[19] However, following dermal absorption, miosis can be absent or delayed after other systemic signs and symptoms. Dark adaptation is lost due to pupillary inability to dilate. Miosis persists for a variable period that depends on the amount of exposure, with pupillary constriction reportedly lasting up to 45 days.[20] Patients will frequently complain of eye pain, headache, nausea, and vomiting due to ciliary spasms that are exacerbated by attempting to focus on close objects.

The sweat glands are innervated by sympathetic muscarinic receptors. After AChE inhibitor intoxication, profuse diaphoresis occurs. This effect can be diffuse after systemic absorption or localized only to the area of dermal droplet exposure.

Muscarinic receptors stimulate secretion from the salivary glands, pancreas, and small and large intestinal goblet cells. As a result, profuse watery salivation and gastrointestinal hyperactivity with resultant nausea, vomiting, abdominal cramps, tenesmus, and uncontrolled defecation are characteristic of systemic AChE blockade. Even with exposure to vapor, as opposed to ingestion and dermal absorption, the Tokyo sarin gas victims reportedly experienced nausea (67%), vomiting (41%), and diarrhea (6%).

Cholinergic stimulation of the detrusor muscle causes contraction of the urinary bladder and relaxation of the trigone and sphincter muscles. The overall effect is involuntary urination.

Atropine administration dries secretions and resolves bronchoconstriction following exposure to organophosphates. The use of this therapy with clinical improvement may help the healthcare team make the correct diagnosis early after exposure.

ANALYTIC DETECTION

A physician's bedside observations of end-organ toxicity are most helpful for making clinical decisions about organophosphate poisoning. The toxicology laboratory is useful but has limitations. Of note, 25% of the moderately to severely poisoned patients in the Tokyo sarin attack had normal admission plasma cholinesterase activity.[13]

Most clinical laboratories cannot measure serum or urine concentrations of organophosphates or their metabolites. Instead, the nervous system's AChE activity is approximated by measuring plasma and erythrocyte cholinesterase activity. Plasma cholinesterase, or "pseudocholinesterase," is made in the liver and is inactivated by organophosphates. The liver regenerates the enzyme rapidly. Erythrocyte cholinesterase, also called RBC (red blood cell) cholinesterase or "true" cholinesterase, is similar to the enzyme found at the neuronal synapse. However, its regeneration depends on replacing RBCs in the circulation. It regenerates at approximately 1% per day and is slower than neuronal enzyme regeneration. Therefore, RBC and plasma cholinesterase activity may not always reflect neuronal enzyme activity.

In general, systemic signs and symptoms have been reported when RBC enzyme activity falls below 40%. The correlation between RBC enzyme activity and clinical effects is hindered by: (1) wide normal range, (2) route of exposure (vapor or dermal), (3) exposure dose, and (4) selective inhibition of RBC or plasma cholinesterase activity. The wide normal range for RBC enzyme activity makes interpretation of mild to moderate exposures difficult without a baseline measurement.[21] Cholinesterase activity correlates poorly with severity of local effects after vapor exposures. On the other hand, when RBC enzyme activity is depressed to 20–25% of normal, it tends to correlate with severe systemic toxic effects.[13,21]

CONCLUSION

The threat of organophosphate poisoning using either pesticides or nerve agents has become a greater concern since the terrorist attacks occurred in Japan. Healthcare professionals and law enforcement should be familiar with the mechanisms of action and clinical course of organophosphate intoxication to enable teams to make the correct diagnosis early.

REFERENCES

1. Okumura T, Suzuki K, Fukuda A, et al. The Tokyo subway sarin attack: disaster management, Part 3: National and international responses. *Acad Emerg Med.* 1998;5(6):625–628.

2. Okumura T, Suzuki K, Fukuda A, et al. The Tokyo subway sarin attack: disaster management, Part 2: Hospital response. *Acad Emerg Med.* 1998;5(6):618–624.

3. Okumura T, Suzuki K, Fukuda A, et al. The Tokyo subway sarin attack: disaster management, Part 1: Community emergency response. *Acad Emerg Med.* 1998;5(6):613–617.

4. Holstege CP, Kirk M, Sidell FR. Chemical warfare. Nerve agent poisoning. *Crit Care Clin.* 1997;13(4):923–942.

5. Newmark J. The birth of nerve agent warfare: lessons from Syed Abbas Foroutan. *Neurology.* 2004;62(9):1590–1596.

6. Black RM, Clarke RJ, Read RW, et al. Application of gas chromatography-mass spectrometry and gas chromatography-tandem mass spectrometry to the analysis of chemical warfare samples, found to contain residues of the nerve agent sarin, sulphur mustard and their degradation products. *J Chromatogr A.* 1994;662(2):301–321.

7. Okudera H. Clinical features on nerve gas terrorism in Matsumoto. *J Clin Neurosci.* 2002;9(1):17–21.

8. Gray GC, Smith TC, Knoke JD, et al. The postwar hospitalization experience of Gulf War Veterans possibly exposed to chemical munitions destruction at Khamisiyah, Iraq. *Am J Epidemiol.* 1999;150(5):532–540.

9. Holstege CP, Dobmeier SG. Nerve agent toxicity and treatment. *Curr Treat Options Neurol.* 2005;7(2):91–98.

10. Emerson GM, Gray NM, Jelinek GA, et al. Organophosphate poisoning in Perth, Western Australia, 1987–1996. *J Emerg Med.* 1999;17(2):273–277.

11. Sidell FR. Soman and sarin: clinical manifestations and treatment of accidental poisoning by organophosphates. *Clin Toxicol.* 1974;7(1):1–17.

12. Grob D, Harvey JC. Effects in man of the anticholinesterase compound sarin (isopropyl methyl phosphonofluoridate). *J Clin Invest.* 1958;37(3):350–368.

13. Okumura T, Takasu N, Ishimatsu S, et al. Report on 640 victims of the Tokyo subway sarin attack. *Ann Emerg Med.* 1996;28(2):129–135.

14. Haruki M. *Underground.* New York: Vintage Books, Random House, Inc; 2001.

15. De Letter EA, Cordonnier JA, Piette MH. An unusual case of homicide by use of repeated administration of organophosphate insecticides. *J Clin Forensic Med.* 2002;9(1):15–21.

16. Grob D. The manifestations and treatment of poisoning due to nerve gas and other organic phosphate anticholinesterase compounds. *AMA Arch Intern Med.* 1956;98(2):221–239.

17. Auta J, Costa E, Davis J, et al. Imidazenil: a potent and safe protective agent against diisopropyl fluorophosphate toxicity. *Neuropharmacology.* 2004;46(3):397–403.

18. Letienne R, Julien C, Barres C, et al. Soman-induced hypertension in conscious rats is mediated by prolonged central muscarinic stimulation. *Fundam Clin Pharmacol.* 1999;13(4):468–474.

19. Ohbu S, Yamashina A, Takasu N, et al. Sarin poisoning on Tokyo subway. *South Med J.* 1997;90(6):587–593.

20. Rengstorff RH. Accidental exposure to sarin: vision effects. *Arch Toxicol.* 1985;56(3):201–203.

21. Coye MJ, Barnett PG, Midtling JE, et al. Clinical confirmation of organophosphate poisoning by serial cholinesterase analyses. *Arch Intern Med.* 1987;147(3):438–442.

16 | Plants and Herbals

R. Brent Furbee and Jou-Fang Deng

INTRODUCTION

Plants have provided the basis for most of the pharmaceutical compounds throughout the past several centuries, so it is not surprising that they have also been employed in criminal activities. There are numerous plant toxins that have been utilized for criminal poisoning. Some of these plant toxins, such as ricin, strychnine, curare, and opium, are discussed in separate chapters in this book. This chapter will focus on five plant toxins: cardiac glycosides, aconitine, nicotine, anticholinergics, and cicutoxin.

CARDIAC GLYCOSIDES

CASE STUDY

In 1859, Edmond de la Pommerais started a homeopathic medical practice in Paris. Unfortunately, his practice did not support his habits of gambling, womanizing, and drinking. He found a young woman of means and promptly married her, but his mother-in-law was suspicious of his motives and kept a tight rein on her daughter's inheritance. A few months after his marriage, de la Pommerais invited his wife's mother to dinner. A short time after the meal, she became ill. Days later, she died. He paid off his bills and resumed his affair with a former beautiful but impoverished lover.

By November of 1863, he was again deeply in debt. His mistress, Madame de Pauw, was suffering from a mysterious illness that baffled doctors, but she insisted it was a mild case of cholera that would respond to de la Pommerais's homeopathic remedies. Her vomiting, abdominal pain, and erratic heartbeat ended in death. Fortunately for her chosen physician, de la Pommerais, she was recently well-insured, and he was the benefactor. Once again, his fortune changed. The insurance company paid but was surprised by the grieving man's aggressive pursuit of compensation.

When detectives interviewed Madame de Pauw's sister, their concerns increased. She related that de la Pommerais had approached her sister with a scheme to defraud the insurance company by having her take out an insurance policy naming him as beneficiary. She would then claim to suffer from a terminal condition and settle with the company for an annuity just before her miraculous cure by her homeopathic physician.

The police stepped in, but they were unsure how to prove this was a murder by poison. With no gastric contents available for testing, Auguste Ambroise Tardieu, a professor of forensic medicine at Paris University, developed a plan. He made an extract from the decedent's organs and injected it into a dog. The animal immediately began to vomit and to suffer from an erratic heart beat much as de Pauw had suffered before her death. This virtually assured that she had been poisoned. A small amount of vomitus was found on the floor of her sickroom, enabling confirmation of digitalis poisoning. Edmond de

la Pommerais was found guilty of murder and went to the guillotine in 1864.[1]

History

The medicinal properties of the cardiac glycosides were known to the ancient Egyptians as well as the Romans, who used them as an emetic, heart tonic, and diuretic.[2] In 1785, William Withering published *An Account of the Foxglove and Some of Its Medical Uses: With Practical Remarks on Dropsy and Other Diseases*, thus popularizing the plant's use. In 1890, Sir Thomas Fraser introduced *Strophanthus* and its digitalis-like effects. Worldwide, these plants have been used as abortifacients; in the treatment of leprosy, venereal disease, and malaria; and as suicide agents.[3] More than 200 naturally occurring cardiac glycosides have been identified to date. Ingestion of *Digitalis* sp. is seldom reported. *Convallaria majalis* (lily of the valley) exposures are associated with minimal morbidity and, in a recent review of 10 years of data from regional poison centers, have had no associated mortality.[4] Of the many plants containing cardiac glycosides, *Nerium oleander* is responsible for the greatest number of toxic exposures each year.[5]

Plants

   Digitalis purpurea, D. lanata (foxglove)
   (Figures 16.1 and 16.2)
   Nerium oleander (oleander) (Figure 16.3)
   Strophanthus gratus (ouabain)
   Thevetia peruviana sp. (yellow oleander)
   (Figure 16.4)
   Convallaria majalis (lily of the valley)
   (Figure 16.5)
   Urginea maritima, U. indica (squill)
   Other plants containing cardiac glycosides: *Asclepias* (milkweed), *Calotropis* (crown flower),[6] *Euonymus europaeus* (spindle tree), *Cheiranthus, Erysimum* (wall flower), and *Helleborus niger* (henbane).

Toxic Parts

All parts of the plant are toxic. Seeds are said to contain more glycoside than other parts of the plant.

Toxicologic Mechanism

Oleandrin (*N. oleander*) and thevetin (*T. peruviana*) are structurally similar to digitoxin. Because of this and the similarity of clinical

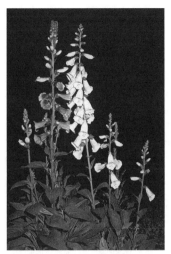

FIGURE 16.1 *Digitalis purpurea* (foxglove)
(See Color Plate 12.)

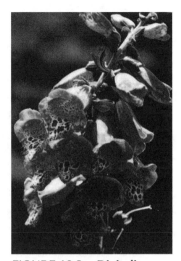

FIGURE 16.2 *Digitalis purpurea* (foxglove)
(See Color Plate 13.)

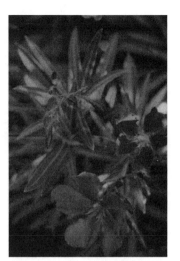

FIGURE 16.3 *Nerium oleander* (oleander)
(See Color Plate 14.)

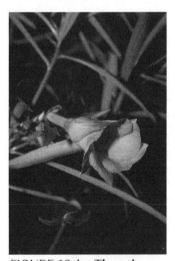

FIGURE 16.4 *Thevetia peruviana* (yellow oleander)
(See Color Plate 15.)

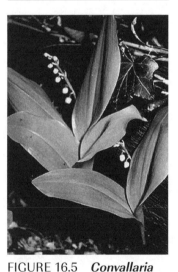

FIGURE 16.5 *Convallaria majalis* (lily of the valley)
(See Color Plate 16.)

automaticity typical of cardiac glycoside poisoning. Depolarization of baroreceptors innervated by the ninth cranial nerve triggers afferent reflexes, which increase vagal tone and produce bradycardia and heart blocks.[7] Severe poisoning results in hyperkalemia because the ability to pump potassium into the muscle is curtailed.

Clinical Effects

Gastrointestinal (GI) irritation is common with ingestion of *N. oleander* or *T. peruviana*. The latter was studied as a potential antiarrhythmic agent in the 1930s but was not marketed because it caused more GI irritation than digitalis.[8] Saravanapavananthan et al. reviewed 170 cases of *T. peruviana* ingestion and found that vomiting was the most common presenting complaint (68.2%). Other symptoms are shown in Table 16.1. Electrocardiographic effects occurred in 61.8% of patients[9] (Table 16.2). PR prolongation, QT shortening, and P- or T-wave flattening may occur.[10] Hyperkalemia occurs in more serious poisonings.[10-12] CNS depression may occur as a direct effect of the toxin,[12] but it is frequently associated with bradycardia and hypotension. Death has been reported.[9,10]

presentation, they are considered to act similarly. The toxin attaches to the β subunit of the Na^+/K^+-ATPase pump to inhibit its action. Because this pump exchanges intracellular sodium ions for extracellular potassium ions, inhibition leads to an overall increase in intracellular sodium ions. Rises in intracellular sodium concentration result in secondary rises in intracellular calcium levels, explaining the positive inotropic effect of cardiac glycosides. In toxic amounts, the increases in intracellular sodium and calcium depolarize the cell after repolarization to cause late after depolarizations and increased

TABLE 16.1 Relative Frequency of Signs
and Symptoms Associated with
Oleander Poisoning

Symptom	Percentage
Vomiting	68.2%
Dizziness	35.9%
Diarrhea	38.0%
Abdominal discomfort	5.9%
Pain or numbness of tongue, throat, lips	4.1%
No symptoms	12.9%

TABLE 16.2 Relative Frequency of Dysrhythmias
Associated with Oleander
Poisoning

Electrocardiogram change	Percentage
AV block	52.4%
Bradycardia	49.5%
T-wave changes	35.2%
ST depression	23.8%
Ventricular ectopy	6.6%
Atrial ectopy	2.8%

Analytic Detection

Osterloh described cross-reactivity of oleander glycosides on radioimmunoassay for digoxin.[11] The test may serve as confirmation of the presence of cardiac glycosides, however, clinical symptoms and electrocardiographic findings are more indicative of toxicity. Postmortem serum concentrations are known to increase and do not predict the premortem levels.[10]

ACONITINE

CASE STUDY

Found about 60 miles from his home, a middle-aged man at first appeared to have died in the accident that put his car in a ditch. A partially burned fuse, however, hung from the open gas tank. Multiple bruises and contusions further complicated the investigation. His blood alcohol was only 23 mg/dL, and no drugs or toxins were detected. The break in the case came when DNA testing was done on the stamp of a suicide letter that was thought to have been sent by the victim. Instead, his wife's DNA was discovered on the stamp. When confronted, she confessed to his murder.

She had taken the leaves and stems of three *Aconitum napellus* plants and boiled them. She mixed the liquid with a few triazolam tablets in a bottle of red wine. Three and a half hours after consuming the wine, her husband was dead. His injuries were due to being dragged up and then down the stairs when she decided to move his body out of the house. Sitting in her dead husband's lap, she drove the car to its point of discovery and pushed it into the ditch. She attempted to set the vehicle ablaze and left the scene to hail a taxi for her return home. Liquid chromatography-tandem mass spectrometry (LC-MS/MS) demonstrated the presence of aconitine in his urine, liver, and kidneys.[13]

History

Members of this genus grow throughout the world. Exposures are commonly associated with the overzealous consumption of herbal preparations containing aconitine. Though a number of fatal poisonings have been reported, aconitine is still readily available at many nutrition or herbal medicine stores.

Plants

    A. napellus (monkshood) (Figure 16.6)

    A. vulparia (wolfsbane)

Several species are also used in herbal preparations, including *A. carmichaeli* ("chuanwu") and *A. kusnezoffii* ("caowu").[14] The latter two appear to account for more fatalities than ingestion of monkshood. *Delphinium* sp. (Larkspur) have similar toxicity.[15]

Toxic Parts

All parts are toxic, with roots possessing greater toxicity than the flowers, leaves, and stems.[16]

Toxicologic Mechanisms

Like grayanotoxins and veratrum alkaloids, aconitine effects its toxicity through action on sodium channels. Aconitine appears to increase sodium entry into muscle, nerve, baroreceptors, and Purkinje fibers to produce a positive inotropic effect, enhanced vagal tone, neurotoxicity, and increased automaticity and torsade de pointes.[17] During late repolarization of the Purkinje fibers (late phase 4), aconitine attaches to a limited number of the sodium channels and increases Na⁺ influx,[18-20] causing *late* (or delayed) afterdepolarizations and increased

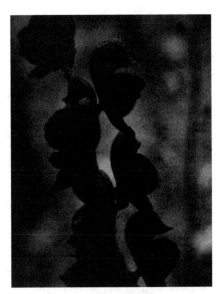

FIGURE 16.6 *Aconitum napellus* (monkshood) (See Color Plate 17.)

automaticity (e.g., premature ventricular beats). However, aconitine-induced sodium accumulation may also lead to *early* afterdepolarization during late phase 2 or early phase 3 of the action potential. These early afterdepolarizations produce lengthening of the QT interval and are thought to explain reports of torsade de pointes in patients poisoned with aconitine.[18, 20-22] Bifascicular ventricular tachycardia, a dysrhythmia most frequently associated with digitalis toxicity, has also been reported in patients poisoned with aconitine.[23]

Clinical Effects

The majority of case reports of aconitine poisoning have come from ingestion of herbs containing aconitine.[14,24] In one series of cases, onset of symptoms was reported within 3 minutes to 2 hours of exposure; the median time elapsed was only 30 minutes.[22] Symptoms may persist for 30 hours.[25] Neurologic complaints include initial visual impairment, dizziness, limb paresthesias, weakness,[26] and ataxia.[16] Coma may follow. Chest discomfort, dyspnea, tachycardia, and diaphoresis may also occur.[26] Hyperglycemia, hypokalemia, bradycardia (with hypotension), atrial and nodal ectopic beats, supraventricular tachycardia, bundle branch block, intermittent bigeminy, ventricular tachycardia, ventricular fibrillation, and asystole have been

reported.[16,18,26,27] Death is usually due to ventricular arrhythmia.[26,28] Ingestion of delphinium root has also resulted in ventricular dysrhythmias and cardiac arrest.[15,26,28]

Analytic Detection

The presence of aconitine has been demonstrated by high-performance liquid chromatography (HPLC) at autopsy.[28]

NICOTINE AND RELATED COMPOUNDS

CASE STUDY

Count Hyppolyte de Bocarmé was not a man of means, but he had a plan. In 1843, he married Lydie Fougnies, the daughter of a local businessman whom the count had hoped would be a source of wealth. Unfortunately, she was no better off than he. However, when her father died, the couple inherited some of his wealth. Lydie's brother Gustave gained most of the inheritance. The will, however, stipulated that if Gustave did not marry, Lydie would be the sole beneficiary in the event of his death. As her brother was in rather poor health, the couple thought it only a matter of time before their fortunes would improve, but Gustave's announcement of marriage caused them to panic.

In celebration of Gustave's impending marriage, the couple invited him to join them at Chateau Bocarmé. Lydie dismissed the servants and served dinner herself. Later that evening, the staff heard a loud thud, and Lydie cried out that Gustave had fallen ill and died of a stroke. The servants were troubled by the events and the couple's behavior. A priest was summoned, then a magistrate. When Gustave's body was examined, several black marks and deep wheals were discovered on his face, leading the magistrate and examining doctors to the inescapable conclusion that this was not a natural death. An autopsy was performed in the coach house, revealing corrosive injury to the mouth, throat, and stomach. Organ samples were sent to Jean Servais Stas, a highly respected chemistry professor at the École Royale Militaire in Brussels. Bocarmé had been working under the assumption that plant alkaloids were virtually impossible to identify at autopsy, but he did not realize that Stas had perfected a method to do just that. Nicotine was identified as the probable poison, and at Stas's recommendation, the chateau was searched. The investigation led to a secluded laboratory used to extract nicotine from tobacco leaves. Local pharmacists recalled answering Bocarmé's questions about toxic doses. The jury would not execute a woman, so Lydie was set free. Bocarmé was not so fortunate and was executed in July of 1851.[29]

History

The pyridine and piperidine alkaloids (nicotine, coniine, anabasine, cystisine, arecoline, lobeline, and many others) all have a similar mechanism of action. Plants containing these alkaloids are widely distributed today but are thought to have originated in South America. *Nicotiana rustica*, which contains up to 18% nicotine, is thought to have been the first tobacco export from the New World. Much more potent than *Nicotiana tabacum* (0.5–9% nicotine), it is still smoked in Turkey and serves as a source for commercial nicotine production. *Nicotiana tabacum* is planted throughout the American southeast as a source of cigar and cigarette tobacco. Because the toxicity of smoked tobacco has been widely discussed elsewhere, only dermal and gastrointestinal absorption will be addressed in this chapter. Small quantities of nicotine are also found in plants from the family *Solanaceae*, such as tomatoes, potatoes, and egg plant. These plants are of little consequence in terms of poisoning.[30,31] Several of the *Nicotiana* and *Lobelia* species are cultivated as flowering plants. Of the uncultivated plants in this group, *Nicotiana glauca* (tree tobacco) and *Conium maculatum* (poison hemlock) are the most common sources of poisoning.

Plants

    Nicotiana tabacum (tobacco) (Figure 16.7)

    N. glauca (tree tobacco) (Figure 16.8)

    N. trigonophylla (desert tobacco)

    N. attenuata (coyote tobacco)

    Conium maculatum (poison hemlock) (Figures 16.9 and 16.10)

    Aethusa cynapium (fool's parsley)

    Lobelia inflata (Indian tobacco)

    L. cardinalis

    Laburnum anagyroides (golden chain tree)

    Sophora secundiflora (mescal bush bean)

    S. tomentosa (necklace pod *Sophora*)

    Gymnocladus dioicus (Kentucky coffee bean) (Figure 16.11)

    Arecoline: Areca catechu (betel palm, betel nut)[32]

Toxic Parts

    All parts of these plants are poisonous.

Toxicologic Mechanisms

Nicotine, coniine, anabasine, lobeline, and related pyridine/piperidine alkaloids cause similar toxicity. Their primary action is activation and then blockade of nicotinic acetylcholine receptors. Activation of nicotinic receptors in the cortex, thalamus, interpeduncular nucleus, and other locations in the central nervous system (CNS) accounts for coma and seizures. Nicotine has been shown to enhance fast excitatory neural transmission in the CNS by triggering presynaptic cholinergic receptors that increase presynaptic calcium and stimulate both cholinergic and glutamatergic transmission.[33] Nicotinic receptor activation facilitates the release of many neurotransmitters, including acetylcholine, norepinephrine, dopamine, serotonin, and beta-endorphins. Activation of nicotinic receptors at autonomic ganglia produces varied effects in the sympathetic and parasympathetic nervous system. These effects most commonly include nausea, vomiting, diarrhea, bradycardia, tachycardia, and miosis. Nicotine alkaloids act as depolarizing neuromuscular blocking agents and produce fasciculations and paralysis.

Clinical Effects

Ingestion or dermal exposure to nicotine and related compounds can result in any or all of the signs and symptoms listed in Table 16.3. Though rare, severe poisonings do occur.[34,35] Curry et al. reported nine cases of ingestion of *N. glauca*, which had been mistaken for collard and turnip greens. Three fatalities occurred. Symptoms included leg cramps, paresthesias, dizziness, and headache. Onset was within 1 hour, and resolution in the surviving patients ranged from 3 hours to several hours.[36] Mellick et al. reported two cases of *N. glauca* ingestion resulting in neuromuscular blockade and

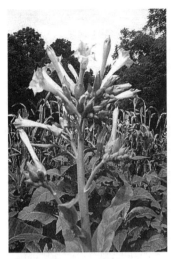

FIGURE 16.7 *Nicotiana tabacum* (tobacco) (See Color Plate 18.)

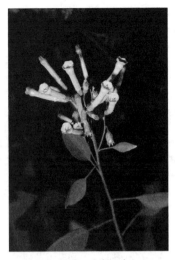

FIGURE 16.8 *Nicotiana glauca* (tree tobacco) (See Color Plate 19.)

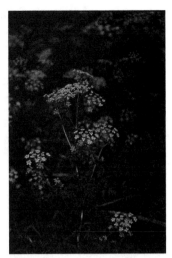

FIGURE 16.9 *Conium maculatu* (poison hemlock) (See Color Plate 20.)

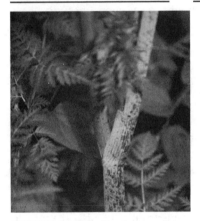

FIGURE 16.10 *Conium maculatum* (poison hemlock) (See Color Plate 21.)

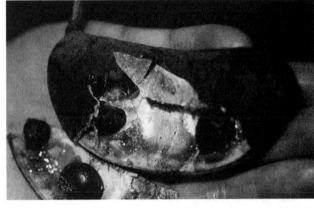

FIGURE 16.11 *Gymnocladus dioicus* (Kentucky coffee bean) (See Color Plate 22.)

eventual complete recovery.[37] Frank reported a *C. maculatum* ingestion in a 4-year-old that resulted in miosis, vomiting, and coma. The onset of symptoms was 30 minutes after ingestion with resolution in about 9 hours.[38] Drummer et al. reported three fatalities from *C. maculatum*.[31] Foster et al. reported the accidental ingestion of *C. maculatum* by a 14-year-old child that resulted in respiratory failure, asphyxia, and eventual death. Another child who ingested a smaller amount of the same *C. maculatum* plant had symptoms of nausea, malaise, and tingling of the extremities and survived.[39] The 2002 American Association of Poison Control Center Annual Report describes a 13-year-old child who developed ascending paralysis, a seizure, and then death after ingestion of *C. maculatum* that was mistaken for parsley.[40]

TABLE 16.3 **Muscarinic and Nicotinic Effects of Nicotine and Related Compounds**

Muscarinic	Nicotinic
Salivation	Weakness
Lacrimation	Fasciculations
Urination	Paralysis
Gastrointestinal cramping	Tachycardia
Emesis	Coma
Miosis	Seizures
Bronchospasm	
Bradycardia	

Green tobacco sickness commonly occurs in the tobacco growing states. Workers handling leaves can absorb nicotine through the skin. It occurs almost exclusively in workers who are cropping leaves from the plant.[41] Symptoms include nausea, vomiting, diarrhea, diaphoresis, and weakness that usually resolve with symptomatic treatment.

The effects of betel quid, which is popular in India, Southeast Asia, and the East Indies,[33] have been reported in people who have immigrated to the United States from those countries. The quid is a betel nut wrapped in a betel vine leaf and smeared with a paste of burnt lime.[42] It contains arecoline and several other cholinergic pyridine alkaloids. Rhabdomyolysis has been reported from the ingestion of *C. maculatum*, although the reports are somewhat confusing in that "hemlock poisoning" is attributed to exposure to both *Cicuta* and *Conium* species.[43,44]

Analytic Detection

Nicotine, coniine, and other alkaloids may be measured in urine by various methods, including gas chromatography,[45] mass spectrometry,[32] and thin-layer chromatography.[46]

ANTICHOLINERGICS (TROPANE ALKALOIDS)

CASE STUDY

Probably the most famous case involving the criminal use of a tropane alkaloid is that of Hawley Harvey Crippen. Born in 1862 in Coldwater, Michigan, he received a diploma from the Homeopathic Hospital in Cleveland, Ohio, which was endorsed by the faculty of the Medical College of Philadelphia. In 1885, he became qualified as an eye and ear specialist at the Ophthalmic Hospital in New York. Over the following years, he practiced medicine throughout the United States. His first wife, Charlotte Belle, died while they were living in Salt Lake City, Utah, in 1890. Crippen returned to New York and married his second wife and ultimate victim, Cora Turner. Cora was an aficionado of the opera but not a diva. After failed attempts in New York and Great Britain, she became honorary treasurer of the Music Hall Ladies Guild in London.

In the early 1900s, Crippen became a "homeopathic" physician, consulting for Dr. Munyon's Homeopathic Company. In London, he and Cora took in borders to supplement his reduced income. Their marriage deteriorated and both found love interests. Harvey became involved with Ethel le Neve, a young typist in his office, while Cora spent most of her time with the theater. Cora became upset after discovering his affair and threatened Crippen that if he did not terminate the affair, she would divorce him and take his money. Cora's death probably took place around February 1, 1910. Cora was last seen around 1:30 that morning by departing visitors. A few days later, Crippen told friends that she had gone to America. He reported a short time later that she was ill and later that she had died. His relationship with Ethel le Neve became public. Eventually, Cora's friends called in Scotland Yard. Police questioned Crippen. In a panic he took Ethel, disguised as a boy, and traveled by ship for Canada. The captain of the ship heard about the case and, spotting an unusual couple aboard (a man hugging and kissing his son, who was obviously a woman), reported the matter via wireless telegraphy to London authorities. Scotland Yard's Chief Inspector Dew boarded a faster ship and arrested Harvey at the entrance of the St. Lawrence River.

Back in England, police found several human body parts under the cellar floor of Harvey and Cora's house. An abdominal scar helped identify Cora's body. Liver and kidney tissue yielded hyoscyamine in high concentration. It was then determined that Crippen had purchased hyoscine hydrobromide from a chemist. The jury deliberated less than 30 minutes before convicting him. He was hanged on November 23, 1910. Ethel le Neve was tried as an accessory and acquitted.[47] To this day, Crippen's guilt or innocence remains the subject of study and controversy.

History

A number of plants and mushrooms exhibit anticholinergic properties. The best known of these are the members of the *Solanaceae* family. Of the anticholinergic plants, the genera *Atropa*, *Datura*, and *Hyoscyamus* produce hyoscyamine (atropine). Other members of this group produce scopolamine. The members of both groups are provided in the following list, but for the sake of this discussion, *Datura* sp. will be this chapter's focus because they account for more hospitalizations than the others. The first recorded *Datura* poisoning occurred in 1676 during the Bacon Rebellion when soldiers under Captain John Smith made a salad of *Datura stramonium* leaves and began to hallucinate. The name "Jamestown weed" was given to this plant, and its name has been corrupted over the years to "Jimson weed."

Plants

 Atropa belladonna (deadly nightshade)

 Brugmansia sp. (angel trumpet) (Figure 16.12)

 Datura meteloides (sacred datura) (Figures 16.13 and 16.14)

 D. stramonium (jimson weed) (Figure 16.15)

 D. arborea (trumpet lily)

 D. candida

 D. suaveolens (angel trumpet)

 Hyoscyamus niger (henbane)

 Lycium barbarum (matrimony vine)

 Mandragora officinarum (mandrake)

Toxic Parts
The entire plant is toxic. The flowers, fruits, and seeds are especially toxic.

Toxicologic Mechanism
The members of the genus *Datura* contain varying amounts of hyoscyamine (atropine) and scopolamine. Young plants tend to contain mostly scopalamine, but as they mature, hyoscyamine predominates. The toxicity of these compounds results from competitive blockade of acetylcholine at peripheral and central muscarinic receptors.

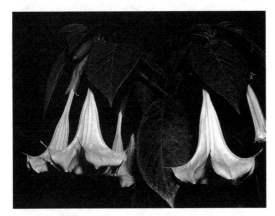

FIGURE 16.12 *Brugmansia* sp. **(angel trumpet)** (See Color Plate 23.)

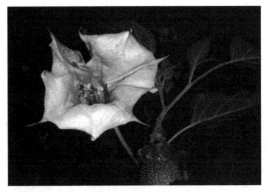

FIGURE 16.13 *Datura meteloides* **(sacred datura)** (See Color Plate 24.)

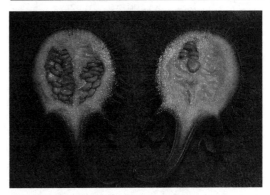

FIGURE 16.14 *Datura meteloides* **(sacred datura)** (See Color Plate 25.)

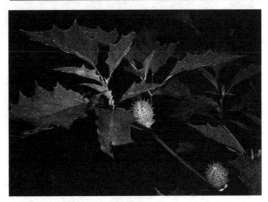

FIGURE 16.15 *Datura stramonium* **(jimson weed)** (See Color Plate 26.)

Clinical Effects
Onset of symptoms is usually within 30 to 60 minutes of ingestion and may last for 24 to 48 hours. Both central and peripheral syndromes may be seen. Levy et al. described 27 cases in which every patient had altered mental status and mydriasis (Figure 16.16).[48] CNS excitation often manifests as agitation and hallucinations.

CNS depression and coma may follow. Hallucinations are generally visual but may be auditory. Speech has a characteristic mumbling quality and is often incomprehensible. Patients frequently answer questions with appropriate one word answers, but if prompted (and able) to speak in sentences, a fragmented speech pattern becomes obvious. Undressing behavior is not uncommon. Tachycardia and mydriasis are common findings. Flushed skin may be more difficult to detect. Fever is occasionally noted. Bowel sounds may be depressed or absent but usually persist. Bladder motility may be decreased as well. Although dry mucous membranes (Figure 16.17) may be associated with hyperventilation, dry axillae, in association with the other signs, indicates anticholinergic poisoning and helps distinguish it from increased adrenergic activity. *Datura* sp. account for many admissions to critical care units each year. Although children are occasionally poisoned, the most frequent exposure occurs in patients who have ingested seeds or a tea brewed from the seeds in an attempt to induce hallucinations. Death is rare and is more often the result of impaired judgment than direct toxicity. A few death reports do seem to indicate potentially fatal toxicity in high-dose

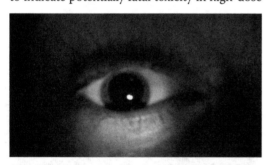

FIGURE 16.16 **Mydriasis (dilated pupil) in a patient intoxicated with *Datura stramonium*.**
(See Color Plate 27.)

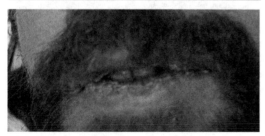

FIGURE 16.17 **Dry mouth in a patient intoxicate with *Datura stramonium*.**
(See Color Plate 28.)

exposures.[49,50] Petechial hemorrhages of the endocardium and hyperemia and edema of the lungs were reported in both cases.

Analytic Detection

Atropine may be detected by radioimmunoassay, gas chromatography-mass spectrometry, thin-layer chromatography,[51] and liquid chromatography. Scopolamine has been analyzed in plasma and urine by radioreceptor assay and gas chromatography-mass spectrometry.[45]

CICUTOXIN

CASE STUDY

Arguably the most toxic of plants, it is surprising that little documentation of the criminal use of water hemlock exists. It has certainly enjoyed great popularity as a homicidal agent in a number of novels. One of the few documented accounts of potential criminal use of *Cicuta* sp. occurred in the 17th century. Near Jamestown, the Powhatan Indian alliance coordinated an attack that killed 350 settlers. In the summer preceding the attack, Opechancanough, the tribal leader, had attempted to get members of the Accomack tribe to poison the settlers with what was later determined to be water hemlock. The Accomacks, however, viewed the English more favorably, and the plan was thwarted.[52]

History

The first reports of toxic effects from *Cicuta* sp. occurred in 1697. In 1814, Stockbridge reported the first case of poisoning in the United States.[53] In a review of deaths reported to poison centers between 1986 and 1996, Krenzelok et al. found reports of 19 deaths; of these, *Cicuta* sp. accounted for more than any other plants.[54] Exposure to *Cicuta* and *Oenanthe* sp. may be accidental, as in most pediatric cases, but more commonly, the fatal cases involve misidentification of the plant as a foodstuff or as a hallucinogen.

Plants
    Cicuta maculata (water hemlock) (Figures 16.18 and 16.19)
    Cicuta douglasii (western water hemlock)
    Oenanthe crocata (hemlock water dropwort)

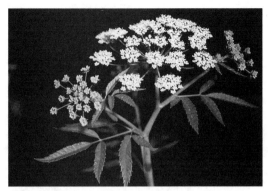

FIGURE 16.18   *Cicuta maculata*
(water hemlock) flowers (See Color Plate 29.)

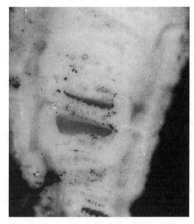

FIGURE 16.19   *Cicuta maculata*
(water hemlock) root (See Color Plate 30.)

Toxic Parts
All parts of these plants are toxic, especially the roots.

Toxicologic Mechanism

Though nausea and vomiting are considered to be the most consistent findings, seizure activity followed by cardiac arrest is the common sequence in fatal exposures.[55] An exact mechanism for the proconvulsant activity of cicutoxin has not been determined. Starreveld et al. suggested that seizure activity might be due to cholinergic overstimulation of the reticular formation or basal ganglia.[56] Nelson et al. performed a series of experiments in mice to explore the efficacy of anticholinergic agents in the prevention of cicutoxin-induced seizures. They found that anticholinergic agents failed to protect the animals and pretreatment with cholinergic agents did not appear to lower seizure threshold.[57]

By 1979, a more appealing theory for cicutoxin's proconvulsant activity had arisen. Carlton et al. suggested that cicutoxin is structurally similar to picrotoxin, an indirect antagonist at GABA-A receptors.[58] GABA-A receptors serve as ion channels to allow the passage of chloride ions into the neuron. These ions hyperpolarize the neuron, moving it away from its threshold for firing. Many anticonvulsants, such as the benzodiazepines and barbiturates, act as indirect agonists at the GABA receptor. By preventing the action of GABA, picrotoxin hyperpolarizes the neuron, moving it closer to its threshold for firing. If cicutoxin acts on the GABA receptor at the picrotoxin site, seizure activity would be expected as it is with picrotoxin. This would also be consistent with Nelson's findings that seizures were better controlled in animals treated with diazepam or barbiturates than with other agents.[57-59]

Clinical Effects
Case reports of *Cicuta* sp.[55,56,61-63] and *Oenanthe* sp.[50,63-66] ingestions are similar in presentation. Ingestion is followed by nausea, vomiting, and diaphoresis. While these signs and symptoms have led some authors to speculate about increased cholinergic activity as the mechanism for seizure activity,[56] the frequent reports of mydriasis detract from this theory.[61-63] The initial convulsion often occurs within the first hour. Repeated convulsions, with intermittent lethargy, ensue for the next several hours. Fatalities usually occur within about 10 hours and are almost invariably associated with repeated seizure activity. *O. crocata* poisoning has been estimated to be 70% fatal in one small series.[65] Rhabdomyolysis and renal failure have been reported.[58] Although some toxins may cause rhabdomyolysis directly, the presence of prolonged seizure activity may well be the etiology.

Analytic Detection
Although clinically useful means of determining cicutoxin or oenanthotoxin are not available, methods of identifying the latter are described by King et al.[65] These methods include ultraviolet absorption, thin-layer chromatography, high-pressure liquid chromatography, and mass spectrometry, which may be useful for later confirmation of exposure.

CONCLUSION

The use of plants to deliberately harm others is uncommon but does occur on occasion. When it does, discovery can be difficult because assays are few and are not available in most hospital laboratories. Plant tissue taken from the GI tract can be very helpful in identifying the source.

When plants are suspected in a criminal poisoning, police should consider that the killer is someone who likely possesses an intimate knowledge of the toxicity of the suspected plant either through their vocation or avocation. Efforts should be made to locate and seize samples of plants used to either harm or kill a victim and to gather evidence that the suspect was aware of the plant's potential toxicity.

REFERENCES

1. Hyppolyte EC, de Bocarme L. *Murder 2: The Second Casebook of Forensic Detection.* Vol 2. Hoboken, NJ: John Wiley & Sons; 2004:208–210.
2. Gilman A, Rall T, Nies A, et al. *Goodman and Gilman's the Pharmacological Basis of Therapeutics.* New York: Macmillan; 1990.
3. Langford SD, Boor PJ. Oleander toxicity: an examination of human and animal toxic exposures. *Toxicology.* 1996;109:1–13.
4. Knutsen OH, Paszkowski P. New aspects in the treatment of water hemlock poisoning. *Clin Toxicol.* 1984;22(2):157–166.
5. Shaw D, Pearn J. Oleander poisoning. *Med J Aust.* 1979;2:267–269.
6. Radford DJ, Gillies AD, Hinds JA, et al. Naturally occurring cardiac glycosides. *Med J Aust.* 1986;144:539–540.
7. Ayachi S, Brown A. Hypotensive effects of cardiac glycosides in spontaneously hypertensive rats. *J Pharmacol Exp Ther.* 1980;213:520.
8. Middleton WS, Chen KK. Clinical results from oral administration of thevetin, a cardiac glycoside. *Am Heart J.* 1936;11:75–88.
9. Saravanapavananthan N, Ganeshamoorthy J. Yellow oleander poisoning—study of 170 cases. *Forensic Sci Int.* 1988;36:247–250.
10. Haynes BE, Bessen HA, Wightman WD. Oleander tea: herbal draught of death. *Ann Emerg Med.* 1985;14(4):350–353.
11. Osterloh J, Herold S, Pond S. Oleander interference in the digoxin radioimmunoassay in a fatal ingestion. *JAMA.* 1982;247:1596–1597.
12. Safadi R, Levy I, Amitai Y, et al. Beneficial effect of digoxin-specific Fab antibody fragments in oleander intoxication. *Arch Intern Med.* 1995;155:2121–2125.
13. Van Landeghem A, De Letter E, Lambert W, et al. Aconitine involvement in an unusual homicide case. *Int J Legal Med.* 2007;121:214–219.
14. C Lin CC, Chan TY, Deng JF. Clinical features and management of herb-induced aconitine poisoning. *Ann Emerg Med.* 2004;43(5):574–579.
15. Tomassoni AJ, Snook CP, McConville BJ, et al. Recreational use of delphinium—an ancient poison revisited. *J Toxicol Clin Toxicol.* 1996;34(5):598.
16. Fatovich DM. Aconite: a lethal Chinese herb. *Ann Emerg Med.* 1992;21(3):309–311.
17. Chan TYK, Tse LKK, Chan J, et al. Aconitine poisoning due to Chinese herbal medicines: a review. *Vet Human Toxicol.* 1994;36(5):452–455.
18. Adaniya H, Hayami H, Hiraoka M, et al. Effects of magnesium on polymorphic ventricular tachycardias induced by aconitine. *J Cardiovasc Pharmacol.* 1994;24:721–729.
19. Pennec JP, Aubin M. Effects of aconitine and veratrine on the isolated perfused heart of the common eel (*Anguilla anguilla L.*). *Comp Biochem Physiol.* 1984;77C(2):367–369.
20. Sawanobori T, Hirano Y, Hiraoka M. Aconitine-induced delayed afterdepolarization in frog atrium and guinea pig papillary muscles in the presence of low concentrations of Ca++. *Jpn J Physiol.* 1987;37:59–79.
21. Leichter D, Danilo P, Boyden P, et al. A canine model of torsade de pointes. *PACE.* 1988;11:2235–2245.
22. Tai YT, But PPH, Young K, et al. Cardiotoxicity after accidental herb-induced aconite poisoning. *Lancet.* 1992;340:1254–1256.
23. Tai YT, Lau CP, But PPH, et al. Bidirectional tachycardia induced by herbal aconite poisoning. *PACE.* 1992;15:831–839.
24. Chan TYK. Aconitine poisoning: a global perspective. *Vet Human Toxicol.* 1994;36(4):326–328.
25. Chan TYK, Critchley JAJH. The spectrum of poisonings in Hong Kong: an overview. *Vet Human Toxicol.* 1994;36(2):135–137.
26. But PPH, Tai YT, Young K. Three fatal cases of herbal aconite poisoning. *Vet Human Toxicol.* 1994;36(3):212–215.
27. Chan TYK. Aconitine poisoning following the ingestion of Chinese herbal medicines: a report of eight cases. *Aust NZ J Med.* 1993;23:268–271.
28. Dickens P, Tai YT, But PPH, et al. Fatal accidental aconitine poisoning following ingestion of Chinese herbal medicine: a report of two cases. *Forensic Sci Int.* 1994;67:55–58.
29. Hyppolyte EC, de Bocarme L. *Murder 2: The Second Casebook of Forensic Detection.* Vol 2. Hoboken, NJ: John Wiley & Sons; 2004:30–32.
30. Domino E, Hornbach E, Demana T. The nicotine content of common vegetables. *N Eng J Med.* 1993;329(6):437.
31. Drummer OH, Roberts AN, Bedford PJ, et al. Three deaths from hemlock poisoning. *Med J Aust.* 1995;162:592–593.
32. Kunkel DB. Tobacco and friends. *Emerg Med.* 1985:142–158.
33. McGehee DS, Heath MJS, Gelber S, et al. Nicotine enhancement of fast excitatory synaptic transmission in CNS by presynaptic receptors. *Science.* 1995;269:1692–1696.
34. Litovitz TL, Normann SA, Veltri JC. 1985 annual report of the American Association of Poison Control Centers National Data Collection System. *Am J Emerg Med.* 1986;4(5):427–458.

35. Smolinske SC, Spoerke DG, Spiller SK, et al. Cigarette and nicotine chewing gum toxicity in children. *Hum Toxicol.* 1988;7:27–31.

36. Curry S, Bond R, Kunkel D. Acute nicotine poisonings after ingestions of tree tobacco. Vet Hum Toxicol 1988, 30:369

37. Mellick LB, Makowski T, Mellick GA, et al. Neuromuscular blockade after ingestion of tree tobacco (*Nicotiana glauca*). *Ann Emerg Med.* 1999;34(1):101–104.

38. Frank BS, Michelson WB, Panter KE, et al. Ingestion of Poison Hemlock (*Conium maculatum*). *West J Med.* 1995;163:573–574.

39. Foster PF, McFadden R, Trevino R, et al. Successful transplantation of donor organs from a hemlock poisoning victim. *Transplantation.* 2003;76(5):874–876.

40. Watson WA, Litovitz TL, Rodgers GC Jr, et al. 2002 annual report of the American Association of Poison Control Centers Toxic Exposure Surveillance System. *Am J Emerg Med.* 2003;21(5):353–421.

41. Hipke ME. Green tobacco sickness. *South Med J.* 1993;86(9):989–992.

42. Taylor RFH, Al-Jarad N, John LME, et al. Betel-nut chewing and asthma. *Lancet.* 1992;339:1134–1136.

43. Rizzi D, Basile C, Di Maggio A, et al. Rhabdomyolysis and acute tubular necrosis in coniine (hemlock) poisoning [letter]. *Lancet.* 1989:1461–1462.

44. Scatizzi A, Di Maggio A, Rizzi D, et al. Acute renal failure due to tubular necrosis caused by waildfoul-mediated hemlock poisoning. *Renal Failure.* 1993;15(1):93–96.

45. Baselt RC, Cravey RH. *Disposition of Toxic Drugs and Chemicals in Man.* Vol 4. Foster City, California: Chemical Toxicology Institute; 1995.

46. Cromwell BT. The separation, micro-estimation and distribution of the alkaloids of hemlock (*Conium maculatum L.*). *Biochem J.* 1956;64:259–266.

47. Maltby JR. Criminal poisoning with anaesthetic drugs: murder, manslaughter, or not guilty. *Forensic Sci.* 1975;6(1-2):91–108.

48. Levy R. Jimson seed poisoning—a new hallucinogen on the horizon. *J Am Coll Emerg Physicians.* 1977;6(2):58–61.

49. Michalodimitrakis M. Discussion of "*Datura stramonium:* a fatal poisoning." *J Forensic Sci.* 1984:961–962.

50. Ulrich RW, Bowerman DL, Levisky JA, et al. *Datura stramonium:* a fatal poisoning. *J Forensic Sci.* 1982;27(4):948–954.

51. Smith EA, Meloan CE, Pickell JA, et al. Scopolamine poisoning from homemade "moon flower" wine. *J Anal Toxicol.* 1991;15(4):216–219.

52. Theobald M. The tyme appointed. *Colonial Williamsburg.* 2005:1–6.

53. Stockbridge J. Account of the effect of eating, a poisonous plant called *Cicuta maculata. Boston Med Surg J.* 1814;3:334–337.

54. Krenzelok EP, Jacobsen TD, Aronis JM. Hemlock ingestions: the most deadly plant exposures. *J Toxicol Clin Toxicol.* 1996;34(5):601–602.

55. Landers D, Seppi K, Blauer W. Seizures and death on a white river float trip: report of water hemlock poisoning. *West J Med.* 1985;142:637–640.

56. Starreveld E, Hope CE. Cicutoxin poisoning (water hemlock). *Neurology.* 1975;25:730–734.

57. Nelson RB, North DS, Kaneriya M, et al. The influence of biperiden, benztropine, physostigmine and diazepam on the convulsive effects of *Cicuta douglasii. Proc West Pharmacol Soc.* 1978;21:137–139.

58. Carlton BE, Tufts E, Girard DE. Water hemlock poisoning complicated by rhabdomyoslysis and renal failure. *Clin Tox.* 1979;14(1):87–92.

59. Nelson RB, Cole FR. The convulsive profile of *Cicuta douglasii* (water hemlock). *Proc West Pharmacol Soc.* 1976;19:193–197.

60. Applefeld JJ, Caplan ES. A case of water hemlock poisoning. *J Am Coll Emerg Physicians.* 1979;8(10):401–403.

61. Costanza DJ, Hoversten VW. Accidental ingestion of water hemlock: report of two patients with acute and chronic effects. *Calif Med.* 1973;119(May):78–82.

62. Egdahl A. A case of poisoning due to eating poison-hemlock (*Cicuta maculata*). *Archives of Int Med.* 1911;7:348–356.

63. Robson P. Water hemlock poisoning. *Lancet.* 1965;2:1274–1275.

64. Ball MJ, Flather ML, Forfar JC. Hemlock water dropwort poisoning. *Postgraduate Medical J.* 1987;63:363–365.

65. King LA, Lewis MJ, Parry D, et al. Identification of *Oenanthotoxin* and related compounds in hemlock water dropwort poisoning. *Human Toxicol.* 1985;4:355–364.

66. Mitchell MI, Routledge PA. Hemlock water dropwort poisoning—a review. *Clin Toxicol.* 1978;12(4):417–426.

17 | Potassium

R. Brent Furbee

CASE STUDY

Mary Ann Alderson was a 69-year-old with severe chronic obstructive lung disease. Despite her disease, she managed to live independently. She presented to Vermillion County Hospital's emergency department at 11:00 PM in November of 1994 with a complaint of epigastric discomfort after consuming pizza and beer. The physician decided to admit her to rule out a possible cardiac cause. She spent about 8 hours in the intensive care unit before being transferred to a medical-surgical floor wearing a telemetry pack. During nearly 2 days of her hospitalization, her course was uncomplicated. In fact, when her intravenous line failed during the second night, it was removed and not replaced. A cardiac cause for her discomfort was ruled out, and she was to be discharged the following day. At approximately 4:00 PM the day before her planned discharge, Orville Lynn Majors entered her room and informed Alderson that she was required to have an intravenous line. She protested that she did not need one because she was going home. Majors pressed, and Alderson acquiesced. He started her new line at 4:20 PM. Twenty minutes later, she was in cardiac arrest. A nurse responding to the code saw Majors standing at Alderson's bedside with a 3 cc syringe in his left hand.

Following exhumation, an autopsy showed no cause for sudden death. The pathologist, John A. Heidingsfelder, excluded a pulmonary embolus as the cause. The cardiac pathologist, Bruce Waller, ruled out contributing coronary artery disease. Cardiac electrophysiologist Eric Prystowsky opined that her death was not consistent with her pre-arrest clinical course but that it was consistent with an injection of potassium. Her caution regarding her health and her physician's prudence to further evaluate her symptoms cost Mary Ann Alderson her life. She would not be the last to die at the hands of Majors at Vermillion County Hospital.[1]

HISTORY

Potassium, most often in the form of potassium chloride, has been employed in numerous homicides. It has been used almost exclusively in medical settings. Some cases arguably involved euthanasia, but many were clearly performed for other more sinister and nefarious reasons. One of the more notorious cases involved a licensed practical nurse, Orville Lynn Majors, who was convicted of killing six patients in a rural hospital by administering potassium chloride intravenously. Though tried on only seven cases, investigators estimated that he killed over 100 patients during his employment between the fall of 1993 and spring of 1995. Several cases of murder by potassium chloride are documented in medical literature and the press.[2-7] Yorker et al. performed an exhaustive review of medical murders from 1971 to 2005. They excluded cases where the motivation was euthanasia. Of 90 healthcare providers charged, 45 were convicted of serial murder, 4 were convicted of attempted murder or assault, and 5 pleaded guilty to lesser charges.[7]

Whether criminal or accidental, potassium (K+) injection or infusion has been responsible for a number of adverse events, including death, over the years. Hospital pharmacies have moved potassium chloride (KCl) from open drawers on the hospital floors back to the pharmacy and more recently to computer-driven, on-site, locked dispensers that require proper identification of the healthcare provider, patient, and even the indication for a drug. While these precautions will almost certainly lead to a marked reduction in medication errors, they are not fool-proof.[8-10] They also make criminal use more difficult, but not impossible.

Potassium has distinct advantages as a criminal poison. First, despite potassium access being more tightly controlled in certain environments, it is still readily available from hospitals, veterinary suppliers, and chemical companies, and through various Internet sources. Second, potassium is an essential element in humans and is present and measurable in everyone, living and dead. Finally, it is present in abnormally high concentrations when measured after cellular death occurs, making detection of exogenously administered potassium difficult.

When employed as a poison, potassium has been used historically by physicians, nurses, and other medical personnel to kill patients. It has also been used in lethal injection for execution. Its use outside these settings has been rare.

POTENTIAL DELIVERY METHODS

Potassium can be administered intravenously or by the oral route. Reported cases of potassium's use for murder have occurred by the intravenous route.

TOXICOLOGIC MECHANISMS

Cardiac

Cardiac effects of potassium have been studied since the early 1900s. The action of potassium on cardiac function is dictated by the route and speed of its administration. In the conductive system of the heart, the sinoatrial (SA) node appears to be highly resistant to a gradual increase in potassium, such as seen in renal failure. Rapid administration, however, can result in SA arrest or SA block. Patients may note generalized weakness prior to the onset of changes on electrocardiogram (ECG). As potassium levels rise, there is an initial shortening of the QT interval. The development of tall peaked or pointed T waves (Figure 17.1) is most often the earliest detected sign of elevated serum potassium, also known as hyperkalemia. This sign is usually not noted until the serum concentration of potassium exceeds 5.5 mmol/L. Note that for potassium and other univalent ions, units of millimoles/L (mmol/L) are equal to milliequivalents/L (mEq/L). Tall, steep, narrow T waves, however, are only present in 22% of hyperkalemic patients.[11] Such T-wave morphology may be seen with myocardial ischemia, stroke, or left ventricular diastolic overload. In those settings, peaked T waves are usually accompanied by a wide corrected QT interval (QTc) but, at lower concentrations, hyperkalemia may not be.[12]

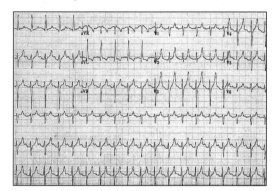

FIGURE 17.1   An electrocardiogram of a patient who presented with hyperkalemia, demonstrating tall, peaked T waves.

Intra-atrial conduction disturbance is considered a characteristic feature of advanced hyperkalemia. It usually occurs before dramatic QRS alterations appear because atrial excitability is abolished at lower concentrations than ventricular activity. The PR interval increases, and the P-wave amplitude is diminished to the point of disappearance.

Intraventricular conduction delays lead to QRS widening as potassium climbs (Figure 17.2). Changes in QRS morphology may begin to occur when the potassium concentration exceeds 6.5 mEq/L, and while some manifestations are commonly seen at potassium concentrations above 8 mEq/L, ECG alterations may not occur until even higher concentrations are reached.[13,14] When QRS widening is observed, it differs from the ECG pattern of bundle branch block or preexcitation because both initial and terminal portions of the complex are affected.[12] This observation would also help differentiate the changes from sodium channel-blocking drugs (i.e., tricyclic antidepressants), in that those drugs commonly impact only the terminal 40 ms of the QRS complex. As potassium concentration increases, atrioventricular (AV) block occurs. As a result, second-degree and third-degree heart block occur, potentially causing profound bradycardia and eventually a

"sine wave" rhythm (Figure 17.3). When potassium is administered as a bolus, AV block and cardiac arrest can occur within seconds. Thus, the "classic" presentation of hyperkalemia is not always apparent.

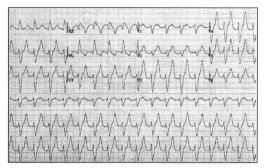

FIGURE 17.2   The electrocardiogram from the same patient depicted in Figure 1, showing progression of hyperkalemia: the T waves have become increasingly peaked, the QRS complex has widened, and there is a loss of P waves.

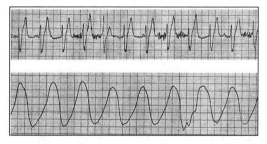

FIGURE 17.3   These two tracings are from a patient fatally injected with potassium chloride. The top tracing demonstrates peaked T waves, a wide QRS, and the absence of P waves. The lower tracing demonstrates the development of the classic sine wave pattern associated with hyperkalemia.

There are a number of reasons for the electrocardiographic changes associated with hyperkalemia (Figure 17.4). The increase in extracellular potassium concentration causes a drop in the transmembrane potassium gradient of conductive cells.[13] This results in a decrease in the resting membrane potential, which is reflected in the diminution of the QRS deflection. In other words, as hyperkalemia worsens, the QRS amplitude decreases. A second product of the decrease in transmembrane potassium gradient is a decrease in the velocity of phase

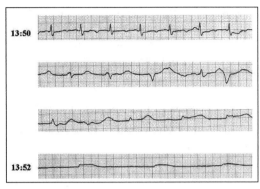

FIGURE 17.4   **Prior to open heart surgery, a cardioplegic infusion begins at 1:50 PM. Subsequent loss of P waves, tall, peaked T waves, widen QRS with decreased amplitude are all evident. Changes in the morphology of the QRS and T waves results in the sine wave at 1:52 PM.**

0 of the action potential. This leads to a slowing of conduction that is seen as widening of the QRS complex. Potassium also causes an increase in the permeability of the conductive cell membrane leading to more rapid passage of potassium ions out of the cell in phase 3. Thus, repolarization occurs more rapidly. On the ECG, this is seen as a narrower, taller T wave. As these changes progress, the QRS gets wider and shorter, and the T wave becomes taller and narrower. The combination of these changing morphologies results in a blurring of the QRS and T waves, known more commonly as "sine waves." This dysrhythmia is almost always a terminal event if not quickly reversed.

It is important to note that rapid administration of potassium may present with only some of the cardiac features that have come to be expected in the typical hyperkalemic paradigm known to healthcare providers, such as the changes seen in renal failure. Bolus injection subjects cardiac conductive cells to an abrupt spike in potassium concentration. Thus, arrest may occur in seconds. Review of pre-arrest ECG tracings would likely show no signs of hyperkalemia, while tracings at the time of arrest might only reflect ventricular tachycardia, profound bradycardia, and asystole. In other words, the lack of P- or T-wave changes does not rule out potassium as an etiology.[14]

Finally, it should be noted that electrocardiographic changes induced by hyperkalemia may be misdiagnosed by clinicians for other causes.

For example, elevation of ST segments has led to the misdiagnosis of myocardial infarction and Brugada syndrome. Also, hyperkalemia may result from poisoning sources other than injected potassium (i.e., digoxin)

Nerve and Musculoskeletal

As potassium concentration increases in the extracellular fluid, the transmembrane potential decreases and the neuron or myocyte becomes partially depolarized, manifesting clinically as weakness initially and potentially progressing to paralysis. If the onset is rapid with intravenous injection of a large dose of potassium, paralysis is more likely due to nerve conduction impairment. Kuwabara et al. demonstrated that higher potassium concentration tended to be associated with longer relative refractory periods in patients whose potassium concentrations were measured over time. It is noteworthy that these subjects' serum potassium concentrations did not exceed 5.0 mEq/L.[15]

Potassium can act as a paralytic agent. In medical cases where potassium rises slowly, weakness may be the first symptom to develop and may be the clinical sign that initiates medical investigation and intervention. While weakness is frequently seen with slow-onset hyperkalemia in renal failure or oral ingestion, intravenous administration most commonly follows a rapid and catastrophic course of weakness, paralysis, cardiac dysthymia, and death in a very few minutes or even seconds. For investigators of such events, there is a very important point: Potassium paralyzes but does not cause amnesia. Therefore, if a patient survives an injection of potassium, that person may fully recall the preceding events. Surprisingly, a number of healthcare workers are not cognizant of the difference between a paralytic agent (as potassium chloride can be) and a sedative hypnotic, believing the paralyzed patient is also comatose.[16]

CLINICAL EFFECTS

In patients with slow increases in serum potassium, the initial complaint is often weakness. The onset of weakness and early ECG changes, such as T-wave elevation, will often occur when serum concentrations reach 6.5–8.0 mEq/L. With increasing serum concentrations, ECG changes become more severe and may lead to cardiac arrest and death.

Oral administration of potassium is not frequently associated with criminal poisoning. However, numerous reports of fatal or near fatal hyperkalemia[16-20] have occurred as a result of ingestion of potassium supplements, such as salt substitutes, which contain as high as 90% potassium chloride.[20]

Rapid intravenous administration, which commonly occurs in criminal poisoning, frequently has a decidedly different look. Pain at the site of injection is a common complaint even with dilute infusions. This pain may be due to chemical or osmotic irritation of the intima and/or mechanical distention of the vessel. Bolus injections or high-concentration infusions subject the vessel wall to considerably higher potassium content.[22] Erythema and phlebitis may also occur.[23] Clinical studies in the late 1980s and early 1990s demonstrated that pretreatment of the blood vessel with lidocaine decreased pain at least for the initial 30 minutes. Two studies demonstrated that inclusion of lidocaine in the infusion significantly reduced pain associated with potassium administration.[23] Some murderers, such as Beverly Allitt, were suspected to have used lidocaine to prevent the pain induced by intravenous injection of potassium.[24]

The clinical presentation of patients deliberately poisoned by a bolus of intravenous potassium is uncommonly reported. Accidental administration in the healthcare setting has, unfortunately, occurred with relative frequency in the past. In a review of medication errors, Emmett and Ranson stated, "Potassium chloride for injection concentrate has been involved in more fatal medication errors than any other drug."[25] With regard to bolus injection, logic would seem to dictate that the administered dose would undergo significant dilution from the peripheral injection site to the aortic root where it enters the coronary arteries. In fact both animal and human studies demonstrated that the bolus traveled from its site of injection to the coronary arteries and even into the arterial system relatively intact. This was confirmed by measurement of the potassium concentration at specific intervals until the concentration spiked and rapidly returned to normal, indicating the passing of the bolus.[26, 27]

One of the most enlightening reviews regarding clinical effects comes from the *Clinical Journal of Oncology Nursing.* Sixteen cases of accidental potassium administration were reviewed. In most cases, the errors involved potassium substitution for sodium chloride or furosemide in similar ampules and were administered in bolus form. While the outcome in some cases is not clear, 11 of the 16 suffered cardiac arrest. Seven deaths were reported. At least five patients clearly received potassium chloride intravenous bolus and did not arrest. Two patients complained of pain immediately upon injection, and administration was stopped. They suffered no injury. A 10-year-old received a 2–3 mL bolus and complained of burning at the injection site but suffered no complications. Two patients appeared to have had more neuromuscular compromise than cardiac effect, probably due to a smaller dose of potassium chloride. The patients became cyanotic, then appeared to have altered mental status, followed by complete recovery in a matter of minutes. This case series also suggests a dose–response relationship. It appears that 4–6 mEq may cause significant symptoms but may not be fatal. Three milliliters (6 mEq) of medical-grade potassium chloride (2 mEq/mL) may be fatal in weaker hearts, particularly in patients with congestive heart failure.[28] Increased doses have increased likelihood of fatal outcome, and 10 mL is nearly always lethal.

Hyperkalemia frequently presents as weakness, particularly if it occurs gradually as in renal failure. Intravenous administration may also cause weakness and paralysis but in a significantly more rapid fashion. Bolus administration may cause cardiac arrest so quickly that musculoskeletal complaints would not be noted.

ANALYTIC DETECTION

Premortem

Potassium is usually measured in bodily fluids by flame photometry or ion-selective potentiometry. The normal reference range for potassium is 3.5–4.9 mEq/L. Concentrations may be altered by malnutrition, diuretics, sympathomimetics, tissue necrosis, or renal insufficiency. Concentrations in red blood cells are higher (105 mEq/L), accounting for serum potassium elevations in hemolyzed specimens. Serum potassium increases 0.5 mEq/L for every 0.5% hemolysis of whole blood.

Potassium During Resuscitation

Electrolytes are often drawn during attempted resuscitation and may be particularly important in criminal investigations involving a question of potassium administration. Unfortunately, the validity of serum potassium drawn during cardiorespiratory resuscitation (CPR) is dependent on the time from arrest to initiation of resuscitation, the extent of circulation produced by cardiac compressions, the drugs that are administered during the resuscitation attempt, and the pre-arrest serum potassium. These factors may vary significantly between prehospital and in-hospital arrests, particularly in emergency or critical care areas. Fish et al. found that in 15 emergency department patients who failed resuscitation attempts, potassium ranged from 2.6 to 12.2 mEq/L. All of these patients arrested outside the hospital, and it is not clear which received potassium-lowering drugs such as sodium bicarbonate or epinephrine.[29] Johnston et al. compared the arterial and venous potassium concentrations of 50 patients presenting to the emergency department in cardiac arrest. Again, drug therapy during resuscitation is not documented. All patients appear to have suffered prehospital arrests, but the arterial potassium concentrations ranged from 2.7 to 6.7 mEq/L (only two patients exceeded 6 mEq/L). The venous concentrations ranged from 2.5 to 6.3 mEq/L (only one patient exceeded 6 mEq/L).[30] Geddes et al. studied multiple parameters, including potassium in pigs with induced ventricular fibrillation (VF). There appears to be no significant delay between VF and onset of CPR, but the sustained blood pressure was only 20–25 mm Hg. Of the 14 animals, only 2 had potassium concentrations in excess of 7.0 mEq/L.[31] These and other studies seem to suggest that with rapid onset of CPR, with or even without potassium-lowering drugs, potassium concentrations during CPR usually remain in the low or normal range.

Postmortem

Potassium is the predominate intracellular ion. Of the body's potassium, 98% is found within the cell. Upon death, cellular membranes and pumps, such as the ATPase driven sodium/potassium pumps, begin to fail. Because the purpose of these structures is to contain potassium within the cell or return it to the cell's interior from the extracellular (and intravascular) space, their failure in death releases large amounts of potassium into the blood. This accounts for the relatively rapid rise in serum potassium that begins within an hour or two following death. Therefore, postmortem blood samples are not indicative of premortem serum concentrations. While vitreous potassium increases at a slower rate, it is also subject to a wide margin of error.[32,33]

CONCLUSION

Potassium has been used to commit murder, primarily in the healthcare setting. In such cases, the intravenous route of administration has been employed. Electrocardiographic changes may be useful in the diagnosis of such poisonings. However, rapid administration of a large, single dose may result in sudden cardiovascular collapse and death prior to the development or capture of classic electrocardiographic changes. The correct diagnosis may be difficult to discern, especially since potassium serum levels rise postmortem as cells die.

REFERENCES

1. *Indiana* v *Orville Lynn Majors*, Cause No. 83CO 1-971 2 CF 0074. 1997, Dec 29. (Vermillion Circuit Court).
2. Alpers A. Criminal act or palliative care? Prosecutions involving the care of the dying. *J Law Med Ethics*. 1998;26(4):308–331.
3. Dyer C. Two doctors confess to helping patients to die. *BMJ*. 1997;315(7102):206.
4. Park GR, Khan SN. Murder and the ICU. *Eur J Anaesthesiol*. 2002;19(9):621–623.
5. Robb N. Death in a Halifax hospital: a murder case highlights a profession's divisions. *CMAJ*. 1997;157(6):757–762.
6. Yorker BC. Nurses accused of murder. *Am J Nurs*. 1988;88(10):1327–1328.
7. Yorker BC, Kizer KW, Lampe P, et al. Serial murder by healthcare professionals. *J Forensic Sci*. 2006;51(6):1362–1371.
8. Schmidt CE, Bottoni T. Improving medication safety and patient care in the emergency department. *J Emerg Nurs*. 2003;29(1):12–16.
9. Webber T, Hupp S. Infant deaths put focus on nurses. *Indianapolis Star*. 2006:B01.
10. Davis RH, Fisch C. Potassium and arrhythmias. *Geriatrics*. 1970;25(11):108–116.
11. Braun HB, Surawicz B, Bellet S. T waves in hyperpotassemia. *Am J Med Sci*. 1955;230:147–156.
12. Surawicz B. Relationship between electrocardiogram and electrolytes. *Am Heart J*. 1967;73(6):814–834.

13. Martinez-Vea A, Bardají A, Garcia C, et al. Severe hyperkalemia with minimal electrocardiographic manifestations: a report of seven cases. *J Electrocardiol.* 1999;32(1):45–49.

14. Szerlip HM, Weiss J, Singer I. Profound hyperkalemia without electrocardiographic manifestations. *Am J Kidney Dis.* 1986;7(6):461–465.

15. Kuwabara S, Misawa S, Kanai K, et al. The effects of physiological fluctuation of serum potassium levels on excitability properties in healthy human motor axons. *Clin Neurophysiol.* 2007;118(2):278–282.

16. Loper KA, Butler S, Nessly M, et al. Paralyzed with pain: the need for education. *Pain.* 1989;37(3):315–316.

17. Bacon C. Letter: death from accidental potassium poisoning in childhood. *BMJ.* 1974;1(5904):389–390.

18. Colledge NR, Northridge B, Fraser DM. Survival after massive overdose of slow-release potassium. *Scott Med J.* 1988;33(3):279.

19. Hoyt RE. Hyperkalemia due to salt substitutes. *JAMA.* 1986;256(13):1726.

20. Kallen RJ, Rieger CH, Cohen HS, et al. Near-fatal hyperkalemia due to ingestion of salt substitute by an infant. *JAMA.* 1976;235(19):2125–2126.

21. Su M, Stork C, Ravuri S, et al. Sustained-release potassium chloride overdose. *J Toxicol Clin Toxicol.* 2001;39(6):641–648.

22. Lim ET, Khoo ST, Tweed WA. Efficacy of lignocaine in alleviating potassium chloride infusion pain. *Anaesth Intensive Care.* 1992;20(2):196–198.

23. Pucino F, Danielson DB, Carlson JD, et al. Patient tolerance to intravenous potassium chloride with and without lidocaine. *Drug Intell Clin Pharm.* 1988;22(9):676–679.

24. Marks V, Richmond C. Beverly Allitt: the nurse who killed babies. *J R Soc Med.* 2008;101:110–115.

25. Emmett SL, Ranson DL. Medication errors: inadvertent administration of potassium chloride. *J Law Med.* 2003;11(2):146–147.

26. McCall BB, Mazzei WJ, Scheller MS, et al. Effects of central bolus injections of potassium chloride on arterial potassium concentration in patients undergoing cardiopulmonary bypass. *J Cardiothorac Anesth.* 1990;4(5):571–576.

27. Tanaka K, Pettinger WA. Pharmacokinetics of bolus potassium injections for cardiac arrhythmias. *Anesthesiology.* 1973;38(6):587–589.

28. Anonymous. Intravenous potassium predicament. *Clin J Oncology Nurs.* 1997;1(2):45–49.

29. Fish RM, Louie L. Laboratory tests during resuscitation. *J Emerg Med.* 1989;7(5):451–456.

30. Johnston HL, Murphy R. Agreement between an arterial blood gas analyser and a venous blood analyser in the measurement of potassium in patients in cardiac arrest. *Emerg Med J.* 2005;22(4):269–271.

31. Geddes LA, Roeder RA, Rundell AE, et al. The natural biochemical changes during ventricular fibrillation with cardiopulmonary resuscitation and the onset of postdefibrillation pulseless electrical activity. *Am J Emerg Med.* 2006;24(5):577–581.

32. Coe JI. Postmortem chemistry of blood, cerebrospinal fluid, and vitreous humor. *Leg Med Annu.* 1977;1976:55–92.

33. Coe JI. Postmortem chemistry update: emphasis on forensic application. *Am J Forens Med Pathol.* 1993;14(2):91–117.

18 | Quinuclidinyl Benzilate (QNB)

Christopher P. Holstege

CASE STUDY

On July 11, 1995, approximately 15,000 people assembled in the village of Jaglici, situated in the Republika Srpska of Bosnia and Herzegovina. This group had fled from Srebrenica (15 km away) after Bosnian Serb forces began to shell the town. In order to flee the Bosnian Serbs, the assembled column started to leave Jaglici on July 12 at 12:30 AM, with the last members of the column leaving 12 hours later. The reported progress of the column was slow because of concern for minefields. Individuals were required to walk in single file holding hands to avoid getting lost in the forest at dark and to enable them to walk in each other's footsteps to avoid landmines. Only a fraction of the members of the column eventually reached safe territory on July 16, after coming under fire from Bosnian Serb forces on a number of occasions.[1]

According to eyewitness accounts, the Bosnian Serbs used different shells; some exploded and others gave out a "strange smoke" that did not rise in the air but rather spread toward the column at the height of a man. Reportedly, a large number of those on the march suffered from hallucinations during the 5-day trek. It was subsequently suspected that the Bosnian Serb forces had used a chemical warfare agent to disorient the marchers, prompting Human Rights Watch to visit the location in March of 1996. During the course of the investigation, marchers were interviewed. Subsequent testimony suggested that unusual munitions may have been utilized by the Bosnian Serbs and that those interviewed had experienced themselves or witnessed others with marked hallucinations. The agent suspected to have caused these effects was 3-quinuclidinyl benzilate.

HISTORY

Quinuclidinyl benzilate, also known as QNB or BZ, is a Chemical Warfare Convention Schedule 2 agent (CAS No. 13004-56-3). QNB is a molecular member of a larger chemical family known as the glycolates (glycolic acid esters).[2] QNB is classified as a hallucinogenic chemical warfare agent. It is a potent anticholinergic agent that affects both the peripheral nervous system and the central nervous system (CNS).[3] It is reportedly 25 times more potent centrally than atropine and 3 times more potent than scopolamine. The minimally effective dose for mild cognitive impairment in 50% of the exposed population (MED$_{50}$) is approximately 2.5 µg/kg.[4] The dose that incapacitates 50% of the exposed population (ID$_{50}$) for QNB is 6.2 µg/kg, compared to 140 µg/kg for atropine.[4]

Use of QNB has been suggested, but not confirmed, in two international conflicts. In addition to the case already noted, an incident occurred on January 16, 1992, when Mozambican government forces (approximately 400 soldiers) attacked one of the largest Renamo strongholds in southern Mozambique, close to the South African border.[1,5] As they approached the camp on foot, an unidentified light aircraft was seen flying above the area. They came under limited small arms fire and took cover when an explosion occurred above their heads, releasing a dense cloud of black smoke that then dissipated. The wind was blowing toward the rear of the formation. Fifteen minutes later, the first complaints occurred. "It became very hot," one witness reported. "Some of us were going crazy." They felt severe chest pains, were tired and thirsty, and when they drank water the next morning, some

of them vomited. Others said they had difficulty seeing. As a consequence, the troops became disorganized. The United Nations' report on this incident concluded that the effect on the troops was consistent with the use of a chemical warfare agent such as QNB; however, in the absence of analytic data, they could not conclude that a chemical warfare agent was used in the attack because a considerable delay occurred between the attack (January 1992) and the formal investigation (March 1992).[6]

In 2002, the world's media initially reported that Russian troops pumped QNB into the Dubrovka Theater Center in Moscow, Russia, when Chechen rebels held patrons hostage at that site. These reports as to the gas used were rapidly disproved based on the clinical effects witnessed.

POTENTIAL DELIVERY METHODS

The intramuscular route of QNB exposure is equally as effective as the intravenous. Oral administration is 80% as effective as the parenteral routes. QNB was developed for aerosol dissemination with the primary route of absorption by aerosol through the respiratory system. By inhalation, if particle size is optimal at 1.0 µm, QNB is approximately 50% as effective as by the parenteral route.[4] QNB is also odorless. When applied to the skin in a propylene glycol solution, absorption is only 5–10%, and the effects may be delayed for 24 hours.

The effects of QNB by any route are slow in onset and long in duration. Depending on the exposure dose and route, performance decline is usually barely measurable at 1 hour, reaches a peak at 8 hours, and subsides gradually over the following 48–72 hours.[4]

TOXICOLOGIC MECHANISMS

QNB acts by competitively inhibiting muscarinic receptors.[7,8] Muscarinic receptors primarily are associated with the parasympathetic nervous system, which innervates numerous organ systems, including the eyes, heart, respiratory system, skin, gastrointestinal tract, and bladder.[9,10] Sweat glands, innervated by the sympathetic nervous system, also are modulated by muscarinic receptors.

CLINICAL EFFECTS

Most of the literature on the effects of QNB on humans is either classified or in military archives.[1] Following exposure to QNB, the physical examination is consistent with an anticholinergic syndrome. Characteristics of the anticholinergic syndrome have long been taught using the old medical adage "dry as a bone, blind as a bat, red as a beet, hot as a hare, and mad as a hatter," which corresponds with a symptomatic person's anhydrosis, mydriasis, flushing, fever, and delirium, respectively.

Depending on the dose and time since exposure, a number of CNS effects may manifest.[11] Restlessness, apprehension, abnormal speech, confusion, agitation, tremor, picking movements, ataxia, stupor, and coma have all been described following exposure to various anticholinergics. When manifesting delirium, the individual will often stare into space and mutter and fluctuate between occasional lucid intervals with appropriate responses and then descriptions of vivid hallucinations. Phantom behaviors, such as plucking or picking at the air or at garments, is characteristic.[4] Hallucinations are prominent, and they may be benign, entertaining, or terrifying to the patient. Exposed patients may have conversations with hallucinated figures, and/or they may misidentify persons they typically know well. Simple tasks typically performed well by the exposed person may become difficult. Motor coordination, perception, cognition, and new memory formation are altered.

Mydriasis causes photophobia. Impairment of near vision occurs because of loss of accommodation and reduced depth of field secondary to ciliary muscle paralysis and pupillary enlargement. Tachycardia may occur. Exacerbated heart rate responses to exertion are also expected. Systolic and diastolic blood pressure may show moderate elevation. A decrease in capillary tone may cause skin flushing. Intestinal motility slows, and secretions from the stomach, pancreas, and gallbladder decrease.[10,12] Nausea and vomiting may occur. Decreased or absent bowel sounds are noted on examination. All glandular cells become inhibited, and dry mucous membranes of the mouth and throat are noted. Inhibition of sweating results in dry skin. Urination may be difficult, and urinary retention may occur. The exposed patient's temperature may become elevated from the inability to sweat and dissipate heat. In warm climates, such as the desert, this may result in marked hyperthermia.

ANALYTIC DETECTION

Most of the QNB that enters the body is excreted by the kidneys, either as the parent compound or as metabolites, making urine the choice for detection.[13] QNB undergoes hydrolysis to produce benzilic acid (BA) and 3-quinuclidinol (Q). A solid-phase extraction of the urine and isotope dilution in conjunction with gas chromatography-mass spectrometry (GC-MS) has been used for detection of QNB.[13]

CONCLUSION

QNB is a potent anticholinergic agent that was developed for chemical warfare. Exposure to this agent can result in delirium that can last for days. Its actual use has not been definitively confirmed but has been suggested in a number of international conflicts.

REFERENCES

1. Hay A. Surviving the impossible: the long march from Srebrenica. An investigation of the possible use of chemical warfare agents. *Med Confl Surviv.* 1998;14(2):120–155.
2. Bering B, Muller WE. Stereospecific 3H-QNB binding to human erythrocyte membranes associated with muscarinic cholinergic receptors. *J Neural Transm.* 1987;68:97–111.
3. Mashkovsky MD, Yakhontov LN. Relationships between the chemical structure and pharmacological activity in a series of synthetic quinuclidine derivatives. *Prog Drug Res.* 1969;13:293–339.
4. Ketchum JS, Sidell FR. Incapacitating Agents; In: Zajtchuk R, Bellamy R, eds. *Textbook of Military Medicine.* United States of America: Office of the Surgeon General, Department of the Army 1997:287–305.
5. *The Chemical Warfare Case:* Research Department of the Truth and Reconciliation Commission by the Netherlands Institute for Southern Africa; November 1997.
6. *United Nations Report of the Investigations into the Allegations of the Use of Chemical Warfare in Mozambique.* New York: UN; 1992.
7. Hiramatsu Y, Eckelman WC, Baum BJ. Interaction of iodinated quinuclidinyl benzilate enantiomers with M3 muscarinic receptors. *Life Sci.* 1994;54(23):1777–1783.
8. Gibson RE, Rzeszotarski WJ, Jagoda EM, et al. [125I] 3-quinuclidinyl 4-iodobenzilate: a high affinity, high specific activity radioligand for the M1 and M2-acetylcholine receptors. *Life Sci.* 1984;34(23):2287–2296.
9. Lambrecht G. Structure and conformation activity relationships of heterocyclic acetylcholine analogues. The inhibitory effect of 3-quinuclidinyl benzilates on cardiac muscarinic receptors. *Arzneimittelforschung.* 1980;30(12):2113–2115.

10. Morisset J, Geoffrion L, Larose L, et al. Distribution of muscarinic receptors in the digestive tract organs. *Pharmacology.* 1981;22(3):189–195.

11. Albanus L. Central and peripheral effects of anticholinergic compounds. *Acta Pharmacol Toxicol (Copenh).* 1970;28(4):305–326.

12. Ng KH, Morisset J, Poirier GG. Muscarinic receptors of the pancreas: a correlation between displacement of (3 H)-quinuclidinyl benzilate binding and amylase secretion. Pharmacology. 1979;18(5):263–270.

13. Byrd GD, Paule RC, Sander LC, et al. Determination of 3-quinuclidinyl benzilate (QNB) and its major metabolites in urine by isotope dilution gas chromatography/mass spectrometry. *J Anal Toxicol.* 1992;16(3):182–187.

19 | Saxitoxin

Christopher P. Holstege

CASE STUDY

Nine people, aged 38 to 80 years, presented to the emergency department over a 12-hour period. They complained of acute onset dizziness, staggering gait, and oral-facial and distal extremity paresthesias ("pins and needles" sensation). The individuals did not complain of digestive or intestinal symptoms. Six patients had progressive impairment of gait requiring confinement to a wheelchair after 6 to 8 hours. All patients had normal body temperature, blood pressure, and heart rate. The patients developed progressive axial ataxia, impairing unaided walk. They demonstrated bilateral dysmetria consisting of a lack of coordinated movement, with undershoot/overshoot of intended position with the limbs, which was not significantly increased by closing the eyes. Bilateral nystagmus (involuntary eye movement) was found in four patients. Three others, who had more severe incoordination, developed poor speech articulation. All patients examined had distal sock-and-glove superficial sensory impairment, as well as bilateral moderate position and vibration sense impairment. All nine were admitted to the hospital for further study and supportive treatment. The patients remained hospitalized for 1 to 3 days, all subsequently improved, and none had any long-term sequelae. It was later discovered that saxitoxin was present in shell-fish they had eaten.[1]

HISTORY

Saxitoxin (STX) is a potent toxin associated with the syndrome known as paralytic shellfish poisoning (PSP).[2,3] STX is formed by dinoflagel-lates that cause a phenomenon known as a red tide. Marine life (mollusks, crabs, and fish) may feed on these and bio-accumulate the dino-flagellates' toxins. Humans may inadvertently consume intoxicated seafood.[2,4] Numerous out-breaks of PSP have been reported worldwide. PSP is caused by not only STX but also by other chemical variations of STX, including decar-bamoyl STX (dc-STX) and N-sulfocarbamoyl (B1) toxin. Current U.S. Food and Drug Admin-istration (USFDA) guidelines require that all shellfish sold in the United States be tested for PSPs. The mouse bioassay is the current gold standard approved by the USFDA for detection and quantification of paralytic shellfish toxins in shellfish marketed to human consumers.[5]

Governments reportedly began experiment-ing with STX in the 1950s. In 1969, President Richard Nixon banned biologic weapons. Sub-sequently, nearly all the U.S. STX produced was destroyed. However, in 1975, approximately 10 grams of STX was discovered in a U.S. storage facility, triggering a U.S. Senate investigation and a redistribution of the remaining STX to universities for research purposes.

In recent years, terrorist events have resulted in increased regulations of STX.[6] The U.S. De-partment of Health and Human Services and the U.S. Department of Agriculture published final rules that implement the provisions of the USA PATRIOT Act and Public Health Security and Bioterrorism Preparedness and Response Act of 2002. These rules set forth the require-ments for possession, use, and transfer of select agents and toxins. The select chemical toxins identified in the final rules have the potential to pose a severe threat to public health and safety, to animal and plant health, or to animal and plant products. The Centers for Disease Control and Prevention (CDC) regulates the possession,

use, and transfer of the select agents and toxins that have the potential to pose a severe threat to public health and safety. The CDC Select Agent Program oversees these activities and registers all laboratories and other entities in the United States that possess, use, or transfer a select agent or toxin.

STX is currently listed as Schedule 1 by the Chemical Weapons Convention and is consid-ered one of the most potent toxins known. STX and ricin are the only two naturally occurring toxins classified as Schedule 1 by the Chemical Weapons Convention.

STX is a naturally occurring toxin but has also been synthesized using a variety of differ-ent methods.[7] STX is water soluble and heat stable, and is unaffected by cooking.[4] The LCt_{50} (the lethal concentration of exposure by inhala-tion that would kill about 50% of unprotected people) of STX is 5 mg-min/m^3, and STX is reportedly 2000 times more toxic than sodium cyanide by weight.[8,9]

POTENTIAL DELIVERY METHODS

STX toxicity can occur by either ingestion or in-halation. Contamination of food or water with STX is viewed as a viable concern for mass hu-man exposure.[10] In animal experiments, inhala-tional routes of administration are more potent than oral routes, causing death within minutes compared to hours for oral.[9,11]

TOXICOLOGIC MECHANISMS

STX is a specific high-affinity blocking ligand of voltage-dependent sodium channels, similar to tetrodotoxin.[12] STX binds competitively to a site on the external surface of the channel, named toxin site 1.[13] This binding inhibits sodium flux through these ion channels, rendering excitable tissues such as nerves and muscle nonfunctional.

CLINICAL EFFECTS

There are no published reports of STX being used by terrorists or other criminals, though concern remains high pertaining to its potential use, its marked toxicity, and its natural availabil-ity. In addition to the previously presented case, there are numerous reports in the literature of STX being ingested in contaminated food, which shed light on the clinical manifestations of STX toxicity.

In two separate outbreaks reported in 1990, nine fishermen developed symptoms within 2 hours of consuming STX-contaminated shellfish.[4] Reported symptoms included numbness of the mouth (in 6 of 9), vomiting (in 4 of 9), paresthesias of the extremities (in 7 of 9), numbness and tingling of the tongue (in 2 of 9), numbness of the face (in 5 of 9), lower back pain (in 6 of 9), and periorbital edema (in 1 of 9). Two hours following the onset of symptoms, one of the fishermen suffered a "cardiopulmonary arrest" and died. Of the remaining eight, only two required hospitalization. The duration of neurologic symptoms was less than 24 hours, and lower back pain lasted approximately 3 days. Of those who survived, all recovered uneventfully.

In 2000, a 65-year-old woman reportedly ingested STX-contaminated blowfish and within minutes developed tingling of her lips and tongue, which intensified over the ensuing 2 hours.[14] She developed increasing chest pain and had mild tachycardia and hypertension (160/70 mm Hg), requiring treatment with topical nitroglycerin.[15] Six to eight hours after ingestion, she developed ascending paralysis and declining pulmonary function requiring intubation. Over the following day she regained reflexes and voluntary movement and was extubated 72 hours later.

In 2002, two fishermen died after eating STX-contaminated shellfish.[16] Symptoms prior to demise included lip paresthesias, nausea, extremity weakness, and "tongue immobilization." The forensic examination of both victims did not show pathologic abnormalities with the exception of the lungs, which revealed pulmonary edema. STX was detected in gastric contents, body fluids, and tissue samples.

In summary, following oral exposure, STX causes prominent paresthesias, often beginning circumorally and spreading to the limbs. Symptoms can then progress to paralysis with retention of reflexes.[11] Cranial nerve dysfunction, hypersalivation, diaphoresis, respiratory failure, hypertension, and hypotension have all been reported. There have been no published reports of human exposure to aerosolized STX. STX toxicity is nearly indistinguishable from tetrodotoxin toxicity. There is no known antidote for STX toxicity. The majority of patients will recover if they receive adequate and timely supportive care.

ANALYTIC DETECTION

Measuring levels of STX in human samples requires early acquisition of samples. STX undergoes minimal metabolism but is rapidly excreted in the urine. STX can also concentrate in the liver, spleen, and central nervous system tissues.[17] Due to the extremely rapid excretion profile of STX compounds, urine samples are preferred rather than serum samples. Testing for STX can be performed using high-performance liquid chromatography-tandem mass spectroscopy (HPLC-MS/MS). These HPLC-MS/MS methods can provide STX fingerprint analyses to determine if the STX agent was derived from an organic source (shellfish ingestion) or a purified STX source (biologic warfare agent). Any individuals suspected of STX exposure should have urine specimens collected within 24 hours of exposure. Higher levels of STX exposure can extend detection times for several days.[18] Alternatively, less sensitive methods, such as HPLC and receptor-binding assays, are available for detecting STX in human samples.[19,20]

CONCLUSION

STX is a potent natural toxin. All published reports of human exposure have involved oral ingestion of STX. However, it is an effective aerosolized toxin also. It is associated with neuromuscular weakness and the potential progression to complete paralysis requiring life support. Its action is similar to the effects of tetrodotoxin. No reports of use in criminal poisoning have been published, but the potential for such use certainly exists.

REFERENCES

1. de Carvalho M, Jacinto J, Ramos N, et al. Paralytic shellfish poisoning: clinical and electrophysiological observations. *J Neurol.* 1998;245(8):551–554.
2. Landsberg JH, Hall S, Johannessen JN, et al. Saxitoxin puffer fish poisoning in the United States, with the first report of *Pyrodinium bahamense* as the putative toxin source. *Environ Health Perspect.* 2006;114(10):1502–1507.
3. Holstege CP, Bechtel LK, Reilly TH, et al. Unusual but potential agents of terrorists. *Emerg Med Clin North Am.* 2007;25(2):549–566.
4. Paralytic shellfish poisoning—Massachusetts and Alaska, 1990. *MMWR* 1991;40(10):157–161.
5. Van Egmond HP, Van Den Top HJ. *Worldwide regulations for marine phycotoxins.* Paper presented at: CNEVA, Proceedings of Symposium of Marine Biotoxins; January 30–31, 1991; Paris.

6. Llewellyn LE. Saxitoxin, a toxic marine natural product that targets a multitude of receptors. *Nat Prod Rep.* 2006;23(2):200–222.

7. Fleming JJ, Du Bois J. A synthesis of (+)-saxitoxin. *J Am Chem Soc.* 2006;128(12):3926–3927.

8. Wang J, Salata JJ, Bennett PB. Saxitoxin is a gating modifier of HERG K⁺ channels. *J Gen Physiol.* 2003;121(6):583–598.

9. Franz D, ed. Defense against toxic weapons. In: Sidell F, Takafuji E, Franz D, eds. *Medical Aspects of Chemical and Biological Warfare.* Falls Church, VA: Office of the Surgeon General; 1997.

10. Gleick P. Water and terrorism. *Water Policy.* 2006;8:481–503.

11. Donaghy M. Neurologists and the threat of bioterrorism. *J Neurol Sci.* 2006;249(1):55–62.

12. Penzotti JL, Fozzard HA, Lipkind GM, Dudley SC Jr. Differences in saxitoxin and tetrodotoxin binding revealed by mutagenesis of the Na⁺ channel outer vestibule. *Biophys J.* 1998;75(6):2647–2657.

13. Llewellyn LE. Sodium channel inhibiting marine toxins. *Prog Mol Subcell Biol.* 2009;46:67–97.

14. Wong M, Ruck B, Shih R, et al. Two cases of suspected saxitoxin poisoning from puffer fish ingestion. *J Toxicol Clin Toxicol.* 2002;40(5).

15. Neurologic illness associated with eating Florida pufferfish—2002. *Can Commun Dis Rep.* 2002;28(13):108–111.

16. Garcia C, del Carmen Bravo M, Lagos M, et al. Paralytic shellfish poisoning: post-mortem analysis of tissue and body fluid samples from human victims in the Patagonia fjords. *Toxicon.* 2004;43(2):149–158.

17. Andrinolo D, Michea LF, Lagos N. Toxic effects, pharmacokinetics and clearance of saxitoxin, a component of paralytic shellfish poison (PSP), in cats. *Toxicon.* 1999;37(3):447–464.

18. Stafford RG, Hines HB. Urinary elimination of saxitoxin after intravenous injection. *Toxicon.* 1995;33(11):1501–1510.

19. Bell P, Gessner B, Hall G, Mosczydlowski E. Assay of saxitoxin in samples from human victims of paralytic shellfish poisoning by binding competition to saxiphilin and block of single sodium channels. *Toxicon.* 1996;34(3):337.

20. Doucette M, Logan F, Dolah F, et al. Anlaysis of samples from a human PSP intoxication event using a saxitoxin receptor assay and HPLC. *Toxicon.* 1996;34(3):337.

20 | Sedative-Hypnotics

Laura K. Bechtel

CASE STUDY

Awoman met a male coworker in a cafe. She briefly left their meeting to use the lavatory and, when she returned, ingested an open soft drink that she had already partially consumed. Approximately 40 minutes later, she developed a feverish sensation of the entire body accompanied by progressive loss of consciousness. She was amnestic to the ensuing 7 hours and found herself in the home of the male coworker. She attempted to drive home, reported being extremely drowsy, collided with a wall approximately 7 hours after consuming the drink, and eventually returned to her home. The following day, she sought medical attention and was found to have little recollection of the 19-hour period following the consumption of the beverage. An initial urine drug screen was negative for any substance, but more extensive forensic evaluation by the police discovered 7-aminoflunitrazepam, the major metabolite of flunitrazepam, in her urine. It was later discovered that the assailant, her male coworker, had dissolved a 1-mg tablet of flunitrazepam in her soft drink while she was using the lavatory.[1]

HISTORY

The sedative-hypnotics are a diverse group of chemical classes that share similar characteristics—all have the potential to produce sedation, hypnosis, and potential anterograde amnesia (Table 20.1). These effects often rapidly incapacitate victims, and the effects can be intensified when they are willingly or involuntarily taken with another agent in the group, such as the combination of diazepam with ethanol.[2,3] Because of the sedative and amnesic properties of these drugs, victims may have no memory of what occurred following the exposure to these agents, making them susceptible to criminals. This chapter will review some of the more commonly encountered sedative-hypnotics reported to facilitate crime.

ETHANOL

The most common agent associated with crime is ethanol. For example, ethanol is commonly associated with drug-facilitated sexual assaults. Due to the prevalence of ethanol consumption by college students, numerous institutions across the United States offer health information programs focused on increasing the awareness of ethanol-associated sexual assaults.[4,5]

Clinical Effects

The clinical effects of ethanol are dose and time dependent. Ethanol metabolism is complex. Although the rate of metabolism varies from person to person due to phenotypic differences in alcohol dehydrogenase and metabolic "tolerance" in chronic drinkers, the reported average rate of metabolism is approximately 15 mL/dL/hour.[6,7] The clinical effects of ethanol intoxication include impaired judgment, incoordination, behavioral changes, ataxia, cognitive slowing, memory impairment, nausea, vomiting, diplopia, and lethargy. Depending on a person's preexisting tolerance, respiratory depression, coma, and death may occur at levels of 300–400 mg/dL. It takes little volume to intoxicate a person. To achieve levels of intoxication of 200 mg/dL requires consumption of about 100 mL of absolute ethanol in a 70-kg (154-lb.) adult. Many liquors contain 40–50% ethanol, therefore six to seven shots (30 mL/shot) of liquor in rapid succession may result in an ethanol level of 200 mg/dL.[8] Significantly lower concentrations of ethanol are required to incapacitate a smaller-framed victim or a person who voluntarily or unwillingly coingests drugs with sedative and/or psychotropic effects.

TABLE 20.1 **Samples of Sedative-Hypnotics Utilized in Criminal Poisoning**

Acetone	Barbiturates
Anticholinergics	Amobarbital (Amytal)
Antihistamines	Pentobarbital (Nembutal)
	Phenobarbital (Luminal)
Atypical benzodiazepine receptor ligands	Secobarbital (Seconal)
Zopiclone (Imovane)	Thiopental (Pentothal)
Eszopiclone (Lunesta)	Chloral hydrate
Zolpidem (Ambien)	Clonidine
Zaleplon (Sonata)	Dextromethorphan
Baclofen (Lioresal)	Ethanol
Benzodiazepines	Ethchlorvynol (Placidyl)
Alprazolam (Xanax)	Gamma-hydroxybutyrate
Chlordiazepoxide (Librium)	Kava
Clonazepam (Klonopin)	Ketamine
Clorazepate (Tranxene)	Meprobamate (Miltown)
Diazepam (Valium)	Methaqualone
Flunitrazepam (Rohypnol)	Opioids
Estazolam (ProSom)	Oxymetazoline
Flurazepam (Dalmane)	Tetrahydrozoline
Lorazepam (Ativan)	Valerian
Midazolam (Versed)	
Oxazepam (Serax)	
Temazepam (Restoril)	
Triazolam (Halcion)	

Laboratory Monitoring

Ethanol levels from urine and blood specimens are commonly evaluated in clinical, private, and state laboratories. Blood and urine ethanol is screened using enzymatic analyses (e.g., Architecht, Abbott; EMIT, by Dade-Behring). Blood alcohol and urine analysis confirmation is performed using headspace gas chromatography-flame ionization detector (GC-FID) or gas chromatography-mass spectrometry (GC-MS).[9,10] Although most clinical laboratories set the limit of detection (LOD) at 10 mg/dL, published reports document the limits of detection for ethanol using GC-FID and GC-MS as low as 1 mg/dL and 0.02 mg/dL, respectively.[7,9] "Backtracking" calculations (15 mg/dL/hour) are often performed by physicians to estimate the blood ethanol level at a given time prior to the actual time the blood sample was taken. Caution must be used with this method of reverse extrapolation because chronic ethanol abusers and heavy drinkers metabolize ethanol faster than social or naïve drinkers.[7]

CHLORAL HYDRATE

Anecdotal reports about individuals combining drugs and ethanol to assault their victims date back to the early 19th and 20th centuries. An infamous example is Mickey Finn, the proprietor of Chicago's Lone Star Saloon at the turn of the 20th century. He was alleged to have added chloral hydrate to the saloon's ethanol-based beverages to drug and rob his customers. Subsequently, chloral hydrate has become known as "Mickey Finn."

Chloral hydrate is classified as a nonbarbiturate hypnotic. It is an inexpensive transparent crystalline compound that can be easily dissolved in beverages. It was first synthesized in 1832 and was one of the original "depressants" developed for the specific purpose of inducing sleep. At therapeutic single doses, chloral hydrate has a rapid onset (30 minutes), produces minimal side effects, and is useful in alleviating sleeplessness due to pain or insomnia in a relatively short time. The abuse and misuse of this drug and the subsequent introduction of newer sedatives (i.e., barbiturates and benzodiazepines) led to its decline for medicinal purposes.

Clinical Effects

The diagnosis of chloral hydrate can be difficult to differentiate from ethanol, benzodiazepine, and barbiturate intoxication, as all share similar clinical effects. Although the exact mechanism of action of chloral hydrate has not been determined, it is a general central nervous system (CNS) depressant that has sedative effects with minimal analgesic effects when administered independently. At low doses (< 20 mg/kg), symptoms may include relaxation, dizziness, slurred speech, confusion, disorientation, euphoria, irritability, and hypersensitivity rash. At higher doses (> 50 mg/kg), chloral hydrate can cause hypotension, hypothermia, hypoventilation, tachydysrhythmias, nausea, vomiting, diarrhea, headache, and amnesia.[11] The elimination half-life ($t_{1/2}$) of chloral hydrate is 4 to 12 hours.[11,12] If coingested with ethanol, chloral hydrate metabolism may be seriously impaired. Because ethanol and chloral hydrate are both metabolized by CYP2E1 and alcohol dehydrogenase, coingestion may not only exacerbate their clinical effects but may also prolong their duration of action.[12,13]

Laboratory Monitoring

Chloral hydrate is not detected by routine, commercially available drug screens. Quantification of chloral hydrate and its metabolites trichloroethanol (TCE), TCE-glucuronide, and trichloroacetic acid (TCA) can be detected in plasma or urine using capillary gas chromatography–electron-capture detection (GC-ECD), GC-MS, or liquid chromatography-tandem mass spectrometry (LC-MS/MS).[14-16] Limit of detection for chloral hydrate is 5 ng/mL and 10 ng/mL for its metabolites using GC-ECD.[16]

BENZODIAZEPINES

Benzodiazepines are a large class of drugs that bind to specific receptor sites on gamma-amino butyric acid (GABA)-mediated receptor synapses in the brain. Benzodiazepines are thought to increase GABA-mediated chloride conduction into the postsynaptic neuron, prolonging hyperpolarization of the cell, diminishing synaptic transmission, and thereby inducing sedation. Drugs within this class vary in their affinity and efficacy at their receptor, resulting in differences in the degree of their clinical effects, time of onset, and rate of metabolism. Ultimately, with a faster rate of onset, there tends to be greater abuse potential.[17]

Flunitrazepam (Rohypnol) is a frequently reported (4% of sexual assault cases) "date rape" drug that belongs to the benzodiazepine class.[18] Flunitrazepam is a fast-acting sedative–hypnotic and categorized as a Schedule I drug by the U.S. Drug Enforcement Administration. Flunitrazepam is more potent than diazepam because of its slower dissociation from the GABA receptor.[19-21] It is rapidly absorbed and distributed into tissues upon oral administration. The onset of its sedative, amnesic, hypnotic, and disinhibitory effects can occur within 20 to 30 minutes.[19] Although the effects of flunitrazepam occur rapidly when used alone, it is often coingested with alcohol, which amplifies its effects.[22,23] Because it is still licensed for use in Europe, Asia, and Latin America for sedation and treatment of insomnia, sexual predators can acquire this drug through illegal trafficking.[24] On the street, flunitrazepam is known as roofies, forget pills, rubies, ruffies, rope, roopies, ropies, rib, R-2, roaches, papas, Mexican Valium, and circles. Sexual assault predators use flunitrazepam because it can be easily dissolved into a beverage, is relatively tasteless and odorless, will quickly incapacitate victims, and is not detected on routine drug screens. However, flunitrazepam is not the only benzodiazepine associated with crime. Other benzodiazepines have also been reported in victims of crime, such as diazepam, triazolam, temazepam, tetrazepam, clonazepam.[25-29]

Clinical Effects

Initial symptoms of benzodiazepine intoxication may include dizziness, disorientation, lack of coordination, and slurred speech—all of which mimic alcohol intoxication. Other unique effects are anterograde amnesia as early as 15 minutes after oral administration.[30] Rapid alternation of hot and cold flashes may precipitously be followed by loss of consciousness. Large doses (>2 g) have produced aspiration, muscular hypotonia, hypotension, bradycardia, coma, and death.[27,29,31,32] The clinical diagnosis of benzodiazepine intoxication can be difficult to differentiate from alcohol intoxication.

Laboratory Monitoring

Commonly marketed drug screens turn positive for most benzodiazepines, but not all (i.e., flunitrazepam and other benzodiazepines marketed outside the United States). Point-of-care testing is available for benzodiazepines, but clinical samples should be confirmed and documented using more accurate techniques (e.g., OnTrak, Roche Diagnostic Systems; Triage, Biosite).[33] Specific benzodiazepines have different time windows for detection. For example, flunitrazepam metabolites can be detected for up to 60 hours in the urine using an automated immunoassay system (e.g., EMIT II), which is categorized as a general "toxicological screen" and is available in many hospital laboratories. Flunitrazepam metabolites can be detected as early as 7 days in hair samples (using HPLC-MS/MS).[29]

ATYPICAL BENZODIAZEPINE RECEPTOR LIGANDS

Zopiclone, eszopiclone (Lunesta), zolpidem (Ambien), and zaleplon (Sonata) belong to a new generation of sedative-hypnotics that are structurally different from benzodiazepines. Like benzodiazepines, these drugs modulate the GABA-A-receptor chloride channel by binding to the benzodiazepine (BZ) receptors, otherwise known as the omega (ω_1) receptors, in the brain[34] without binding to peripheral BZ receptors.[35,36] Therefore, these drugs have significantly fewer muscle-relaxant properties.[36] The rapid-onset and amnesic properties of this class of drugs can result in disinhibition, passivity, and retrograde amnesia. These drugs require only a low dosage to cause an effect and are rapidly metabolized. Due to the amnesic properties of these drugs, victims are often confused following a criminal assault and may delay reporting the event.[18] Commonly utilized drug screens also do not test for these substances. Therefore, suspected amnesic drug use must be documented to justify more elaborate drug testing. All these characteristics make these drugs potential agents in crime.

Recognition of these new-generation sleep aids as potential agents for facilitating assault has only recently been reported in the United States, the United Kingdom, and France.[18,32,37-39]

Most of the nonbenzodiazepine sleep aids are available through a prescription as a Schedule IV drug and are readily available in North American social circles (e.g., college campuses). These highly prescribed insomnia drugs are available in a tablet form that may be crushed and dissolved into the beverage or food of an unsuspecting victim. All may produce additive CNS-depressant effects when coadministered with other psychotropic medications such as anticonvulsants, antihistamines, ethanol, and other drugs that themselves produce CNS depression.

Clinical Effects and Drug Characteristics

Zolpidem (Ambien)

Zolpidem is available as an immediate- or extended-release tablet. An average oral dose of 10–15 mg has a rapid onset of clinical symptoms between 10 and 30 minutes. Clinical effects peak at approximately 1.5 hours for immediate-release preparations. For both immediate- and extended-release preparations, duration lasts about 6 to 8 hours and the $t_{1/2}$ is approximately 2.5 hours.[40] Clinical effects may include dizziness, psychomotor dysfunction, confusion, nervousness, amnesia, and hallucinations. There is evidence of minimal respiratory depression when used as a single agent, but it may produce additive CNS-depressive effects and death when coadministered with other sedatives.[41]

Zaleplon (Sonata)

Zaleplon is available as an immediate-release tablet or capsule. An average oral dose of 10–15 mg has a rapid onset of clinical symptoms of approximately 10–30 minutes. Although the $t_{1/2}$ for zaleplon is about 1 hour, the duration of clinical effects may persist for longer than 6 hours. This may be due to the higher affinity of zaleplon for specific α_2 and α_3 subunits of the GABA receptor, unlike that seen for zolpidem or zopiclone.[42] Clinical effects may include somnolence, dizziness, psychomotor dysfunction, confusion, nervousness, rebound amnesia, and hallucinations. Higher doses (> 40–60 mg) may cause increased CNS effects and impaired motor skills.[11]

Eszopiclone (Lunesta)

The precise mechanism of action of eszopiclone is unknown, but its effect is believed to result from its interaction with GABA-A-receptor complexes at binding domains located close to or allosterically coupled to BZ receptors. An average dose of 2–3 mg has a rapid onset of clinical symptoms occurring in approximately 30 minutes. Both immediate- and extended-release preparations are available. Clinical effects include dizziness, psychomotor dysfunction, confusion, nervousness, amnesia, and hallucinations. Nausea, vomiting, and anticholinergic effects have been reported in less than 10% of patients.[43] By itself, eszopiclone has not been reported to cause respiratory depression, but it may produce additive CNS-depressant effects when coadministered with other sedatives. The clinical effects of eszopiclone are longer in duration than those of zopiclone or zolpidem, with a $t_{1/2}$ of 6 hours.[35]

Zopiclone

Zopiclone is not currently available in the United States. It is the racemic mixture of two stereoisomers; the active stereoisomer is eszopiclone. Therefore, clinical effects are similar to eszopiclone.

Laboratory Monitoring

Due to the amnesic properties of these drugs, victims often may not report their assault for several days. Therefore, sensitive analytic techniques are necessary to detect these drugs and their metabolites in urine or hair samples. Unfortunately, the drug screens found in most hospital laboratories do not detect the new generation of short-acting sleep aids called nonbenzodiazepine hypnotics. Although many private facilities are capable of detecting nonbenzodiazepine drugs, most state forensic laboratories integrate these tests into their repertoire of available "toxicology screens."[44]

KETAMINE

Ketamine (ketamine hydrochloride), an analgesic and general anesthetic, produces a rapid-acting dissociative effect. It was first synthesized in 1962 as a medical anesthetic for both humans and animals. Today ketamine is approved for use in emergency medicine, critical care, and veterinary medicine. The prosecution of a ketamine-facilitated sexual assault perpetrator in 1993 and the increase in its illicit use prompted the U.S. Drug Enforcement Administration (DEA) to restrict ketamine as a Schedule III drug in August 1999.[44] Ketamine is outlawed in the United Kingdom and classified as a Schedule I narcotic in Canada. Ketamine (Ketanest, Ketaset, and Ketalar) is available by prescription as a tablet or a parenteral solution. On the street, ketamine is sold under a variety of names including K, ket, special K, super acid, super C, spesh, vitamin K, smack K, kit-kat, keller, Barry Keddle, HOSS, the hoos, hossalar, kurdamin, kiddie, wonk, regreta, and tranq. Ketamine generally is sold illegally as a colorless and odorless liquid or as a white or off-white powder. Either liquid or powder form can be disguised in beverages. Liquid ketamine can be rapidly injected intramuscularly. Ketamine powder can even be sprinkled onto marijuana or tobacco and smoked.

Clinical Effects

The onset of action after oral ingestion can be as little as 20 minutes.[45] Its hallucinatory effects may be short-acting (< 1 hour) but so intense that the victim may have trouble discerning reality.[46] Ketamine produces effects similar to phencyclidine and dextromethorphan. The onset of clinical effects is rapid and dependent on route of administration. Anesthesia effects take as little as 20–30 seconds via intramuscular injection, 30 minutes via oral ingestion, and approximately 10 minutes via nasal insufflation.[11,47,48] The $t_{1/2}$ for ketamine is 2 to 3 hours.[49] Duration of anesthetic effects is dose dependent (usually < 1 hour), and effects on the senses, judgment, and coordination can have a longer duration (~ 6–24 hours). Ketamine can cause amnesia, dissociative anesthesia hallucinations, delirium, hypersalivation, nystagmus, impaired motor function, hypertension, and potentially fatal respiratory problems. Effects on blood pressure and respiratory depression can be significantly enhanced when coingested with alcohol.

Laboratory Monitoring

No clinical immunoassays are available to detect ketamine at this time. Ketamine and its active metabolites, norketamine and dehydronorketamine, can be detected in urine samples using GC-MS or LC-MS analyses. The limit of detection is 1 ng/mL.[50,51]

BARBITURATES

Barbiturates can produce a variety of CNS-depressant effects, ranging from mild sedation to general anesthesia. Depending on their duration of clinical effects, they are categorized as ultra-short-acting, short-acting, medium-acting, or long-acting. Barbiturates are classified as Schedule II–IV drugs, based on their rapid onset, duration, and abuse potential. They can inhibit excitatory or enhance inhibitory synaptic transmission. Barbiturates inhibit excitatory by reducing glutamate-induced depolarizations.[52] They enhance the effectiveness of GABA transmission by directly activating chloride channels and depressing synaptic transmission at virtually all synapses. Barbiturates affect the duration, not frequency, of GABA channel opening, thereby hyperpolarizing and decreasing the firing rate of neurons.[53] The slang names for these drugs are barbs, barbies, sleepers, blue bullets, nembies, pink ladies, and red devils.

Clinical Effects

Onset of clinical symptoms varies (15–40 minutes), and the degree of symptoms is dose and drug dependent. Clinical effects may consist of CNS and respiratory depression, hypothermia, bullous skin lesions, aspiration pneumonia, nystagmus, dysarthria, ataxia, drowsiness hypothermia, renal failure, muscle necrosis, hypotension, hypoglycemia, coma, and death.[11] Coingestion with alcohol and/or other CNS depressants enhances toxic effects. Duration of effects depends on the dose and the specific drug itself.

Laboratory Monitoring

Detection periods for barbiturates vary greatly depending on the specific barbiturate being used. Each barbiturate has a different half-life in the body. Ultra-short- and short-acting (thiopental, secobarbital) may only be detected in the urine for 1 to 4 days, while longer-duration barbiturates (phenobarbital) can be detected for 2 to 3 weeks. Many larger hospitals can detect most barbiturates from urine samples using an extensive toxicology screen and automated clinical immunoassay systems.[54] Detection is dependent upon the dose and half-life of the specific drug being tested. State forensic laboratories have extremely sensitive assays, such as high-performance liquid chromatography-tandem mass spectrometry (HPLC-MS/MS) and gas chromatography mass spectrometry (GC-MS), that are capable of detecting very low concentrations of barbiturates from urine and hair samples. Such tests expand the window of detection greatly.[55]

DEXTROMETHORPHAN

Dextromethorphan is sold as an over-the-counter antitussive agent alone or in combination with other cough aids (pseudoephedrine, acetaminophen, chlorpheniramine). It is the d-isomer of the potent opiate analgesic 3-methoxy-N-methylmorphine (levorphanol). Although dextromethorphan is structurally related to opioids, it is devoid of analgesic or sedative effects at therapeutic doses. Dextromethorphan is metabolized by CYP2D6 to a more potent metabolite, dextrorphan.[56,57] Dextrorphan is a stronger noncompetitive antagonist than dextromethorphan for the N-methyl-D-aspartate (NMDA) glutamate receptor.[58] These properties promote its use in treatment of neuropathic and postoperative pain management.[58-62]

Clinical Effects

Even though dextromethorphan has a strong safety profile at therapeutic concentrations, it is abused for its sedative, hallucinogenic, dissociative, and euphoric properties at high doses. Large doses can impair a victim's sensory and motor skills, as well as cause short-term memory loss, making it a potential drug for assault. Dextromethorphan is widely available over the counter in liquid, tablet, and gel capsule formulations, and it is available via the Internet in a white powder form.[63] Although liquid dextromethorphan has a reported bad taste, crystallized and powder forms can be disguised in drinks and consumed by victims. Street names for dextromethorphan are dex, DXM, tuss, robo, skittles, triple-C, and syrup.

Despite the safety of dextromethorphan when used at the recommended dosage (< 120 mg/day), higher doses can result in nausea, vomiting, seizure, loss of consciousness, irregular heartbeat, and death.[64,65] Serotonin syndrome may develop in patients on other serotonergic drugs, due to additive inhibition of serotonin reuptake by dextromethorphan.[66] Patients with genetic variations in CYP2D6, causing rapid metabolism of dextromethorphan, may present with greater clinical effects.[67-69]

Laboratory Monitoring

Analysis of blood or urine dextromethorphan levels is not typically performed in healthcare settings. Therapeutic doses of dextromethorphan do not cross-react with most clinically available immunoassays for opioid compounds. Detection and confirmation protocols for dextromethorphan are available using GC-MS.

ANTIHISTAMINES

Antihistamines are typically used in the treatment of allergies or insomnia. First-generation antihistamines (diphenhydramine, chlorpheniramine) readily cross the blood–brain barrier, producing greater CNS effects than second-generation antihistamines (fexofenadine). First-generation antihistamines are agonists of both central and peripheral histamine (H1 and H2) receptors but are still widely used because they are effective and inexpensive.[70] Few cases have documented the use of diphenhydramine in assaults.[71]

Clinical Effects

First-generation antihistamines can cause CNS depression and anticholinergic symptoms such as sedation, hallucinations, confusion, agitation, and psychosis. Onset of action is 15–60 minutes, and clinical symptoms typically last 4 to 6 hours.[72] Large doses can exacerbate these effects and can even result in cardiotoxicity, coma, and seizures.[73] Coingestion with alcohol or other sedative–hypnotic drugs may increase some or all of these clinical symptoms. Victims may have difficulty distinguishing events of an assault due to the anticholinergic effects of the drugs. Therefore, a victim may not present for hours or days after the assault due to the clinical effects of the drugs themselves.

Laboratory Monitoring

Analysis of blood or urine antihistamine levels is not typically performed in the healthcare setting. Because these nonprescription drugs are commonly used by the public, interpretation of a "positive" test result is problematic. Most antihistamines are detected using GC-MS. Urine specimens are sufficient for the highly specific GC-MS and LC-MS/MS analyses.[14,74]

CONCLUSIONS

Numerous agents are used to incapacitate a victim. The presence of ethanol or a positive routine drug screen in a victim does not exclude the potential presence of another drug. In addition, a negative routine drug screen does not exclude all potential agents that are used by criminals to incapacitate victims. It is imperative for healthcare and law enforcement personnel to clearly document the history as well as the presenting clinical effects to help laboratory personnel hone in on the agent used in a crime, which will in turn help to identify and prosecute the offender(s).

REFERENCES

1. Ohshima T. A case of drug-facilitated sexual assault by the use of flunitrazepam. *J Clin Forensic Med.* 2006;13(1):44–45.

2. Kintz P, Villain M, Cirimele V. Chemical abuse in the elderly: evidence from hair analysis. *Ther Drug Monit.* 2008;30(2):207–211.

3. Kintz P, Villain M, Ludes B. Testing for the undetectable in drug-facilitated sexual assault using hair analyzed by tandem mass spectrometry as evidence. *Ther Drug Monit.* 2004;26(2):211–214.

4. Mohler-Kuo M, Dowdall GW, Koss MP, Wechsler H. Correlates of rape while intoxicated in a national sample of college women. *J Stud Alcohol.* 2004;65(1):37–45.

5. Cole TB. Rape at US colleges often fueled by alcohol. *JAMA.* 2006;296(5):504–505.

6. Holford NH. Clinical pharmacokinetics of ethanol. *Clin Pharmacokinet.* 1987;13(5):273–292.

7. Smith GD, Shaw LJ, Maini PK, et al. Mathematical modeling of ethanol metabolism in normal subjects and chronic alcohol misusers. *Alcohol.* 1993;28(1):25–32.

8. Taylor P. The time course of drug action. In: Pratt WB, ed. *Principles of Drug Action.* 3rd ed. Philadelphia: Churchill Livingstone; 1990.

9. Wasfi IA, Al-Awadhi AH, Al-Hatali ZN, et al. Rapid and sensitive static headspace gas chromatography-mass spectrometry method for the analysis of ethanol and abused inhalants in blood. *J Chromatogr B Analyt Technol Biomed Life Sci.* 2004;799(2):331–336.

10. Macchia T, Mancinelli R, Gentili S, et al. Ethanol in biological fluids: headspace GC measurement. *J Anal Toxicol.* 1995;19(4):241–246.

11. Rumack B, Toll L, Gelman C. Micromedex healthcare series. In: *Thomson. Healthcare.* Vol 129. Englewood CO: Micromedex, Inc; 2006.

12. Breimer DD. Clinical pharmacokinetics of hypnotics. *Clin Pharmacokinet.* 1977;2(2):93–109.

13. Ni YC, Wong TY, Lloyd RV, et al. Mouse liver microsomal metabolism of chloral hydrate, trichloroacetic acid, and trichloroethanol leading to induction of lipid peroxidation via a free radical mechanism. *Drug Metab Dispos.* 1996;24(1):81–90.

14. Miyaguchi H, Kuwayama K, Tsujikawa K, et al. A method for screening for various sedative-hypnotics in serum by liquid chromatography/single quadrupole mass spectrometry. *Forensic Sci Int.* 2006;157(1):57–70.

15. Schmitt TC. Determination of chloral hydrate and its metabolites in blood plasma by capillary gas chromatography with electron capture detection. *J Chromatogr B Analyt Technol Biomed Life Sci.* 2002;780(2):217–224. .

16. Humbert L, Jacquemont MC, Leroy E, Leclerc F, Houdret N, Lhermitte M. Determination of chloral hydrate and its metabolites (trichloroethanol and trichloracetic acid) in human plasma and urine using electron capture gas chromatography. *Biomed Chromatogr.* 1994;8(6):273–277.

17. Roset PN, Farre M, de la Torre R, et al. Modulation of rate of onset and intensity of drug effects reduces abuse potential in healthy males. *Drug Alcohol Depend.* 2001;64(3):285–298.

18. ElSohly MA, Salamone SJ. Prevalence of drugs used in cases of alleged sexual assault. *J Anal Toxicol.* 1999;23(3):141–146.

19. Mattila MA, Larni HM. Flunitrazepam: a review of its pharmacological properties and therapeutic use. *Drugs.* 1980;20(5):353–374.

20. Chiu TH, Rosenberg HC. Comparison of the kinetics of [3H]diazepam and [3H]flunitrazepam binding to cortical synaptosomal membranes. *J Neurochem.* 1982;39(6):1716–1725.

21. Mattila MA, Säilä K, Kokko T, et al. Comparison of diazepam and flunitrazepam as adjuncts to general anaesthesia in preventing arousal following surgical stimuli. *Br J Anaesth.* 1979;51(4):329–337.

22. Seppala T, Nuotto E, Dreyfus JF. Drug-alcohol interactions on psychomotor skills: zopiclone and flunitrazepam. *Pharmacology.* 1983;27(Suppl 2):127–135.

23. Drummer OH, Syrjanen ML, Cordner SM. Deaths involving the benzodiazepine flunitrazepam. *Am J Forensic Med Pathol.* 1993;14(3):238–243.

24. Waltzman ML. Flunitrazepam: a review of "roofies." *Pediatr Emerg Care.* 1999;15(1):59–60.

25. Joynt BP. Triazolam blood concentrations in forensic cases in Canada. *J Anal Toxicol.* 1993;17(3):171–177.

26. Negrusz A, Gaensslen RE. Analytical developments in toxicological investigation of drug-facilitated sexual assault. *Anal Bioanal Chem.* 2003;376(8): 1192–1197.

27. Marc B, Baudry F, Vaquero P, et al. Sexual assault under benzodiazepine submission in a Paris suburb. *Arch Gynecol Obstet.* 2000;263(4):193–197.

28. Adamowicz P, Kala M. Date-rape drugs scene in Poland. *Przegl Lek.* 2005;62(6):572–575.

29. Cheze M, Duffort G, Deveaux M, et al. Hair analysis by liquid chromatography-tandem mass spectrometry in toxicological investigation of drug-facilitated crimes: report of 128 cases over the period June 2003-May 2004 in metropolitan Paris. *Forensic Sci Int.* 2005;153(1):3–10.

30. Goulle JP, Anger JP. Drug-facilitated robbery or sexual assault: problems associated with amnesia. *Ther Drug Monit.* 2004;26(2):206–210.

31. Kintz P, Villain M, Dumestre-Toulet V, et al. Drug-facilitated sexual assault and analytical toxicology: the role of LC-MS/MS. A case involving zolpidem. *J Clin Forensic Med.* 2005;12(1):36–41.

32. Scott-Ham M, Burton FC. Toxicological findings in cases of alleged drug-facilitated sexual assault in the United Kingdom over a 3-year period. *J Clin Forensic Med.* 2005;12(4):175–186.

33. Mastrovitch TA, Bithoney WG, DeBari VA, et al. Point-of-care testing for drugs of abuse in an urban emergency department. *Ann Clin Lab Sci.* 2002;32(4):383–386.

34. Wagner J, Wagner ML, Hening WA. Beyond benzodiazepines: alternative pharmacologic agents for the treatment of insomnia. *Ann Pharmacother.* 1998;32(6):680–691.

35. Sanna E, Busonero F, Talani G, et al. Comparison of the effects of zaleplon, zolpidem, and triazolam at various GABA(A) receptor subtypes. *Eur J Pharmacol.* 2002;451(2):103–110.

36. Lunesta [product information]. Marlborough, MA: Sepracor; 2005.

37. Hindmarch I, ElSohly M, Gambles J, et al. Forensic urinalysis of drug use in cases of alleged sexual assault. *J Clin Forensic Med.* 2001;8(4):197–205.

38. Anderson IB, Kim SY, Dyer JE, et al. Trends in gamma-hydroxybutyrate (GHB) and related drug intoxication: 1999 to 2003. *Ann Emerg Med.* 2006;47(2):177–183.

39. Goulle JP, Cheze M, Pepin G. Determination of endogenous levels of GHB in human hair. Are there possibilities for the identification of GHB administration through hair analysis in cases of drug-facilitated sexual assault? *J Anal Toxicol.* 2003;27(8):574–580.

40. Ambien CR, zolpidem tartrate extended-release tablets [product information]. New York, NY: Sanofi-Synthelabo Inc; 2005.

41. Gock SB, Wong SH, Nuwayhid N, et al. Acute zolpidem overdose—report of two cases. *J Anal Toxicol.* 1999;23(6):559–562.

42. George CF. Pyrazolopyrimidines. *Lancet.* 2001;358(9293):1623–1626.

43. LUNESTA, eszopiclone tablets [product information]. Marlborough, MA: Sepracor Inc; 2004.

44. Woodworth T. DEA Congressional Testimony. House Commerce Committee Subcommittee on Oversight and Investigations; 1999.

45. Green SM, Johnson NE. Ketamine sedation for pediatric procedures: part 2, review and implications. *Ann Emerg Med.* 1990;19(9):1033–1046.

46. Smith KM. Drugs used in acquaintance rape. *J Am Pharm Assoc* (Washington). 1999;39(4):519–525; quiz 581–513.

47. Hersack RA. Ketamine's psychological effects do not contraindicate its use based on a patient's occupation. *Aviat Space Environ Med.* 1994;65(11):1041–1046.

48. Louon A, Lithander J, Reddy VG, et al. Sedation with nasal ketamine and midazolam for cryotherapy in retinopathy of prematurity. *Br J Ophthalmol.* 1993;77(8):529–530.

49. Clements JA, Nimmo WS, Grant IS. Bioavailability, pharmacokinetics, and analgesic activity of ketamine in humans. *J Pharm Sci.* 1982;71(5):539–542.

50. Moore KA, Sklerov J, Levine B, et al. Urine concentrations of ketamine and norketamine following illegal consumption. *J Anal Toxicol.* 2001;25(7):583–588.

51. Anonymous. An overview of club drugs. Drug Intelligence Brief. Drug Inforcement Admnistration, February, 2000: 1–10.

52. Macdonald RL, McLean MJ. Cellular bases of barbiturate and phenytoin anticonvulsant drug action. *Epilepsia.* 1982;23:S7–S18.

53. Gilman A. *The Pharmacological Basis of Therapeutics.* 9th ed. New York: McGraw-Hill; 2002.

54. Schwenzer KS, Pearlman R, Tsilimidos M, et al. New fluorescence polarization immunoassays for analysis of barbiturates and benzodiazepines in serum and urine: performance characteristics. *J Anal Toxicol.* 2000;24(8):726–732.

55. Frison G, Favretto D, Tedeschi L, et al. Detection of thiopental and pentobarbital in head and pubic hair in a case of drug-facilitated sexual assault. *Forensic Sci Int.* 2003;133(1-2):171–174.

56. Kupfer A, Schmid B, Pfaff G. Pharmacogenetics of dextromethorphan O-demethylation in man. *Xenobiotica.* 1986;16(5):421–433.

57. Motassim N, Decolin D, Le Dinh T, et al. Direct determination of dextromethorphan and its three metabolites in urine by high-performance liquid chromatography using a precolumn switching system for sample clean-up. *J Chromatogr.* 1987;422:340–345.

58. Palmer GC. Neuroprotection by NMDA receptor antagonists in a variety of neuropathologies. *Curr Drug Targets.* 2001;2(3):241–271.

59. Price DD, Mao J, Frenk H, et al. The N-methyl-D-aspartate receptor antagonist dextromethorphan selectively reduces temporal summation of second pain in man. *Pain.* 1994;59(2):165–174.

60. Hughes AM, Rhodes J, Fisher G, et al. Assessment of the effect of dextromethorphan and ketamine on the acute nociceptive threshold and wind-up of the second pain response in healthy male volunteers. *Br J Clin Pharmacol.* 2002;53(6):604–612.

61. Ilkjaer S, Bach LF, Nielsen PA, et al. Effect of preoperative oral dextromethorphan on immediate and late postoperative pain and hyperalgesia after total abdominal hysterectomy. *Pain.* 2000;86(1-2):19–24.

62. Sindrup SH, Jensen TS. Pharmacologic treatment of pain in polyneuropathy. *Neurology.* 2000;55(7):915–920.

63. Schwartz RH. Adolescent abuse of dextromethorphan. *Clin Pediatr* (Philadelphia). 2005;44(7):565–568.

64. Hanzlick R. National Association of Medical Examiners Pediatric Toxicology (PedTox) Registry Report 3. Case submission summary and data for acetaminophen, benzene, carboxyhemoglobin, dextromethorphan, ethanol, phenobarbital, and pseudoephedrine. *Am J Forensic Med Pathol.* 1995;16(4):270–277.

65. Carlsson KC, Hoem NO, Moberg ER, et al. Analgesic effect of dextromethorphan in neuropathic pain. *Acta Anaesthesiol Scand.* 2004;48(3):328–336.

66. Navarro A, Perry C, Bobo WV. A case of serotonin syndrome precipitated by abuse of the anticough remedy dextromethorphan in a bipolar patient treated with fluoxetine and lithium. *Gen Hosp Psychiatry.* 2006;28(1):78–80.

67. Li L, Pan RM, Porter TD, et al. New cytochrome P450 2D6*56 allele identified by genotype/phenotype analysis of cryopreserved human hepatocytes. *Drug Metab Dispos.* 2006;34(8):1411–1416.

68. Chen SQ, Cai WM, Wedlund PJ. [Distinguishing CYP2D6 homozygous and heterozygous extensive metabolizers by dextromethorphan phenotyping]. *Yao Xue Xue Bao.* 1997;32(12):924–927.

69. Manaboriboon B, Chomchai C. Dextromethorphan abuse in Thai adolescents: a report of two cases and review of literature. *J Med Assoc Thai.* 2005;88:S242–S245.

70. Tomassoni AJ, Weisman RS. Antihistamines and decongestants. In: Goldfrank L, Hoffman R, Lewin N, Flomenbaum N, Howland M, Nelson L, eds. *Goldfrank's Toxicologic Emergencies.* 8th ed. New York: McGraw-Hill; 2006.

71. Dyer JaK, SY. Drug facilitated sexual assault: a review of 24 incidents. *J Toxicol Clin Toxicol.* 2004;42(4):519.

72. Albert KS, Hallmark MR, Sakmar E, et al. Pharmacokinetics of diphenhydramine in man. *J Pharmacokinet Biopharm.* 1975;3(3):159–170.

73. Sharma AN, Hexdall AH, Chang EK, et al. Diphenhydramine-induced wide complex dysrhythmia responds to treatment with sodium bicarbonate. *Am J Emerg Med.* 2003;21(3):212–215.

74. Hasegawa C, Kumazawa T, Lee XP, et al. Simultaneous determination of ten antihistamine drugs in human plasma using pipette tip solid-phase extraction and gas chromatography/mass spectrometry. *Rapid Commun Mass Spectrom.* 2006;20(4):537–543.

21 | Sodium Monofluoroacetate

Christopher P. Holstege

CASE STUDY

A healthy 47-year-old man with no known medical problems sustained a tonic clonic seizure. He presented to the local hospital with agitation, obtundation, and acidosis (pH 7.3, pCO_2 29 mm Hg, pO_2 92 mm Hg, bicarbonate 14 mEq/L, anion gap 24 mEq/L). His initial serum creatinine was 2 mg/dL. The urine drug screen was only positive for benzodiazepines that were given by the hospital to control his seizures. His toxic alcohol levels were not detectable. At 30 hours postarrival, the patient only responded to noxious stimuli, his head computed axial tomography scan was unremarkable, and electroencephalography showed diffuse slowing. During his stay, he developed hypocalcemia, with a serum ionized calcium level of 3.2 mg/dL (normal is 4.5–5.6 mg/dL), and hypokalemia, with a serum potassium level of 3.0 mEq/L (normal is 3.5–5 mEq/L). It was later discovered that he ingested Compound 1080 (sodium monofluoroacetate). Two days after arrival, he recovered fully and was discharged.[1]

HISTORY

Sodium monofluoroacetate (SMFA) is both chemically and toxicologically identical to the fluoroacetate found in certain poisonous plants found in Australia, South Africa, and South America.[2,3] SMFA is also known as "1080," referring to SMFA's catalogue number, which became its brand name. SMFA was discovered by German military chemists during World War II.[4] President Nixon banned the poison in the United States in 1972, but the Reagan administration re-authorized its use in the mid-1980s for livestock protection collars.[3] SMFA is manufactured by one U.S. company: Tull Chemical Co. in Oxford, Alabama. Tull Chemical has been manufacturing the poison since 1956.[5] Much of Tull's 1080 is exported to other countries such as New Zealand, Mexico, Israel, and Australia for pest control. Accidental cases of ingestion of SMFA are rare but have occurred.[6] Also rare are cases of intentional (suicidal) ingestion.[1] There are no official reports that document the use of 1080 in a criminal manner.[7]

In November 2004, Rep. Peter DeFazio (D-OR) asked the Department of Homeland Security to halt production and use of Compound 1080 due to its potential as a terrorism agent.[8] In May 2005, a U.S. report was released that included a photograph (taken in May 2003) of a Tull 1080 can recovered by coalition troops in Iraq.[5] The FBI, U.S. Air Force, Canadian Security Intelligence Service, and U.S. Homeland Security publicly list 1080 as a poison that terrorists could potentially use to contaminate public water supplies. In December 2005, Rep. DeFazio introduced a bill "to prohibit the manufacture, processing, possession, or distribution in commerce of the poison sodium fluoroacetate," as well as to destroy existing stores of the poison.[9] On December 18, 2007, the Compound 1080 and M-44 Elimination Act was introduced to emend the Toxic Substances Control Act to prohibit the manufacture, processing, possession, or distribution in commerce of sodium fluoroacetate. This act has been referred to the Subcommittee on Horticulture and Organic Agriculture before being voted upon by the House.

POTENTIAL DELIVERY METHODS

The synthetic form of SMFA (CAS No. 62-74-8) exists as a white powder (similar in appearance to flour or powdered sugar) that remains stable. It is odorless, tasteless, and readily dissolves into water.[2] When present in natural water sources, it degrades within 7 days due to its metabolism by microorganisms within those environments. In water devoid of microorganisms, SMFA appears to remain stable.[10] It is relatively insoluble in organic solvents such as ethanol or vegetable oils.[1] The only reported distinguishing characteristic is that it has a weak vinegar taste when mixed with water.[1] It is heat stable; it does not decompose until temperatures approach 200°C (392°F). SMFA is highly toxic to vertebrates, although the sensitivity of different species varies dramatically. In man, the estimated lethal poisoning dose (LD_{50}) ranges from 2 to 5 mg/kg body weight.[1]

Compound 1080 is well absorbed from the gastrointestinal tract, the respiratory tract, open wounds, mucous membranes, and ocular exposure.[2] The majority of human exposures reported in the medical literature have been through ingestion. Toxicity has been reported to be the same whether it is administered orally, subcutaneously, intramuscularly, or intravenously.[2] Dusts containing SMFA are effectively toxic by inhalation.[2]

TOXICOLOGIC MECHANISMS

The toxicologic mechanism of SMFA involves disruption of cellular energy production, resulting in multisystem organ failure.[11] The parent compound, fluoroacetate, has very low cellular toxicity. Once ingested and absorbed, however, enzymatic reactions within cells convert fluoroacetate to fluoroacetyl-CoA. Fluoroacetyl-CoA, in the presence of oxaloacetate, is converted by citrate synthase to fluorocitrate, a potent inhibitor of the enzyme aconitase.[11] Aconitase catalyzes the reversible Krebs cycle reaction, converting citrate to isocitrate. The inhibition of aconitase results in the interruption of the energy-producing Krebs cycle and the buildup of citrate. Fluorocitrate also inhibits transport of citrate in and out of mitochondria, contributing to the buildup of citrate. Elevated citrate levels disrupt energy production via glycolysis, by inhibiting the enzyme phosphofructokinase. Elevated citrate levels may also cause life-threatening hypocalcemia. Because it takes time for the metabolic conversion of fluoroacetate to fluorocitrate, there is a delay from the time the poison is ingested to the initial onset of signs and symptoms.[12]

CLINICAL EFFECTS

Clinical signs and symptoms associated with SMFA poisoning are nonspecific. SMFA poisoning is characterized by a latent period of 30 minutes to 3 hours following the administration of the compound by any route.[12,13] Delayed onset of symptoms, however, has been reported up to 20 hours.[1] Even massive doses do not elicit immediate responses, although the latent period may be reduced. In animal studies, the early stages of poisoning are typically reported to include lethargy, vomiting, trembling, excessive salivation, incontinence, muscular weakness, disorientation, hypersensitivity to nervous stimuli, and respiratory distress. Early neurologic signs include muscular twitches often affecting the face, such as nystagmus and blepharospasm. These reactions progress to generalized seizures, initially tonic and becoming cyclically tonic-clonic with periods of lucidity between seizures.[13] Partial paralysis may occur, lasting prolonged time periods. Death typically results from depression of the respiratory center, cardiovascular failure, and/or ventricular fibrillation.[13,14] On autopsy, there are no characteristic lesions associated with SMFA poisoning.[2]

Numerous human reports exist in the literature. Trabes et al., for example, described a 15-year-old who attempted suicide by ingesting SMFA.[13] She developed nausea, vomiting, and abdominal pain within 30 minutes of ingestion followed by a grand mal seizure 1 hour later with associated tachycardia (150 beats per minute) and profuse diaphoresis. She was described as disorientated, demonstrated signs of psychomotor agitation, and over the ensuing 4 hours had three additional grand mal seizures before becoming comatose. Her cerebral spinal fluid was unremarkable, with normal opening pressures. She recovered but developed a chronic cerebellar ataxia and computerized tomography findings of moderate diffuse brain atrophy.

Reigart et al. described an 8-month-old who developed two episodes of nausea and vomiting after ingesting SMFA but was otherwise asymptomatic.[15] The child abruptly developed seizures 20 hours postingestion.

Chi et al. described two cases of SMFA intoxication.[16] The first involved a 26-year-old woman who attempted suicide by swallowing 32 mL of 1% SMFA solution. She initially developed nausea and vomiting and, upon presentation, was found to have a blood pressure of 80/40 mm Hg, respiratory rate of 32 breaths per minute, and a pulse of 120 beats per minute. Her initial labs were significant for a plasma creatinine of 1.8 mg/dL, potassium of 3.3 mmol/L, alanine aminotransferase 124 U/L, and blood sugar of 248 mg/dL. Her initial arterial blood gas revealed: pH 7.342, pCO_2 32.1 mm Hg, pO_2 74.4 mm Hg, HCO_3^- 17.4, and base excess −7.2 on 40% oxygen. She developed progressive metabolic acidosis and subsequent hypotension and respiratory failure. She expired 48 hours after exposure. In the second case, a 62-year-old woman presented 1 hour after ingestion of 16 mL of 1% SMFA solution. She immediately suffered nausea and vomiting. Her initial vitals signs were blood pressure 167/78 mm Hg, respiratory rate 19 breaths per minute, and pulse 120 beats per minute. Her initial labs were significant for a plasma creatinine of 1.0 mg/dL, potassium of 2.8 mmol/L, alanine aminotransferase 65 U/L, and blood sugar of 478 mg/dL. Her initial arterial blood gas revealed: pH 7.296, pCO_2 39.5 mm Hg, pO_2 123 mm Hg, HCO_3^- 19.4, and base excess −6.0 on 28% oxygen. She developed progressive metabolic acidosis, hypotension, respiratory failure, and gastrointestinal bleeding, but she survived and was discharged without sequelae 21 days after ingestion.

In a retrospective study of 38 human cases of SMFA poisoning, Chi et al. noted the most frequent symptom to be nausea and/or vomiting (74%).[6] Electrocardiograph changes were quite variable, ranging from mild nonspecific ST and T-wave abnormalities (72%), to ventricular tachycardias and asystole. The most common electrolyte abnormalities were hypocalcemia (42%) and hypokalemia (65%). Seven of the 38 patients died in this series (18%). Discriminate analysis identified hypotension, increased serum creatinine, and decreased pH as the most important predictors of mortality, with sensitivity of 86% and specificity of 96%.

There is no specific antidote for SMFA toxicity, and therapy is primarily focused on supportive care. A number of different treatments have been explored for SMFA toxicity. Because SMFA induces hypocalcemia, calcium supplementation through administration of either calcium gluconate or calcium chloride has been shown to be of benefit.[18,19]

ANALYTIC DETECTION

The Centers for Disease Control and Prevention (CDC) has created a multilevel laboratory response network (LRN) to provide surge capacity testing for exposure to chemical or biologic terrorist agents. The LRN links 126 clinical laboratories to public health agencies in all states by providing state-of-the-art facilities that can analyze potential biologic and chemical terrorist agents. At the onset of an event, state laboratories are capable of performing some initial testing. More specialized analyses from one of the seven CDC-funded level 1 facilities may be required. Furthermore, the CDC may directly employ a "rapid toxic screen" to analyze human blood and urine samples for a large number of potential terrorist agents. If medical personnel suspect patient exposure to a chemical or biologic terrorist agent, the healthcare team should immediately contact their respective state or local health department. Chemical detection methods are currently utilized to detect SMFA in human blood specimens. Derivatized extracts are analyzed using gas chromatography-mass spectrometry (GC-MS) or gas chromatography with electron-capture detection. Because the exact mechanism for SMFA metabolism has not been elucidated, blood specimens should be immediately collected and stored at 4°C (39.2°F) in suspected cases.

CONCLUSION

SMFA is a potent toxin. Its physical characteristics (stability, lack of odor and taste, and ease of solubility into water) make it a marked threat as an agent of criminal poisoning. Diagnosing a surreptitious poisoning would be difficult. A victim of SMFA poisoning may present with seizures, progressive renal failure, marked acidosis resistant to therapy, and electrolyte abnormalities consisting of hypocalcemia and hypokalemia.

REFERENCES

1. Robinson RF, Griffith JR, Wolowich WR, et al. Intoxication with sodium monofluoroacetate (compound 1080). *Vet Hum Toxicol.* 2002;44(2):93–95.
2. Egekeze JO, Oehme FW. Sodium monofluoroacetate (SMFA, compound 1080): a literature review. *Vet Hum Toxicol.* 1979;21(6):411–416.
3. Eason C. Sodium monofluoroacetate (1080) risk assessment and risk communication. *Toxicology.* 2002;181–182:523–530.
4. Abraham K. Defazio bill bans poison. *The Eugene Weekly.* January 12, 2006.
5. Milstein M. Iraq's tests of coyote poison surface. *The Oregonian.* May 28, 2005.
6. Chi CH, Chen KW, Chan SH, et al. Clinical presentation and prognostic factors in sodium monofluoroacetate intoxication. *J Toxicol Clin Toxicol.* 1996;34(6):707–712.
7. Holstege CP, Bechtel LK, Reilly TH, et al. Unusual but potential agents of terrorists. *Emerg Med Clin North Am.* 2007;25(2):549–566; abstract xi.
8. Milstein M. Wolf poison raises alarms about its terrorism potential. *The Oregonian.* November 3, 2004.
9. De Fazio P. Sodium Fluoroacetate Elimination Act. In: Congress US, ed. Vol 109th; 2005:H.R. 4567.
10. Booth LH, Ogilvie SC, Wright GR, et al. Degradation of sodium monofluoroacetate (1080) and fluorocitrate in water. *Bull Environ Contam Toxicol.* 1999;62(1):34–39.
11. Twigg LE, Mead RJ, King DR. Metabolism of fluoroacetate in the skink (*Tiliqua rugosa*) and the rat (*Rattus norvegicus*). *Aust J Biol Sci.* 1986;39(1):1–15.
12. Sherley M. The traditional categories of fluoroacetate poisoning signs and symptoms belie substantial underlying similarities. *Toxicol Lett.* 2004;151(3):399–406.
13. Trabes J, Rason N, Avrahami E. Computed tomography demonstration of brain damage due to acute sodium monofluoroacetate poisoning. *J Toxicol Clin Toxicol.* 1983;20(1):85–92.
14. Ando J, Shiozu K, Kawasaki H. A selective blockade of the cardiac inotropic effect of adrenaline by sodium monofluoroacetate. *Bull Osaka Med Sch.* 1966;12(1):1–4.
15. Reigart JR, Brueggeman JL, Keil JE. Sodium fluoroacetate poisoning. *Am J Dis Child* 1975; 129(10): 1224–6.
16. Chi CH, Lin TK, Chen KW. Hemodynamic abnormalities in sodium monofluoroacetate intoxication. *Hum Exp Toxicol.* 1999;18(6):351–353.
17. Omara F, Sisodia CS. Evaluation of potential antidotes for sodium fluoroacetate in mice. *Vet Hum Toxicol.* 1990;32(5):427–431.
18. Taitelman U, Roy A, Raikhlin-Eisenkraft B, Hoffer E. The effect of monoacetin and calcium chloride on acid-base balance and survival in experimental sodium fluoroacetate poisoning. *Arch Toxicol Suppl.* 1983;6:222–227.

22 | Strychnine

Gerald F. O'Malley and Kelli D. O'Donnell

CASE STUDY

A 51-year-old minister, S. A. Berrie, had been married to Fannie Berrie for 29 years. Mr. Berrie was cheating on her and, unbeknownst to her, wanted out of the marriage. On a particular Sunday, Mrs. Berrie went to Sunday school and then returned to her home, drank a cup of coffee, ate no lunch, and took an aspirin capsule, which was her habit. Mrs. Berrie went back to church later in the day but became ill. She was taken home where she began having convulsions at various intervals until her death 30 hours later.[1]

In the months preceding Mrs. Berrie's death, Mr. Berrie had been spending much of his time with his 17-year-old secretary, Miss Bright. He became infatuated with her, writing her suggestive poems and letters. Mrs. Berrie objected to Miss Bright working in the home, so Mr. Berrie took Miss Bright to cafés and hotels, renting rooms under an assumed name. Mr. Berrie and Miss Bright talked about his getting a divorce so they could be married.[1]

Fifty-nine days after his wife's death, Mr. Berrie and Miss Bright were married, raising suspicion about the unusual circumstances of Mrs. Berrie's death. Mrs. Berrie's body was exhumed, and the presence of postmortem strychnine was found via chemical tests for poisons in vital organs. It was also noted that a ring that had previously been removed from her finger was being worn by the new, younger Mrs. Berrie. Mr. Berrie provided false and contradictory statements to the police and to the district attorney. Several weeks after his wife's death, he claimed to have found a suicide note written by her embedded in the pages of his Bible. An investigation, however, conclusively determined the handwriting was not hers.[1]

Testimony from Dr. Rafter, one of the doctors who attended to Mrs. Berrie during the last agonizing 30 hours of her life, strongly suggested that she died from strychnine poisoning. He reported that she appeared apprehensive and that "she was thrown into convulsions by the least noise, the least touch, as by attempting to take off her underclothing, the creak of the stair, the whistling of a train, the touch of her grandchild; that she was conscious during and between convulsions and with her pupils dilated."[1]

Mr. Berrie was convicted of murder, and on appeal, the conviction was upheld.[1]

HISTORY

Strychnine is an alkaloid developed from the seeds and fruit of *Strychnos nux-vomica* and other members of the family *Loganiaceae,* an evergreen tree native to India, Ceylon, and other parts of Southeast Asia and northern Australia. The seeds were first described by Valerius Cordus during the 16th century and are mentioned in Langham's *The Garden of Health* (1578). In *The Herbal* (1597), Gerard also wrote about the drug and sketched the plant and seeds. *Nux vomica* was first used as a rodenticide in the 16th century; it continued to be used as such and was sold as a grey powder in British apothecaries at the beginning of the 19th century for eightpence per ounce.[2-4]

In 1818, Pelletier and Caventou derived strychnine from the St. Ignatius bean (*Ignatia Amara,* another tree of the order *Loganiaceae*).[5] Extract and tincture of strychnine were introduced to the United States Pharmacopeia of 1820; it was produced by Parke-Davis and Mallinckrodt and

sold under several names, including Wampole's preparation (a tonic and stimulant with 0.0125 grams of strychnine per tablespoonful), Easton's syrup, and Aitkin's syrup.[6] In the United States, doctors used strychnine to treat epilepsy, amenorrhea, ague, dysentery, and rheumatism, "beginning with a sixth of a grain, and increasing the dose gradually every other day till muscular twitches are produced."[6] The dosage for medical use was cited as between "1/60th grain [and] 1/10th grain," which is between 1.1 mg and 6.4 mg in modern measures. At that time, lethal dose was cited as half a grain (32 mg), but people have been known to die from as little as 5 mg of strychnine.[7] The U.S. Centers for Disease Control and Prevention quantify the dose of strychnine that is "immediately dangerous to life and health" as 30 mg.

Strychnine ceased to be used as a tonic in the early 20th century. Instead, it was widely used as a rodenticide until 1978 when the U.S. Environmental Protection Agency restricted the use of products containing strychnine in concentrations greater than 0.50% to certified applicators.[8]

POTENTIAL DELIVERY METHODS

Strychnine is most commonly found in the powdered crystalline form, and 1 gram is easily dissolved in 6400 mL of water or 220 mL of alcohol.[7] Because of its bitter taste, strychnine is detectable in food in very low concentrations, making it difficult but not impossible to disguise in food or beverages.[9,10] It has a neutral pH and can be administered through intravenous or intramuscular injection, rubbed on the mucous membranes, or delivered in powder form through inhalation. All routes of exposure result in the development of symptoms, although dermal application typically requires higher dosages.

Strychnine has been implicated in numerous criminal cases.[11-16] There have been cases in which strychnine has been deliberately added to street drugs such as LSD, heroin, and cocaine.[17] It has also been implicated in tainted pharmaceutical and herbal products.[18]

TOXICOLOGIC MECHANISMS

Strychnine alkaloid is derived from the seeds of the *Nux vomica* through a relatively simple extraction using chloroform and sulfuric acid to digest and solubilize the plant material followed by distilled water, ammonia, and sodium hydroxide to raise the pH of the solution.[7] Strychnine sulfate is most often encountered as a translucent or white crystalline powder with a melting point of 268–290°C (514–554°F), depending on the speed of heating.[19] It is odorless and has a bitter metallic taste. Several case reports describe elimination after overdose as following first-order kinetic principles; the elimination half-life of strychnine is 10–16 hours.[20-23]

The principal effect of strychnine in the body is the promotion of muscle spasms. Strychnine interferes with glycine-dependent inhibition of neural transmission at the level of the spinal cord. This interference results in unopposed spinal cord stimulation via reflex arcs and inability to stop muscle contractions once they start.[19,24,25]

Control of muscle contraction and relaxation depends on a fine balance between promotion of stimulatory signals from the brain to the muscles through reflex arcs in the spinal cord and inhibition of those signals. Glycine is an amino acid with unique chemical properties, which make it a principal component of the inhibitory process at the level of the reflex arc in the central nervous system, particularly the spinal cord. The presence of glycine in the receptor allows chloride to enter the neuron, changing the membrane potential and inhibiting promulgation of the neural signal.[26] Strychnine is an antagonist of the glycine receptors and does not allow the development of the inhibitory postsynaptic potential.[27] Stimulation of neurons, therefore, occurs without the counter-regulatory balance of the inhibitory receptor, reulting in muscle contractions and spasms that accelerate out of control.

CLINICAL EFFECTS

Strychnine is a remarkably effective poison. Only small doses of strychnine are required to inhibit critical numbers of glycine receptors and cause profound and lethal physiological consequences.[28]

Ten to twenty minutes following exposure to strychnine, the victim may feel a sense of restlessness and experience a violent convulsion, abrupt myoclonic movements, or muscle pain and stiffness. The generalized muscle spasms typically begin with the head and neck. All the muscles of a given part of the body tend to spasm and convulse at the same time. When the victim loses control of the muscles of the face, the resulting fear, apprehension, pain, and violent, uncontrolled spasm of the masseter, platysma, frontalis, and other facial muscles may cause a characteristic expression called *Risus sardonicus* (from the Latin for scornful laughter) or *Risus caninus* (from the Latin for dog-like laughter or grinning). This facial expression has also been observed among patients with tetanus. *Risus sardonicus* causes a patient's eyebrows to rise, eyes to bulge, and mouth to retract dramatically, resulting in what has been described as an evil-looking grin.

The spasms spread quickly to every muscle in the body, with nearly continuous convulsions. These spasms become worse with the slightest stimulus. The muscles may relax completely between convulsions. Typically, the patient will be awake, in considerable pain, extremely anxious, and anticipating the next series of convulsions. After several minutes, or with the slightest stimulation, such as a loud noise or bumping against the patient's bed, hypersensitivity returns with further convulsions.

As convulsions progress, they usually increase in intensity and frequency until the paraspinal muscles and other muscles of the back contract continuously. Death comes from asphyxiation caused by disinhibition of the neural pathways that control breathing, or by exhaustion from the convulsions.[29] The patient frequently dies within 2 to 3 hours after significant exposure. At the point of death, the body reportedly "freezes" immediately, even in the middle of a convulsion, resulting in instantaneous rigor mortis.[30] Animal studies have also documented this phenomenon.[31] Because strychnine does not cross the blood–brain barrier, victims remain awake and aware of everything around them during the convulsions.[14]

There is no antidote for strychnine. Treatment primarily involves supportive care with minimization of external stimulus and prevention of convulsions.

Strychnine poisoning may be confused with tetanus and epilepsy.[32] Strychnine poisoning can be differentiated from tetanus (infection and toxicity from *Clostridium tetani*) primarily by the length of time and onset of symptoms. While the symptoms of tetanus poisoning usually persist for several days, those involving strychnine poisoning develop over a period of hours. Patients who present with convulsive status epilepticus (persistent seizures) can be differentiated from strychnine patients because they have a depressed, obtunded mental status, whereas patients with strychnine poisoning are awake and aware.[24,29]

ANALYTIC DETECTION

With modern techniques, strychnine can be detected easily in blood, urine, gastric fluid, bile, and fixed liver or kidney samples at autopsy. Early detection of strychnine in biologic fluids via thin-layer chromatography or ultraviolet-spectrophotometric methods can be easily accomplished. More sensitive analyses can be performed on bodily fluids with gas chromatography-mass spectrometry (GC-MS) and high-performance liquid chromatography.[25,33-35] Accuracy and sensitivity of different analyses for strychnine depend on a number of factors, including the body fluid being tested, time since exposure, and presence of compounds that might interfere with the analysis. In one series of three samples, at very low levels of strychnine (0.1 µg/mL), analysis of the urine via GC-MS yielded the highest recovery.[35] Postmortem strychnine levels in fatal cases of poisoning range from 0.4–61 mg/L in whole blood, 0.5–33 mg/L in urine, and 7.5–1000 mg/L in gastric contents.[25,34-37]

CONCLUSION

Strychnine is a highly potent, lethal poison that causes prolonged convulsions in patients who are awake. Because the victims are unable to control their muscles or stop the convulsions and spasms, death is caused by asphyxiation, usually within 1 or 2 hours after ingestion. Strychnine poisoning should not be confused with tetanus or epilepsy.

REFERENCES

1. *Berrie v State of Oklahoma*, OK CR 20, 55 Okl.Cr. 302, 29 P .2d 979 (1934).
2. Simon J. Naming and toxicity: a history of strychnine. *Stud Hist Philos Sci Part C.* 1999;30(4):505–525.
3. McGarry RC, McGarry P. Please pass the strychnine: the art of Victorian pharmacy. *CMAJ.* 1999;161(12):1556–1558.
4. Haller JS. The history of strychnine in the nineteenth-century material medica. *Trans Stud Coll Physicians Phila.* 1973;40(4):226–238.
5. Simon J. The New Pharmacy: The first generation of chemical pharmacists. In: *Chemistry, Pharmacy and Revolution in France, 1777-1809.* Ashgate Publishing; Surrety, United Kingdom 2005:157.
6. Howes PE, Lloyd JU. *Drug Treatise Number VIII: A Treatise on Nux Vomica.* Cincinnati: Lloyd Brothers; 1904:7–8.
7. Felter HW, Lloyd JU. *Strychnine (U.S.P.)—Strychnine in Kings' American Dispensatory.* 18th ed, 3rd rev. Cincinnati: Ohio Valley Co; 1898. http://www.henriettesherbal.com/eclectic/kings/strychnos-nux.html. Accessed September 24, 2009.
8. United States Environmental Protection Agency. Reregistration eligibility document (RED). *Fact sheet on strychnine.* Cincinnati: National Center for Environmental Publications and Information; July 1996.
9. Sukul NC, Ghosh S, Sinhababu SP, et al. *Strychnos nux-vomica* extract and its ultra-high dilution reduce voluntary ethanol intake in rats. *J Altern Complement Med.* 2001:7(2):187–193.
10. Yan W, Sunavala G, Rosenzweig S, et al. Bitter taste transduced by PLC-B2-dependent rise in IP3 and a-gustducin-dependent fall in cyclic nucleotides. *Am J Physiol Cell Physiol.* 2001;280(4)C742–C751.
11. Lynch PP. Poisoning by strychnine; recovery of strychnine from exhumed body; adipocere formation; conviction for murder. *N Z Med J.* 1948;47(261):448–457.
12. Bogan J, Rentoul E, Smith H, et al. Homicidal poisoning by strychnine. *J Forensic Sci Soc.* 1966;6(4):166–169.
13. Oliver JS, Smith H, Watson AA. Poisoning by strychnine. *Med Sci Law.* 1979;19(2):134–137.
14. Reardon M, Duane A, Cotter P. Attempted homicide in hospital. *Ir J Med Sci.* 1993;162(8):315–317.
15. Benomran FA, Henry JD. Homicide by strychnine poisoning. *Med Sci Law.* 1996;36(3):271–273.
16. Ferguson MB, Vance MA. Payment deferred: strychnine poisoning in Nicaragua 65 years ago. *J Toxicol Clin Toxicol.* 2000;38(1):71–77.
17. Shannon M. Clinical toxicity of cocaine adulterants. *Ann Emerg Med.* 1988;17(11):1243–1247.
18. Yamarick W, Walson P, DiTraglia J. Strychnine poisoning in an adolescent. *J Toxicol Clin Toxicol.* 1992;30(1):141–148.
19. Strychnine. International Programme on Chemical Safety Web site. http://www.inchem.org/documents/pims/chemical/pim507.htm. Accessed September 24, 2009.
20. Wood DM, Webster E, Martinez D, Dargan PI, Jones AL. Case report: survival after deliberate strychnine self-poisoning with toxicokinetic data. *Crit Care.* 2002;6(5);456–459.
21. Palatnick W, Meatherall R, Sitar D, Tenenbein M. Toxicokinetics of acute strychnine poisoning. *J Toxicol Clin Toxicol.* 1997;35(6):617–620.
22. Heiser JM, Daya MR, Magnussen AR, et al. Massive strychnine intoxication: serial blood levels in a fatal case. *J Toxicol Clin Toxicol.* 1992;30(2):269–283.

23. Edmunds M, Sheehan TM, Van't Hoff W. Strychnine poisoning: clinical and toxicological observations on a non-fatal case. *J Toxicol Clin Toxicol.* 1986;24(3):245–255.

24. Katz J, Prescott K, Woolf AD. Strychnine poisoning from a Cambodian traditional remedy. *Am J Emerg Med.* 1996;14(5):475–476.

25. Rosano TG, Hubbard JD, Meola JM, Swift TA. Fatal strychnine poisoning: application of gas chromatography and tandem mass spectrometry. *J Anal Toxicol.* 2000;24:643–645.

26. Jursky F, Tamura S, Tamura A, et al. Structure, function and brain localization of neurotransmitter transporters. *J Exp Biol.* 1994;196:283–295.

27. Kuno M, Weakly JN. Quantal components of the inhibitory synaptic potential in spinal mononeurones of the cat. *J Physiol.* 1972;224:287–303.

28. Mackerer CA, Kochman RL, Shen TF, et al. The binding of strychnine and strychnine analogues to synaptic membranes of rat brainstem and spinal cord. *J Pharmacol Exp Ther.* 1977;201:326–331.

29. Smith BA. Strychnine poisoning. *J Emerg Med.* 1990;8:321–325.

30. Teitelbaum D, Ott J. Acute strychnine intoxication. *Clin Toxicol.* 1970;3:267.

31. Krompecher T, Bergerioux, Brandt-Casadevall C, et al. Experimental evaluation of rigor mortis. VI. Effect of various causes of death on the evolution of rigor mortis. *Forensic Sci Inter.* 1983;22:1–9.

32. Lambert JR, Byrick RJ, Hammeke MD. Management of acute strychnine poisoning. *Can Med Assoc J.* 1981;124:1268–1270.

33. Barroso M, Gallardo E, Margalho C, et al. Determination of strychnine in human blood using solid-phase extraction and GC-EI-MS. *J Anal Toxicol.* 2005;29(5):383–386.

34. Wang Z, Zhao J, Xing J, et al. Analysis of strychnine and brucine in postmortem specimens by RP-HPLC: a case report of fatal intoxication. *J Anal Toxicol.* 2004;28(2):141–144.

35. Marques EP, Gil F, Proenca P, Monsanto P, et al. Analytical method for the determination of strychnine in tissues by gas chromotagrophy/mass spectrometry: two case reports. *Forensic Sci Int.* 2000;110:145–152.

36. Lindsey T, O'Hara J, Irvine R, et al. Strychnine overdose following ingestion of gopher bait. *J Anal Toxicol.* 2004 28(2):135–137.

37. Cingolani M, Froldi R, Mencarelli R, et al. Analytical detection and quantitation of strychnine. *J Anal Toxicol.* 1999;23(3):219–221.

23 | Thallium

Daniel E. Rusyniak

CASE STUDY[1]

After a weekend at work as a millwright at an automotive plant, a 58-year-old man developed a persistent painful burning sensation in his feet. The following day, he was seen by his physician and diagnosed as having a muscle strain. His pain worsened, and 7 days after symptom onset, he was evaluated in a local emergency department and admitted to the hospital for pain control. Testing during that admission revealed normal complete blood count, blood chemistry studies, vitamin B_{12} and B_6 levels, antinuclear antibody levels, and sedimentation rate. Liver function tests were normal, except for a mildly elevated gamma-glutamyl-transferase (90 IU/L) level and an elevated total bilirubin level (2 mg/dL). The patient underwent nerve conduction studies, which revealed a sensorimotor peripheral neuropathy. Computed tomography of the brain revealed chronic bilateral subdural hygromas and a magnetic resonance imaging scan of the cervical spine revealed a mild cervical disk bulge with stenosis. This information, along with the patient's history of drinking 2 quarts of beer a day, led to the initial diagnosis of alcoholic peripheral neuropathy. The patient was discharged with pain medications. Over the ensuing 5 days, the pain increased in severity and progressed up his legs and involved his hands. In addition to this pain, the worker developed muscles aches, abdominal pain, nausea, insomnia, and hair loss. Over the same time period, four coworkers developed nearly identical symptoms. Concerned that a workplace exposure was the etiology, a physician screened the 58-year-old man's urine for the heavy metals lead, mercury, and arsenic. When the test revealed elevated urine arsenic concentrations (2130 µg/L), both the company personnel and the U.S. Department of Labor's Occupational Safety and Health Administration officials investigated the workplace for possible exposures. This investigation revealed a low concentration of arsenic in a breakroom coffee can and creamer. Despite this finding, a group of involved medical toxicologists found the worker's symptoms to be inconsistent with arsenic toxicity. This opinion was based on four key findings: low concentrations of arsenic detected in the workplace and the worker, the marked severity and rapid rate at which the neuropathy developed, the lack of associated gastrointestinal (GI) symptoms, and the rapid development of whole body alopecia. The medical toxicologists considered a more likely culprit to be thallium. Examination of the victim's hair revealed the characteristic root changes of thallium toxicity. These suspicions were confirmed later when urine and hair tests from the five men revealed markedly elevated levels of thallium (highest levels were 5885 µg in a 24-hour urine specimen and 1324 ng/g in a hair sample).

A criminal investigation resulted in the identification of a likely suspect who was a coworker of the victims. Police theorized that he had added thallium to the office coffee pot. The 3-week delay in making the correct diagnosis hampered the investigation, giving the culprit adequate time to dispose of the thallium source.

HISTORY

Thallium's Discovery and Early Usage

The development of spectrochemical analysis allowed scientists to detect minute quantities of previously unknown elements. In 1861, one of these scientists, Sir William Crookes, heated a deposit obtained from a sulphuric acid chamber and noted the transient appearance of a bright green line. Crookes identified this line as a new heavy metal. Using the Greek word *thallos*, meaning the green color of young vegetation,[2] Crookes named this new metal thallium.

Although useful in some manufacturing processes and as a radioactive contrast agent in medicine,[3] thallium became known not for its benefits but rather its toxicity. Early on, researchers discovered a unique property of thallium; it caused hair loss (alopecia).[4] This effect was thought to be beneficial in treating adults and children with fungal infections of the scalp.[4] The practice was abandoned in the 1930s after several children's deaths were attributed to thallium.[5] Its pharmacologic and toxic properties made thallium salts excellent rodenticides; these salts are highly toxic, tasteless, odorless, water soluble, and are completely absorbed by the GI tract.[4] Although widely used as a rodenticide, cases of accidental and malicious poisonings caused the United States to ban retail sales of thallium salts in 1973,[3] and by 1984 its production in the United States had ceased altogether.[6] Despite its lack of availability, thallium's toxicity and ease of administration make it a useful agent for murder or suicide.

The Misuse of Thallium: Cases Involving Thallium Poisoning

While most criminal cases of thallium poisoning involve a lone perpetrator, a few highly publicized cases have been linked to governments and political groups. The KGB (Soviet State Security Committee) is suspected of poisoning a KGB defector, Nikolai Khokhlov, with radioactive thallium in 1957.[7-9] Members of Saddam Hussein's party allegedly used thallium as a poison.[10] In 1960, the French Secret Service is reported to have assassinated Dr. Félix-Roland Moumié, the exiled leader of the Cameroonian nationalist movement, with thallium.[11] While Nelson Mandela was in prison, South African police and military officials reportedly plotted to kill him with thallium.[12] The Central Intelligence Agency allegedly plotted to sprinkle thallium in Cuban president Fidel Castro's shoes in an attempt to destroy his beard and subsequently his image.[13]

Thallium's toxicity, ease of administration, and delay in onset have long made it a favorite agent of individual poisoners. Perhaps the most famous of these poisoners was British citizen Graham Frederick Young.[14] From an early age,

Young was obsessed with poisons and began poisoning animals in his neighborhood. Young's father responded by throwing away his son's medical textbooks. The young man retaliated by killing his stepmother with a poison later determined to be thallium. Shortly thereafter, Young's father became ill with identical symptoms (diarrhea, vomiting, and stomach pains). A criminal investigation ensued, and police discovered in Young's possession a notebook containing poems referencing different poisons, poisoners, and bottles of antimony and thallium. In 1962, at 15 years of age, Young was sent to a mental hospital where he remained for 8 years. Upon his release, Young accepted a job at a photographic development company. Shortly thereafter, several of his coworkers became sick; the subsequent deaths of two of them would later be attributed to thallium poisoning. A police investigation revealed a makeshift laboratory in Young's house as well as sadistic drawings and pictures of Hitler. Young was convicted of murder and sentenced to life in prison.[14,15]

In 1988, a family in Florida came down with a mysterious illness characterized by severe pains in their feet and development of alopecia. The mother would eventually die from this illness. Police investigation revealed the presence of thallium in soft drinks inside the family refrigerator. A neighbor, George Trepal, became a suspect after authorities learned that he had argued repeatedly with this family and had reportedly threatened them because they played loud music and rode motorcycles on his property. Investigators believe that Trepal retaliated by breaking into their residence and putting thallium in their soda bottles. Trepal was subsequently convicted of murder based on comments he made to investigators and after a search of his property revealed traces of thallium and a machine designed to recap soda bottles.[16,17]

POTENTIAL DELIVERY METHODS

Thallium salts are odorless, tasteless, and readily dissolve in water, making the primary means of poison delivery a victim's food and drink. Examples include thallium placed in coffee,[1] tea,[14,15,18,19] jelly,[20] and even candies.[21]

TOXICOLOGIC MECHANISMS

Thallium's toxicity involves interrupting several enzyme systems. Thallium, having a similar charge and atomic radii to potassium, interferes with several potassium-dependent enzymes, including pyruvate kinase and Na^+/K^+ ATPase.[22,23] Thallium also has a high affinity for sulfhydryl groups and can therefore inhibit several sulfhydryl-containing enzymes: pyruvate dehydrogenase complex, succinate dehydrogenase, hydrolases, oxidoreductases, and several transferases.[3] The inhibition of potassium and sulfhydryl-dependent enzymes decreases the breakdown of sugars and impairs energy production, resulting, if severe enough, in cell death.

CLINICAL EFFECTS

The earliest symptoms of thallium poisoning, occurring within hours of exposure, affect the GI tract. Unlike those seen with other heavy metals, GI symptoms from thallium are not typically severe and do not dominate the early clinical picture. The GI symptoms most commonly reported are abdominal pain, mild vomiting, and loose stools. These are typically followed within a few days by constipation or obstipation.[1,4,16,21,24]

Early in the course of toxicity, typically within 2 or 3 days of exposure, the most specific finding in thallium poisoning is the development of a rapidly progressive peripheral neuropathy.[25-27] Symptoms of neuropathy, involving the feet and less commonly the hands, manifest as pain. Described as pins and needles, the pain may be excruciating, making even the weight of a bed sheet intolerable.[1,4,21,28] In severe cases, thallium neuropathy may rapidly progress and involve the arms and respiratory muscles, at times necessitating artificial respiration.[4,16,29] In these cases, the clinical picture of rapidly ascending weakness with associated sensory symptoms can be misdiagnosed as the neurologic disorder Guillain-Barré.[28]

The best-known complication of thallium poisoning is hair loss, also known as alopecia (Figure 23.1). Alopecia typically begins at 10–14 days after exposure to thallium; complete hair loss occurs by 3 to 4 weeks. Victims will report that their hair is coming out in clumps and that it can be painlessly removed if pulled.[4] If one survives, hair regrowth typically begins by the fourth month. Hair loss involves the entire body, including axillary hair, pubic hair, and the lateral eyebrows.[24,30-32] Thallium spares the medial part of the eyebrow where the hairs are in a resting, nongrowth phase.[24,33] While the exact cause of thallium-induced hair loss is not

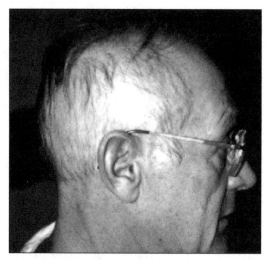

FIGURE 23.1 **Hair loss associated with thallium poisoning** (See Color Plate 31.)
Permission for use from Dr. Dan Rusyniak

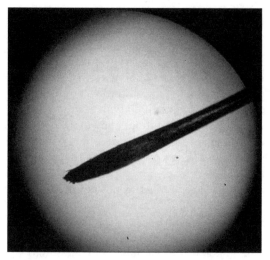

FIGURE 23.2 **Microscopic examination of hair revealing a darkened root associated with thallium toxicity** (See Color Plate 32)
Permission for use from Dr. Dan Rusyniak

known, it likely involves thallium interrupting cysteine in the synthesis of keratin and disturbing energy metabolism in the growing cells of the hair matrix.[32,34] It is important to note that not all thallium-poisoned patients develop alopecia and that thallium neuropathies can occur without hair loss.[1]

In cases of severe poisoning, the CNS may also be affected with the development of some or all of the following: hallucinations, altered mental status, insomnia, psychosis, and coma.[4,16,25,27,35,36] Along with peripheral nerve involvement, cranial neuropathies are also reported in thallium poisoning.[4,16,25,28,36-38]

Other less specific manifestations of thallium poisoning include diffuse myalgias, pleuritic chest pain,[1,21,39] hypertension,[21] nail dystrophy,[35] acne,[24,31] and chronic neuropsychiatric manifestations.[1,4,40]

Thallium poisoning is uncommon. Its initial symptoms may be attributed to other etiologies, making the diagnosis difficult.[1,28] One difficulty in making an early diagnosis is that alopecia, the most recognizable feature of thallium poisoning,[18] may not be evident for up to 14 days after exposure.[32]

One technique that may help in the early diagnosis is visually inspecting a victim's hair under a microscope. When examined under a light-powered microscope, the hair roots of thallium-poisoned patients appear dark (Figure 23.2).[1,24,41] Present in up to 95% of scalp hair, black hair roots from thallium poisoning may be seen as early as 4 days after exposure.[24,41] Several black bands can be seen if multiple episodes of poisoning occur.[24,41] While some authors suggest that the dark roots represent an accumulation of pigment,[24] it is actually gaseous inclusions diffracting the light that cause the appearance of a black stain.[30,32]

In summary, thallium poisoning should be considered in any patient developing any of the following: (1) the acute onset of pain and numbness in the feet, (2) development of alopecia, and (3) blackened hair roots on visual inspection. In patients with severe poisoning, only the painful neuropathy and blackened hair roots may be evident prior to death.

ANALYTIC DETECTION

To make a definitive diagnosis of thallium poisoning, one must identify elevated concentrations of thallium in urine, hair, or tissues. The gold standard of detection, as with other metals, is a 24-hour urine analysis. Normal levels of thallium in a 24-hour urine analysis are less than 20 μg/specimen. Thallium can also be detected in hair, with normal levels being less than 15 ng thallium/gram of hair.[3,19] Hair analysis is not typically as reliable as urine, and a negative hair test should not exclude the possibility of thallium poisoning. Along with hair and urine, postmortem tissues including paraffin tissue blocks and cremated ashes have been used to confirm elevations of thallium in suspected poisoning cases.[19,42]

CONCLUSION

Thallium salts have the qualities of a perfect criminal poison: They are tasteless and odorless, they dissolve completely in liquids, they are rapidly and completely absorbed, and they defy detection on routine toxicologic screens. Thallium, however, leaves a characteristic enough footprint to enable detection. To do so, one must avoid waiting for the development of alopecia before considering thallium, as victims may die prior to developing hair loss. The rapid onset of a progressive peripheral neuropathy with pain and dysesthesias occurring in the feet should alert an investigator to the potential for thallium poisoning. When thallium poisoning is suspected, an investigator should analyze urine for thallium concentrations and visually inspect pulled hair for blackening of the roots. As thallium is no longer available to the public, accidental exposures should rarely, if ever, occur, and all cases of poisoning warrant a criminal investigation.

REFERENCES

1. Rusyniak DE, Furbee RB, Kirk MS. Thallium and arsenic poisoning in a small midwest town. *Ann Emerg Med.* 2002;39(3):307–311.
2. James FA. Of "Medals and Muddles," the context of the discovery of thallium: William Crookes's early spectro-chemical work. *Notes Rec R Soc Lond.* 1984;39(1):65–90.
3. Mulkey JP, Oehme FW. A review of thallium toxicity. *Vet Hum Toxicol.* 1993;35(5):445–453.
4. Prick JJG, Sillevis Smitt WG, Muller L. *Thallium Poisoning.* New York: Elsevier Publishing Company; 1955.
5. Lynch GR, Lond MB. The toxicology of thallium. Lancet. 1930;Dec 20:1340–1344.
6. ATSDR. *Toxicological Profile for Thallium.* Atlanta, GA: U.S. Department of Health and Human Services, Public Health Service; 1992.
7. Khokhlov N. *In the Name of Conscience.* New York: D. McKay Co; 1959.
8. Macintyre B. The spy poisoned by the KGB—but who lived to tell the tale. *The Times.* December 1, 2006.
9. Volodarsky B. The KGB's poison factor. *The Wall Street Journal (Europe).* April 7, 2005.
10. Mcgery J. Inside Saddam's World. *Time.* 2002;59.
11. Faligot R, Krop P. *LA Piscine: The French Secret Service Since 1944.* London: Blackwell Publishing; 1989.
12. What is thallium? BBC News. http://news.bbc.co.uk/1/hi/uk/6163520.stm. Accessed September 25, 2009.
13. US Senate—Select Committee on Governmental Operations. *Interim Report: Alleged Assassination Plots Involving Foreign Leaders.* US Government Printing Office; 1975:72.
14. Holden A. *The. St. Albans Poisoner.* London: Hodder & Stoughton Ltd; 1975.
15. Bowden P. Graham Young (1947-90); the St. Albans poisoner: his life and times. *Crim Behav Ment Health.* 1996;(suppl 6):17–24.
16. Desenclos JC, Wilder MH, Coppenger GW, et al. Thallium poisoning: an outbreak in Florida, 1988. *South Med J.* 1992;85(12):1203–1206.
17. Good J, Goreck S. *Poison Mind.* New York: St. Martin's Paperbacks; 1996.
18. Moore D, House I, Dixon A. Thallium poisoning. Diagnosis may be elusive but alopecia is the clue. *BMJ.* 1993;306(6891):1527–1529.
19. Wecht C, Saitz G. *Mortal Evidence.* New York: Prometheus Books; 2007.
20. McCormack J, McKinney W. Thallium poisoning in group assassination attempt. *Postgrad Med.* 1983;74(6):239–241, 244.
21. Meggs WJ, Hoffman RS, Shih RD, et al. Thallium poisoning from maliciously contaminated food. *J Toxicol Clin Toxicol.* 1994;32(6):723–730.
22. Douglas KT, Bunni MA, Baindur SR. Thallium in biochemistry. *Int J Biochem.* 1990;22(5):429–438.
23. Gehring PJ, Hammond PB. The interrelationship between thallium and potassium in animals. *J Pharmacol Exp Ther.* 1967;155(1):187–201.
24. Moeschlin S. Thallium poisoning. *Clin Toxicol.* 1980;17(1):133–146.
25. Davis LE, Standefer JC, Kornfeld M, et al. Acute thallium poisoning: toxicological and morphological studies of the nervous system. *Ann Neurol.* 1980;10(1):38–44.
26. Malbrain ML, Lambrecht GL, Zandijk E, et al. Treatment of severe thallium intoxication. *J Toxicol Clin Toxicol.* 1997;35(1):97–100.
27. Reed D, Crawley J, Faro SN, et al. Thallotoxicosis. *JAMA.* 1963;183(7):516–522.
28. Misra UK, Kalita J, Yadav RK, et al. Thallium poisoning: emphasis on early diagnosis and response to haemodialysis. *Postgrad Med J.* 2003;79(928):103–105.
29. Hologgitas J, Ullucci P, Driscoll J, et al. Thallium elimination kinetics in acute thallotoxicosis. *J Anal Toxicol.* 1980;4(2):68–75.
30. Feldman J, Levisohn DR. Acute alopecia: clue to thallium toxicity. *Pediatr Dermatol.* 1993;10(1):29–31.
31. Heyl T, Barlow RJ. Thallium poisoning: a dermatological perspective. *Br J Dermatol.* 1989;121(6):787–791.
32. Tromme I, Van Neste D, Dobbelaere F, et al. Skin signs in the diagnosis of thallium poisoning. *Br J Dermatol.* 1998;138(2):321–325.
33. Koblenzer PJ, Weiner LB. Alopecia secondary to thallium intoxication. *Arch Dermatol.* 1969;99(6):777.

34. Cavanagh JB, Gregson M. Some effects of a thallium salt on the proliferation of hair follicle cells. *J Pathol.* 1978;125(4):179–191.

35. Saha A, Sadhu HG, Karnik AB, et al. Erosion of nails following thallium poisoning: a case report. *Occup Environ Med.* 2004;61(7):640–642.

36. Hoffman RS. Thallium toxicity and the role of Prussian blue in therapy. *Toxicol Rev.* 2003;22(1):29–40.

37. Cavanagh JB, Fuller NH, Johnson HRM. The effects of thallium salts, with particular reference to the nervous system changes. A report of three cases. *Q J Med.* 1974;170:293–319.

38. Tabandeh H, Crowston JG, Thompson GM. Ophthalmologic features of thallium poisoning. *Am J Ophthalmol.* 1994;117(2):243–245.

39. Bank WJ, Pleasure DE, Suzuki K, et al. Thallium poisoning. *Arch Neurol.* 1972;26(5):456–464.

40. McMillan TM, Jacobson RR, Gross M. Neuropsychology of thallium poisoning. *J Neurol Neurosurg Psychiatry.* 1997;63(2):247–250.

41. Widy W. Pigment changes in the hair roots in thallium poisoning. *Acta Med Pol.* 1961;2:259–282.

42. Cavanagh JB. What have we learnt from Graham Frederick Young? Reflections on the mechanism of thallium neurotoxicity. *Neuropathol Appl Neurobiol.* 1991;17:3–9.

24 | Toxalbumins

Ayrn D. O'Connor

CASE STUDY

Georgi Markov was a controversial playwright and novelist from Bulgaria. Markov was outspoken in his criticism of the Communist authorities that controlled Bulgaria, and in 1969 he was responsible for the production of a play considered to be dissident by the authorities. Fearful of reprisal, Markov fled Bulgaria for Great Britain. He continued to express his strong anticommunist views by writing programs for broadcasts and by broadcasting for such entities as the Bulgarian Service of the BBC in Britain and Radio Free Europe in Munich. Markov knew that he was unpopular and had made many powerful enemies; consequently, he feared for his life.[1]

On September 7, 1978, Markov was waiting at a bus stop on the Waterloo Bridge when he felt a sharp blow to the back of his right thigh. He turned to find a man picking up an umbrella. The man apologized and quickly disappeared into the nearest taxi. Markov returned to his office and complained to a colleague of pain in the back of his thigh; on further inspection, a red, inflamed lesion was noted. When Markov arrived home that evening, he complained to his wife of weakness. By the next morning he had developed nausea, vomiting, and fever. His symptoms worsened, prompting admission to a local hospital later that night.

On arrival, Markov was noted to be ill-appearing, febrile, and tachycardic, with tender lymph nodes and an area of inflammation on the back of his right thigh approximately 6 cm in diameter. His clinical course worsened the following day. He became hypotensive, his heart rate rose to 160 beats per minute, and he developed an elevated white blood cell count of 26,300 cells per cubic mm. The clinical picture appeared consistent with septic shock, although the etiology remained elusive. His clinical condition continued to worsen, renal failure developed, and vomiting persisted with hematemesis; he ultimately died on September 11 following cardiac arrest.[1]

An autopsy was performed and revealed diffuse interstitial hemorrhages with necrosis involving the intestines, pancreas, myocardium, and lymph nodes. The most intriguing finding was a small metallic foreign body in the soft tissue of his right thigh. An identical pellet was removed from Vladimir Kostov, another Bulgarian dissident who had suffered a similar injury 2 weeks prior to Georgi Markov's attack. Kostov had been waiting for the metro train when he heard a sound like an air pistol being fired and felt a blow to his back. He became ill, developed a fever, and was hospitalized for 12 days. Ultimately he recovered, but x-rays revealed a metallic foreign body in his back. The foreign body was retrieved. When this foreign body was compared with the one found in Georgi Markov, the two appeared nearly identical. The pellet was only 1.52 mm in diameter, had two holes, each about 0.34 mm in diameter, and was believed to hold the toxin responsible for Markov's death and Kostov's illness.[1]

It was concluded that the responsible toxin was ricin, the toxalbumin found in the castor bean plant (*Ricinus communis*). Although ricin was never isolated from the body of Georgi Markov, the similarity in the clinical picture and autopsy findings based on injection of ricin in a pig model satisfied the coroner.[1] According to the U.S. Army Medical Research Institute of Infectious Diseases, this technique was employed in at least five other assassination attempts in the late 1970s and early 1980s.[2]

HISTORY

Toxalbumins are complex proteins found in various plant species, and they are toxic when ingested or administered parenterally. Although numerous species exist, the most toxicologically significant include the castor bean plant (*Ricinus communis*), the jequirity bean plant (*Abrus precatorius*), and the black locust tree (*Robinia pseudoacacia*).[3-6] These plants have been used since antiquity for a multitude of purposes. The seeds of the jequirity bean plant (Figure 24.1), which contain the toxalbumin abrin, are colorful (usually red and black) and have been used primarily in ornaments, jewelry, and rosaries. The castor bean (Figure 24.2), which contains the toxalbumin ricin, has not only been used for decoration but has also served a more functional purpose in several cultures. It has been used as a treatment for syphilis, leprosy, and as a cathartic. Annually, more than a million tons of castor beans are used worldwide in the production of the widely used lubricant castor oil. The waste mash from the process used to make castor oil is 2–5% ricin by weight.[7,8]

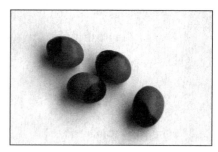

FIGURE 24.1 *Abrus precatorius* seeds
(See Color Plate 33.)

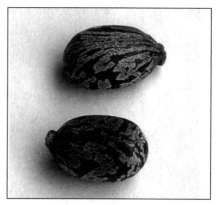

FIGURE 24.2 *Ricinus communis* seeds
(See Color Plate 34.)

Ricin is the most extensively studied and widely encountered toxalbumin in criminal poisoning. Ricin was first isolated in 1889 by Herman Stillmark.[9] Since that time, extensive work has been done concerning its application in the field of immunology and as a possible anticancer agent. Because ricin is a relatively potent toxin that is widely available and relatively easy to produce, it has been targeted as a possible warfare agent and terrorist weapon. Near the end of World War I, the U.S. Chemical Warfare Service began studying ricin (which was given the code name Compound W) as a possible inhalational warfare agent.[8] The war, however, ended before a functional weapon that used ricin was developed. The U.S. military's interest in ricin resurfaced in World War II. In 1944 efforts to manufacture a weapon that produced and used aerosolization of ricin were successful.[8] Field tests were reportedly performed, but the weapon was never used in battle.[8] Currently, ricin is a Schedule 1 chemical under the provisions of the Chemical Weapons Convention and consequently subject to the restrictions and requirements of that provision.[10]

It is apparent from the case of Georgi Markov that ricin has been used as a terrorist weapon. Several more recent instances of ricin procurement for use as a terrorist weapon have been documented. In 1994 and 1995 four members of the Minnesota Patriots Council, a tax-protest group, conspired to murder law enforcement officials and were found in possession of ricin.[2,11] In 1995, Deborah Greene, a Kansas City oncologist, was charged with attempted murder after contaminating her husband's food with ricin.[2,11] In January of 2003, United Kingdom (UK) Scientists at the Defense Science and Technology Laboratories at Porton Down identified ricin in material found in an apartment flat following a police raid of terrorist suspects. In October of 2003, a mail processing and distribution center in Greenville, South Carolina, received a letter threatening to contaminate water supplies along with a sealed container later confirmed by the Centers for Disease Control and Prevention (CDC) to contain ricin.[11,12] A similar incident occurred in February of 2004, when ricin was found on an automatic mail sorter in the Dirksen Senate Office Building that was serving Senate Majority Leader Bill Frist. No clinical cases of ricin-associated illness were identified after subsequent statewide surveillance and investigations of these incidents.

POTENTIAL DELIVERY METHOD

Ricin can be used in its crude form, after being purified into a crystalline structure, or as a dried white powder.[2] In its purified form, it is soluble in water and stable over a wide pH range. It can be inactivated through heating to 80°C (176°F) in an aqueous solution for 10 minutes.[2] Routes of exposure vary and have different levels of potency. The least toxic route is ingestion of contaminated food and water. Ricin can also be dispersed through the air with an aerosolized form of ricin ranging from 1 to 10 micron-sized particles; this method results in inhalational exposure. The most severe toxicity is through parenteral injections of ricin directed at a specific target.

TOXICOLOGIC MECHANISMS

Toxalbumins are similar in structure to other toxins such as cholera, diphtheria, botulinum, and tetanus. Ricin consists of two subunits joined by a disulfide bond. The B subunit binds to glycoproteins on the surface of the cell's membrane, enabling the toxin to enter the cytoplasm (Figure 24.3). The A subunit irreversibly inactivates the eukaryotic ribosome, thereby inhibiting protein synthesis.[1] This ultimately leads to cell death. Cells with higher turnover rates, such as those of the gastrointestinal (GI) tract, are more susceptible. Other mechanisms of toxicity have been noted, including apoptosis (programmed cell death), direct damage to the cell membrane with alteration of its structure and function, as well as the release of inflammatory mediators.[9,13,14] An additional glycoprotein, ricin communis agglutinin, has been identified and has an affinity for red blood cells, resulting in agglutination and subsequent hemolysis; significant hemolysis is typically the result of only parenterally administered ricin.[7,15]

CLINICAL EFFECTS

The clinical picture of a patient exposed to ricin depends on the route of exposure. The clinical signs and symptoms of ricin toxicity following ingestion are based on reports in the medical literature of castor bean ingestion. The degree of toxicity is dependent on a number of factors, including the number of beans ingested; their

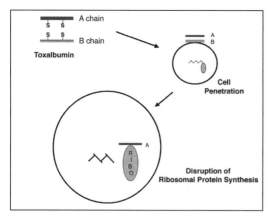

FIGURE 24.3   Mechanism of toxalbumins:
1) The toxin consists of 2 subunits joined
by a disulfide bond. 2) The B subunit binds
to glycoproteins on the surface of the cell's
membrane, enabling the toxin to enter the
cytoplasm. 3) The A subunit irreversibly inactivates the eukaryotic ribosome, thereby
inhibiting protein synthesis.

size, weight, and moisture content; the region
and season of growth; as well as the degree of
mastication, patient age, and comorbidities.
There are no documented cases of ingestion
of purified ricin formulation, although it is believed the clinical course would be similar to
that described in the cases of castor bean ingestion. Oral exposure is considered less toxic than
other routes.

In a review published in 1985 that identified
751 cases of castor bean toxicity, there were 14
deaths, yielding an estimated mortality rate of
1.8%.[3] This rate appears to be significantly lower
than what has been perpetuated in the medical literature. Of the 14 deaths, 12 were prior to
1930 when the medical care was vastly different than today's supportive care. Also, in these
deaths, the number of beans ingested varied
significantly. Consequently, drawing conclusions about the toxic or lethal dose is difficult.
According to Rauber and Heard, the two lethal
cases since 1930 occurred in a 24-year-old man
and a 15-year-old boy who ingested 15–20 and
10–12 beans, respectively.[3]

All of the severe or deadly castor bean intoxications have a similar clinical course. Patients develop nausea, vomiting, and abdominal
cramping within a few hours of ingestion.[3,4,8,16]
These symptoms are followed by profuse watery
diarrhea, often described as cholera-like.[3,4,8,16,17]

Reports of GI bleeding are documented. Ultimately, patients develop electrolyte disturbances, severe dehydration, and hypovolemia over
the course of several days following ingestion.
Evidence of renal impairment and liver dysfunction manifests with increased blood urea
nitrogen, creatinine, and transaminases.[3,4,8,17]
Patients typically develop a leukocytosis. Hypovolemic shock followed by cardiovascular
collapse and death may occur between 3 and 5
days after ingestion.[8,17] Autopsy results following oral intoxication reveal diffuse ulceration of
the mucosa of the GI tract with necrosis of the
lymphoid tissue.[8] Making the diagnosis of ricin
toxicity from ingestion will likely be challenging, as it will strongly resemble gastroenteritis
from a multitude of other causes such as foodborne toxins, chemicals, or infectious causes.

There is less information available character-
izing the clinical course in humans following
inhalational exposure to a purified aerosolized
form of ricin. There are animal studies, including nonhuman primate studies, which shed
some light on the expected clinical manifestations. Severity of toxicity is largely dependent on
dose and particle size, with smaller micron particles reaching deeper into the respiratory tract
resulting in higher mortality.[18] In 1993, a study
describing the effects of inhaled ricin on rhesus monkeys was published by Wilhelmsen and
Pitt. This study described a dose-dependent delay before the onset of symptoms, ranging from
8 to 24 hours.[19] Progressive lethargy and anorexia developed, culminating in death from respiratory failure 36 to 48 hours after exposure.[19]
All of the monkeys developed airway inflammation, variable degrees of bronchial necrosis,
and acute severe fibrinopurulent pneumonia.[19]
Tracheitis, purulent mediastinal lymphadenitis,
and diffuse edema were other notable findings
on histopathologic examination.[19] There is also
a poorly documented account of an accidental
sublethal aerosol exposure in humans that reportedly occurred in the 1940s. Reactions were
characterized by the development of cough,
chest tightness, dyspnea, fever, and arthralgias
4 to 8 hours after exposure.[2] All of the exposed
individuals recovered uneventfully.

Diagnostic features expected following inhalational exposure to ricin include bilateral
infiltrates on chest radiographs, hypoxemia,
possible leukocytosis, and in severe exposures a

clinical picture consistent with acute respiratory distress syndrome. Diagnosis of an attack with aerosolized ricin would likely be made on the basis of consistent clinical findings, as well as sufficient epidemiologic evidence. For example, one should develop a high index of suspicion should a group of previously healthy individuals in the same geographic area develop acute lung injury following a credible attack. One should remain suspicious of other biologic or chemical threats; the differential diagnosis may include tularemia, Q fever, staphylococcal enterotoxin B, plague, or phosgene gas.[8]

Parenteral injection of a specific target is another possible route of exposure to ricin. The clinical effects expected following injection of ricin have been based on a number of animal studies and the rare report of human exposure.[1,20-22] A variable delay, estimated as 10 to 12 hours from the time of exposure to the onset of systemic symptoms, is anticipated, although more immediate discomfort at the injection site may occur.[1,20-22] Patients initially develop nonspecific symptoms such as general malaise, nausea, headache, anorexia, and dizziness resembling a flu-like syndrome.[1,20,21] However, as toxicity progresses, vomiting, abdominal pain, tachycardia, hypotension, enlargement of the lymph nodes, and worsening inflammation at the injection site may develop.[1,20,21] Patients proceed to develop fever, renal insufficiency, and liver dysfunction. Ultimately, the clinical course resembles septic shock and culminates in multisystem organ failure.[1]

Expected lab abnormalities include elevated blood urea nitrogen and creatinine levels, which indicate renal insufficiency; elevated transaminases, reflecting liver injury; elevated creatinine kinase consistent with muscle cell breakdown; and leukocytosis.[1] Postmortem findings reveal hemorrhage, necrosis, and edema of lymphoid tissue, kidneys, and the GI tract including the liver.[1]

Diagnosing parenteral ricin toxicity will undoubtedly prove challenging, not only because it will likely present as an isolated case but also because the differential diagnosis of multisystem organ failure or sepsis is so broad. The resultant clinical picture could be secondary to an extensive list of possible causes including infectious etiology, heavy metal toxicity such as arsenic or mercury, or a multitude of drugs such as colchicine or an antimetabolite neoplastic agent.

In summary, the clinical presentation associated with ricin toxicity is highly dependent on the route of exposure, whether from ingestion, inhalation, or injection (Table 24.1). Furthermore, there will be a variable delay in the time of onset of symptoms, which will be determined not only by the route of exposure but also by the potency and form of ricin used. Oral exposure will result in GI symptoms including nausea, vomiting, abdominal pain, and watery diarrhea 2–8 hours after ingestion. These symptoms can progress to severe dehydration, hypovolemic shock, renal insufficiency, and liver dysfunction 36–72 hours after exposure. If death occurs, it is typically between 3 and 5 days postingestion. An inhalational exposure will primarily cause respiratory symptoms that begin 8–12 hours later. Chest pain, shortness of breath, cough, fever, hypoxia, and acute lung injury are anticipated findings. Injection of ricin is considered the most toxic route of exposure and may culminate in multisystem organ failure or a clinical picture resembling septic shock. Symptoms may begin several hours after exposure and progress over 2–3 days.

ANALYTIC DETECTION

Clinicians who suspect that a patient has been exposed to ricin should collect urine and blood specimens immediately and contact their state health department or the CDC for further guidance. Currently there is limited ability to detect ricin in biologic specimens. The CDC does possess the capability of detecting urinary ricinine, an alkaloid of the castor bean plant used as a marker of ricin exposure.[23,24] Detection of ricinine is done through high-pressure liquid-chromatography–electospray-ionization–mass spectrometry (HPLC-ESI-MS) and may be possible up to 48 hours after exposure.[23] This test is currently available at 10 laboratories through the CDC and its laboratory response network (LRN).[23] There is evidence that immunostaining techniques may offer another way of detecting ricin in biologic specimens. Terazawa, Griffiths, and Leith studied several techniques and found that immunogold silver staining (IGSS) could detect minute amounts (4 ng) of ricin in tissues.[25] Unfortunately, this test is not currently widely available.

Environmental samples suspected of containing ricin can be tested through the CDC

TABLE 24.1 **Route of Ricin Exposure Determines Clinical Presentation**

Ingestion	Inhalation	Injection
Nausea	Cough	Localized pain and Inflammation
Vomiting	Chest Tightness	General Malaise
Abdominal Cramping	Dyspnea	Nausea and Vomiting
Profuse Diarrhea	Nausea	Fever and Leukocytosis
Tachycardia	Fever	Tender Lymphadenopathy
Dehydration	Arthralgias	Tachycardia and Hypotension
Renal Insufficiency	Hypoxemia	Renal Insufficiency and Hepatic Injury
Hypovolemic Shock	ARDS	Multisystem Organ Failure

and LRN using either time-resolved fluorescence immunoassay, which uses an antibody that binds to ricin, or polymerase chain reaction (PCR), which looks for the DNA of the gene that produces ricin.[23] The U.S. Military and Department of Homeland Security are developing techniques that would allow for field testing to detect ricin; however, these "handheld" assays are not commercially available.[17] Although, significant progress is being made and there appears to be an immunochromatographic test (ICT) that can be used to screen various specimens for minute amounts of ricin on the order of 1-2.5 ng/mL.[26] The ICT was found to be accurate using 19 different varieties of *Ricinus communis* and both experienced and inexperienced operators.[26] The test is currently being evaluated in animal models and would prove to be invaluable in the rapid evaluation and triage of individuals in a suspected biologic attack.[26]

CONCLUSION

Ricin toxicity will likely be a challenging diagnosis to make. Maintaining a high index of suspicion in light of a credible threat will be the first step to identifying ricin as the toxin involved. An important pitfall to avoid is failing to recognize that different methods of delivery will result in very different clinical presentations. Using epidemiologic evidence will also be helpful. For instance, the development of either severe GI illness or respiratory illness in a group of previously healthy young military personnel who may be targets of a biologic warfare attack would certainly lead an individual to consider ricin as the culprit.

REFERENCES

1. Crompton R, Gall D. Georgi Markov—death in a pellet. *Med Leg J.* 1980;48(2):51–62.
2. Kortepeter M, Christopher G, Cieslak T. *USAMRID's Medical Management of Biologic Casualties Handbook.* 4th ed. Fort Detrick, MD: U.S. Army Medical Research Institute of Infectious Disease, 2001.
3. Rauber A, Heard J. Castor bean toxicity re-examined: a new perspective. *Vet Hum Toxicol.* 1985;27(6) 498–502.
4. Challoner KR, McCarron MM. Castor bean intoxication. *Ann Em Med.* 1990;19(10):1177–1183.
5. Sahni V, Agarwal SK, Singh NP, et al. Acute demyelinating encephalitis after jequirity pea ingestion (*Abrus precatorius*). *Clin Tox.* 2007;45:77–79.
6. Hui A, Marraffa JM, Stork CM. A rare ingestion of the black locust tree. *Clin Tox.* 2004;42(1):93–95.
7. Balint GA. Ricin: the toxic protein of castor oil seeds. *Toxicology.* 1974;2:77–102.
8. Zajtchuk R. *Textbook of Military Medicine. Part I: Warfare, Weaponry and the Casualty.* Washington DC: Office of the Surgeon General Department of the U.S. Army; 1997.
9. Flexner S. The histological changes produced by ricin and abrin intoxications. *J Exp Med.* 1897;2:197–216.
10. *Organization for the Prohibition of Chemical Weapons (OPCW).* Report of the second session of the scientific advisory board. 1999:1–20.
11. Ackerman G. Chronology of incidents involving ricin. *Center for Nonproliferation Studies (CNS) Reports.* 2004;1–6.
12. Centers for Disease Control and Prevention. Investigation of a ricin-containing envelope at a postal facility—South Carolina, 2003. *MMWR* 2003;52:1129–1131.
13. Robertus J. The structure and action of ricin, a cytotoxic N-glycosidase. *Cell Biol.* 1991; 2:23–30.
14. Hughes JN, Lindsay CD, Criffiths GD. Morphology of ricin and abrin exposed endothelial cells is consistent with apoptotic cell death. *Hum Exp Toxicol.* 1996;15:443–451.

15. Olsnes S, Refsnes K, Phil A. Mechanism of action of the toxic lectins abrin and ricin. *Nature.* 1974;249:627–631.

16. Aplin PJ, Eliseo T. Notable cases: ingestion of castor oil plant seeds. *Med J Aust.* 1997;167: 260–261.

17. Audi J, Belson M, Patel M, et al. Ricin poisoning: a comprehensive review. *JAMA.* 2005;294(18):2342–2351.

18. Griffiths GD, Rice P, Allenby AC, et al. Inhalational toxicology and histopathology of ricin and abrin toxins. *Inhal Toxicol.* 1995;7:269–288.

19. Wilhelmsen C, Pitt L. Lesions of acute inhaled lethal ricin intoxication in rhesus monkeys. *Vet Pathol.* 1993;30:482.

20. Fine DR, Sheperd HA, Griffiths GD, et al. Sub-lethal poisoning by self-injection with ricin. *Med Sci Law.* 1992;32(1);70–72.

21. Fodstad O, Kvalheim G, Godal A, et al. Phase I study of the plant protein ricin. *Cancer Res.* 1984;44:862–865.

22. Christiansen VJ, Hsu CH, Dormer KJ, et al. The cardiovascular effects of ricin in rabbits. *Pharmacol Toxicol.* 1994;74:148–152.

23. Department of Health and Human Services, Centers for Disease Control and Prevention. Fact sheet: laboratory testing for ricin. http://www.bt.cdc.gov/agent/ricin/#. Accessed September 25, 2009.

24. Johnson RC, Lemire SW, Woolfitt AR, et al. Quantitfication of ricinine in rat and human urine: a biomarker for ricin exposure. *J Anal Toxicol.* 2005;29:149–155.

25. Terazawa K, Griffiths GD, Leith AG. Electrophoretic determination of ricin using immunogold silver staining comparison with simple "protein dot" method. *Jap J of Leg Med.* 1989;43(3):303–309.

26. Thullier P, Griffiths G. Broad recognition of ricin toxins prepared from a range of Ricinus cultivars using immunochromatographic tests. *Clin tox.* 2009; 47(7):643–650.

25 | Trichothecene Mycotoxins

Stephen W. Borron and Juan C. Arias

CASE STUDY (FICTITIOUS)

A 47-year-old male police officer presents to the emergency department 3 hours after being sprayed with an oily, yellow substance while responding to a political demonstration. He reports wearing a short-sleeve summer uniform with substance contact limited to his face and arms. Noting some irritation at the time, he simply washed his face and arms with soap and water. He complains of severe eye pain and burning, itching, and redness of his exposed skin. He states that he has vomited twice and that his throat is scratchy and raw. He has a nonproductive cough and feels fatigued and a bit lightheaded. On questioning, he admits to having passed a watery brown stool. Examination reveals mild respiratory distress, with tachypnea and sinus tachycardia. The eye exam reveals blepharospasm and keratoconjunctivitis with evidence of corneal injury. The affected skin is erythematous, with numerous vesicles and a few small bullae. The lung exam reveals fine crackles. The abdomen is mildly tender diffusely, and the stool is brown but positive for occult blood. The remainder of the physical exam is unremarkable. Over the next 72 hours, the patient's dyspnea worsens and gastrointestinal bleeding ensues. Laboratory studies reveal severe leuko-cytopenia and thrombocytopenia. Following a prolonged intensive care stay, complicated by pneumonia with septic shock, hemorrhage requiring multiple transfusions, and a brief episode of seizures, the officer is discharged to a rehabilitation facility.

HISTORY

Tricothecenes compose a large subset of the mycotoxins, formed by fungal metabolism, with some 148 toxins described.[1] Numerous fungal species produce trichothecenes, including *Alternaria, Aspergillus, Claviceps, Fusarium, Cephalosporium, Myrotecium, Penicillium, Stachybotrys, Trichoderma,* and *Verticimonosporium.*[2,3] Poisoning has been reported after natural outbreaks of disease (most often associated with fungal overgrowth on food crops) and after intentional dissemination of the toxin. One of the earliest described incidents of grain-related trichothecene disease occurred in western Siberia in the 1890s. Known as "taumalgetriede" (staggering grains), the disease caused vomiting, headache, and vertigo.[4,5] A similar syndrome referred to as alimentary toxic aleukia occurred in subjects who consumed *Fusarium*-contaminated grain (millet, wheat, and barley) in Orenburg, Russia, between 1942 and 1947. The resulting illness reportedly killed over 10% of the population.[2,3,6] Patients suffered vomiting, diarrhea, skin irritation, leucopenia, and hemorrhage.[7] Subsequent analysis revealed the presence of T-2, a trichothecene mycotoxin.[8] Following World War II, several outbreaks of a syndrome known as Akakabi Byo were reported in Japan and Korea. This condition, reportedly due to toxins from *Fusarium* and *Giberella* species, was comprised of nausea, vomiting, diarrhea, and congestion or hemorrhage of numerous organs. It caused no deaths.[5]

The efficacy of these natural toxins in producing illness and death in the civilian population no doubt created interest in their use as agents of biologic warfare (BW).[2] The development, production, and stockpiling of such toxins for purposes of warfare are prohibited under the Biological and Toxin Weapons Convention of 1972 (BTWC).[9] Nonetheless, the Soviet Union is believed by some to have supplied trichothecenes for the wars in Southeast Asia in the 1970s and Afghanistan in the 1980s. Civilians in Laos described seeing "yellow rain" and provided consistent descriptions of the aftermath. The hallmark of the yellow rain attacks in Southeast Asia was onset, within minutes of contact, of nausea, burning skin, lethargy, and incoordination, followed hours later by cough, dyspnea, chest and abdominal pain, diarrhea, bleeding, and blistering of the skin.[10] Prisoners of war and enemy soldiers in both wars are said to have corroborated the use of these agents.[3] Multiple trichothecene toxins, including T-2, were isolated from environmental samples.[11] Others have discounted the yellow rain story, attributing the phenomenon to bee feces.[12,13] Iraq is reported to have performed research on trichothecenes,[14] and is said to have produced other mycotoxins, such as aflatoxin, for use as weapons.[2,14] In recent years, foodborne outbreaks of trichothecene poisoning have been described in China, where "red mold" was implicated in the human gastrointestinal poisoning of some 130,000 people in Anhui Province in 1991. The trichothecenes deoxynivalenol (DON), nivalenol (NIV), and their esters, zearalenone (ZEA) and fumonisins (FMs), were detected in various samples.[15] Similar outbreaks occurred in the late 1990s in Puyang, Henan Province, in China. The authors attributed this latter outbreak to *Fusarium* species having survived winter combined with unusually high precipitation during wheat flowering, producing a high concentration of *Fusarium* mycotoxins.[16]

POTENTIAL DELIVERY METHODS

Given the natural outbreaks of illness caused by grain contamination, it is evident that trichothecenes could be delivered via food supply. They are quite resistant to light and heat, requiring temperatures of 900°F for 10 minutes or 500°F for 30 minutes for complete inactivation[3]; thus cooking would be expected to have little or no effect on the toxin. The toxins are highly soluble in alcohols and propylene glycol,[3] so delivery through beverages is possible. Water supplies could potentially be used as a route for distribution of mycotoxins,[17] although water solubility is limited. Chlorination and dilution would likely diminish the tactical value of attempted contamination of municipal water systems.[17,18]

Aerosolized fungal spores or fragments are another potential means of dissemination. *Stachybotrys atra* (which produces satratoxin

H and other trichothecene toxins) has been grown on sterile rice, autoclaved, dried, and aerosolized by acoustic vibration. Nearly all the particles were less than 15 μm in diameter, and the mass median diameter was 5 μm, thus making them respirable.[19] Brasel and colleagues have demonstrated that trichothecenes may be found on fungal particles smaller than conidia, in the less than 5 μm range.[20,21] Mycotoxins may be efficiently spread as mold spores or fragments in dust, droplets, smokes, and aerosol, as described in the yellow rain incidents.[2,3,10] Because the toxins are both heat and light resistant, these means of delivery would likely be extremely reliable. This would seem to be confirmed by the reported lethality of their use in Laos and Afghanistan, with more than 9000 deaths occurring after some 350 attacks.[3]

Skin exposure to trichothecenes is likewise a substantial concern, as the toxins may be rapidly absorbed by the skin and mucous membranes. Furthermore, because trichothecene is some 400 times more potent than mustard as a blistering agent, local injury to the skin occurs rapidly with T-2 toxin.[22] On the basis of experimental evidence, Wannamacher and Wiener speculate that dermal exposure played a major role in the systemic toxicity observed after the yellow rain attacks.[3] Stark argues that while mycotoxins may be attractive to terrorists for use in crowded or small areas, they are impractical for large-scale dispersion, estimating that 2.2 million tons of rice would be required to supply the needed amount of T-2 toxin to induce 50% human lethality in a 10-km^2 area.[23] It is difficult to tie this assertion with the reported lethality in the yellow rain incidents.[3] In any case, even limited lethality might be sufficient to instill panic in a target population. One clear advantage of these toxins to terrorists is that they do not require extensive preparation, training, or advanced facilities.[23] Suspicion of the use of trichothecene mycotoxins as biologic weapons should be high in groups of people exposed to yellow smokes or mists who present with characteristic symptoms.[10]

TOXICOLOGIC MECHANISMS

Trichothecene mycotoxins are small (250–500 Da) lipid-soluble molecules.[2,24] They easily traverse biologic membranes and produce their toxic effects at the intracellular level.[2,25] Direct toxicity has been attributed to the presence of a 12,13-epoxide group.[26,27] These toxins inhibit RNA synthesis and interfere with ribosomal 60s subunit function and peptidyl transferase activity,[28,29] leading to inhibition of protein synthesis. As such, cells with rapid rates of turnover are more prone to suffer the toxic effects of trichothecene mycotoxins.[2] The toxins also mediate apoptosis through mitogen-activated protein kinase (MAPk) activation.[30,31] Decreased antibody synthesis is likewise reported,[26,32] leading to immune compromise. Trichothecene mycotoxins are classified in four types: A, B, C, and D.[33] In common among the four types is a 12,13-epoxide group.[34] Type A (T-2 toxin type), Type B (nivalenol type), and Type C (crotocin type) are known as nonmacrolytic.[33] Type A toxins inhibit mitochondrial function, whereas Type B toxins cause apoptosis and disruption of the mitochondrial membrane and are considered much less toxic at a mitochondrial level than Type A toxins, which result in necrosis.[35]

CLINICAL EFFECTS

Trichothecene mycotoxins affect multiple organ systems.[2,3,25,34] The dose and route of exposure to the toxin (i.e., oral, dermal, or respiratory) will determine in part which symptoms predominate, as well as the rapidity of onset.[3] The specific toxin involved and the underlying health of the exposed victim will also influence the clinical presentation. A small inoculum may result in primarily dermatologic manifestations, whereas a large inoculum may lead to systemic illness, with hemorrhage, shock, and death in less than 48 hours.[2] McGovern and colleagues cite earlier literature that reports trichothecene median lethal doses (MLD) in animals of 2 to 12 mg/kg after skin absorption.[22] These doses are far lower than the MLDs for mustard and Lewisite. Microgram doses can cause ocular symptoms, whereas doses of 10–20% the MLD may lead to gastrointestinal symptoms.[22] Other factors that may affect toxicity are age, health, gender, and, to a lesser extent, genetics, dietary status, and toxicologic interactions.[34] Dermatologic manifestations commonly include pruritus, erythema, and edema early after exposure,[24] with subsequent appearance of vesicles, bullae, skin pain, and necrosis as later manifestations of skin toxicity.[2,22] Dermal toxicity is thought to be caused by direct injury to skin capillary vessels.[33] Skin manifestations tend to be more frequent in the lips, fingers, and nose.[36] Dermatologic and topical exposures may cause prolonged symptoms.[2] Ocular exposure may cause ocular tearing, blurred vision, corneal irritation, and conjunctivitis.[2,10] When inhaled, mycotoxins can cause pulmonary tissue destruction in the distal airways.[2,22,37] Frequently observed respiratory symptoms include nose and throat pain, rhinorrhea, cough, dyspnea, wheezing, chest pain, and hemoptysis.[10,36] Mycotoxins, particularly those produced by *Stachybotrys*, have been reported as a causative agent of hemoptysis in children, but other studies have refuted this finding.[22,24,34] A condition called stachybotryotoxicosis, consisting of sore throat, epistaxis, dyspnea, cough, low-grade fever, and chest tightness, can follow *Stachybotrys* exposure.[38] After ingestion, nausea and vomiting are common.[39] More severe presentations may include gastrointestinal hemorrhage.[2,34,39]

Hematologic toxicity in humans and animals might be manifested by petechiae, hemorrhages, anemia, thrombocytopenia, granulocytopenia, and reticuloendothelial organ necrosis.[34,36] Pancytopenia might occur at late stages.[2] Consequences of hematologic toxicity include increased infection and sepsis susceptibility.[5,25,26,39] T-2 is believed to be particularly toxic to hematopoietic cells.[5] The similarity of these effects, in combination with the attendant gastrointestinal toxicity, to acute radiation sickness has led trichothecene toxicity to be referred to as "radiomimetic."

Immunotoxicity may present as increased microbial infections.[27,34] Decreased levels of B and T lymphocytes and increased susceptibility to infection with salmonella, *Listeria monocytogenes*, *Babesia microti*, and *Mycobacterium* were observed in animals after exposure to T-2 toxin.[40,41] Additional studies have shown increased susceptibility to normally nonpathogenic viruses after exposure to T-2 mycotoxin.[41] Nephrotoxicity has been observed in animal models.[4]

In terms of neurologic symptoms, severe manifestations may include ataxia, tremors, seizure, and coma.[3,36] The clinical picture resulting from trichothecene toxicity is distinctive but not pathognomonic. Individual cases without an obvious exposure history might very well be misdiagnosed early as sepsis.

Multiple cases presenting in a specific geographical area will likely provide clues to the occurrence of a toxin-derived illness.[6] Reporting of unusual illnesses to poison control centers and local health departments, whether or not they are suspected to be of toxic origin, may lead to earlier detection.[42] Even when a chemical, biologic, or radiologic (CBR) agent is suspected, recognition of trichothecene mycotoxicity will require clinical acumen. For example, Staphylococcal enterotoxin B, ricin, and trichothecenes can all cause severe respiratory symptoms; of these however, only the trichothecenes are likely to cause dermatologic symptoms.[2] Trichothecenes, like acute radiation sickness (ARS), can lead to severe leukopenia, gastrointestinal bleeding, and resultant decreased resistance to infection. Radiation-related skin injury, however, is generally delayed (days to weeks).[43] Mustard, Lewisite, and other blistering agents can cause bullous or vesicular skin and pulmonary injury, making clinical differentiation from trichothecenes difficult. Sulfur mustard, like trichothecenes, can cause severe leukocytopenia and associated skin lesions that do not typically become painful until several hours after exposure; thus it may closely mimic trichothecenes. A readily available field chemical test may be useful for detecting mustard.[2] Lewisite, like trichothecenes, causes immediately painful skin lesions but does not cause a hematopoietic syndrome.[44]

ANALYTIC DETECTION

Exposure to trichothecene toxins may be established by searching for the toxins or their metabolites, antibodies formed against the toxins, or the source fungi. Because toxins may be rapidly metabolized, analysis of metabolites is often undertaken.[25] Matrices include environmental air and dust samples, suspect foodstuffs, as well as urine, plasma, and blood. Immediate on-site detection of trichothecenes is not yet possible; Schneider et al.[45] and Zheng et al. [46] provide excellent reviews of currently available relatively rapid technologies. The most rapid and simple methods of testing employ enzyme-linked immunoassays (ELISA) for the detection of antibodies to trichothecene toxins (an index of previous exposure) and of toxins themselves.[37,47-50] According to Holstege et al., sensitive modified liquid chromatography can give positive results from blood samples for up to 1 month; this technique, however, requires advanced human and material resources.[25] Liquid chromatography-mass spectrometry (LC-MS) has been used for detection of toxins in blood,[51] urine,[52,53] milk,[54] and various foods and grains.[55-60] Other published methods include detection of fungal DNA by polymerase chain reaction,[61-65] cytotoxicity assays,[66] protein translation assays,[67] electrochemical detection,[68] gas chromatography (most often coupled with mass spectrometry),[39,69-75] high-performance liquid chromatography (HPLC),[76] and thin-layer chromatography (TLC).[77] It should be remembered that detection of molds known to produce toxins is not the equivalent of toxin detection and that although finding antibodies establishes prior exposure, it provides no information regarding the dose of the toxin.

CONCLUSION

The trichothecene mycotoxins are commonly found in the natural environment, occasionally causing epidemic foodborne disease. While mass production might be difficult, their production on a small scale for isolated acts of terrorism would require low technology and little cost. The diagnosis of poisoning by these toxins is complicated by multiple presentations depending on the toxin(s), dose, route, and host. The clinical presentation can mimic simple food poisoning or sepsis, acute radiation sickness, and poisoning by other toxins and blistering agents. Relatively rapid onset of painful blisters as well as pulmonary and hematologic symptoms provide the best clues to the diagnosis. Analysis can be performed in air, soil, foods, and biologic matrices. Simple immunoassays can demonstrate the presence of toxin or provide evidence of exposure. Exposure does not necessarily indicate poisoning. Mass spectrometry in combination with liquid or gas chromatography can provide precise identification and quantization, but such procedures are not readily available in clinical laboratories.

REFERENCES

1. World Health Organization. *Environmental health criteria 105: selected mycotoxins: ochratoxins, trichothecenes, ergot.* Geneva: International Programme for Chemical Safety; 1990.

2. Henghold WB II. Other biologic toxin bioweapons: ricin, staphylococcal enterotoxin B, and trichothecene mycotoxins. *Dermatol Clin.* 2004;22(3):257–262.

3. Wannemacher RW Jr, Wiener SL. Tricothecene mycotoxins. In: Sidell FR, Takafuji ET, Franz DR, eds. *Medical Aspects of Chemical and Biological Warfare.* Bethesda, MD: Office of The Surgeon General; 1997:655–676.

4. Pestka JJ, Smolinski AT. Deoxynivalenol: toxicology and potential effects on humans. *J Toxicol Environ Health B Crit Rev.* 2005;8(1):39–69.

5. Parent-Massin D. Haematotoxicity of trichothecenes. *Toxicol Lett.* 2004;153(1):75–81.

6. Peraica M, Radić B, Lucić A, et al. Toxic effects of mycotoxins in humans. *Bull World Health Organ.* 1999;77(9):754–766.

7. Franz DR, Jahrling PB, McClain DJ, et al. Clinical recognition and management of patients exposed to biological warfare agents. *Clin Lab Med.* 2001;21(3):435–473.

8. Yagen B, Joffe AZ. Screening of toxic isolates of *Fusarium poae* and *Fusarium sporotrichoides* involved in causing alimentary toxic aleukia. *Appl Environ Microbiol.* 1976;32(3):423–427.

9. Toxins: potential chemical weapons from living organisms. Organization for the Prohibition of Chemical Weapons Web site. http://www.opcw.org/resp/html/toxins.html. Accessed October 5, 2009.

10. Blazes DL, Lawler JV, Lazarus AA. When biotoxins are tools of terror. Early recognition of intentional poisoning can attenuate effects. *Postgrad Med.* 2002;112(2):89–92, 95–86, 98.

11. Rosen RT, Rosen JD. Presence of four *Fusarium* mycotoxins and synthetic material in "yellow rain." Evidence for the use of chemical weapons in Laos. *Biomed Mass Spectrom.* 1982;9(10):443–450.

12. Marshall E. Yellow rain evidence slowly whittled away. *Science.* 1986;233(4759):18–19.

13. Nowicke JW, Meselson M. Yellow rain—a palynological analysis. *Nature.* 1984;309(5965):205–206.

14. Stone R. Biodefense. Peering into the shadows: Iraq's bioweapons program. Science. 2002;297(5584):1110–1112.

15. Li FQ, Luo XY, Yoshizawa T. Mycotoxins (trichothecenes, zearalenone and fumonisins) in cereals associated with human red-mold intoxications stored since 1989 and 1991 in China. *Nat Toxins.* 1999;7(3):93–97.

16. Li FQ, Li YW, Luo XY, et al. *Fusarium* toxins in wheat from an area in Henan Province, PR China, with a previous human red mould intoxication episode. *Food Addit Contam.* 2002;19(2):163–167.

17. Wilson SC, Brasel TL, Martin JM, et al. Efficacy of chlorine dioxide as a gas and in solution in the inactivation of two trichothecene mycotoxins. *Int J Toxicol.* 2005;24(3):181–186.

18. Nuzzo JB. The biological threat to U.S. water supplies: toward a national water security policy. *Biosecur Bioterror.* 2006;4(2):147–159.

19. Sorenson WG, Frazer DG, Jarvis BB, et al. Trichothecene mycotoxins in aerosolized conidia of Stachybotrys atra. *Appl Environ Microbiol.* 1987;53(6):1370–1375.

20. Brasel TL, Douglas DR, Wilson SC, et al. Detection of airborne *Stachybotrys chartarum* macrocyclic trichothecene mycotoxins on particulates smaller than conidia. *Appl Environ Microbiol.* 2005;71(1):114–122.

21. Brasel TL, Martin JM, Carriker CG, et al. Detection of airborne *Stachybotrys chartarum* macrocyclic trichothecene mycotoxins in the indoor environment. *Appl Environ Microbiol.* 2005;71(11):7376–7388.

22. McGovern TW, Christopher GW, Eitzen EM. Cutaneous manifestations of biological warfare and related threat agents. *Arch Dermatol.* 1999;135(3):311–322.

23. Stark AA. Threat assessment of mycotoxins as weapons: molecular mechanisms of acute toxicity. *J Food Prot.* 2005;68(6):1285–1293.

24. Cieslak TJ, Talbot TB, Hartstein BH. Biological warfare and the skin I: bacteria and toxins. *Clin Dermatol.* 2002;20(4):346–354.

25. Holstege CP, Bechtel LK, Reilly TH, et al. Unusual but potential agents of terrorists. *Emerg Med Clin North Am.* 2007;25(2):549–566.

26. Revankar SG. Clinical implications of mycotoxins and *Stachybotrys. Am J Med Sci.* 2003;325(5):262–274.

27. Shima J, Takase S, Takahashi Y, et al. Novel detoxification of the trichothecene mycotoxin deoxynivalenol by a soil bacterium isolated by enrichment culture. *Appl Environ Microbiol.* 1997;63(10):3825–3830.

28. Middlebrook JL, Leatherman DL. Binding of T-2 toxin to eukaryotic cell ribosomes. *Biochem Pharmacol.* 1989;38(18):3103–3110.

29. Cannon M, Smith KE, Carter CJ. Prevention, by ribosome-bound nascent polyphenylalanine chains, of the functional interaction of T-2 toxin with its receptor site. *Biochem J.* 1976;156(2):289–294.

30. Yang GH, Jarvis BB, Chung YJ, et al. Apoptosis induction by the satratoxins and other trichothecene mycotoxins: relationship to ERK, p38 MAPK, and SAPK/JNK activation. *Toxicol Appl Pharmacol.* 2000;164(2):149–160.

31. Shifrin VI, Anderson P. Trichothecene mycotoxins trigger a ribotoxic stress response that activates c-Jun N-terminal kinase and p38 mitogen-activated protein kinase and induces apoptosis. *J Biol Chem.* 1999;274(20):13985–13992.

32. Corrier DE. Mycotoxicosis: mechanisms of immunosuppression. *Vet Immunol Immunopathol.* 1991;30(1):73–87.

33. Ueno Y. Toxicological features of T-2 toxin and related trichothecenes. *Fundam Appl Toxicol.* 1984;4(2 Pt 2):S124–S132.

34. Bennett JW, Klich M. Mycotoxins. *Clin Microbiol Rev.* 2003;16(3):497–516.

35. Nasri T, Bosch RR, Voorde S, et al. Differential induction of apoptosis by type A and B trichothecenes in Jurkat T-lymphocytes. *Toxicol In Vitro.* 2006;20(6):832–840.

36. Rosenbloom M, Leikin JB, Vogel SN, et al. Biological and chemical agents: a brief synopsis. *Am J Ther.* 2002;9(1):5–14.

37. Ngundi MM, Qadri SA, Wallace EV, et al. Detection of deoxynivalenol in foods and indoor air using an array biosensor. *Environ Sci Technol.* 2006;40(7):2352–2356.

38. Etzel RA: Mycotoxins. *JAMA.* 2002;287(4):425–427.

39. Schothorst RC, Jekel AA, Van Egmond HP, et al. Determination of trichothecenes in duplicate diets of young children by capillary gas chromatography with mass spectrometric detection. *Food Addit Contam.* 2005;22(1):48–55.

40. Kamalavenkatesh P, Vairamuthu S, Balachandran C, Manohar BM, Raj GD. Immunopathological effect of the mycotoxins cyclopiazonic acid and T-2 toxin on broiler chicken. *Mycopathologia.* 2005;159(2):273–279.

41. Li M, Harkema JR, Islam Z, et al. T-2 toxin impairs murine immune response to respiratory reovirus and exacerbates viral bronchiolitis. *Toxicol Appl Pharmacol.* 2006;217(1):76–85.

42. Wolkin AF, Patel M, Watson W, et al. Early detection of illness associated with poisonings of public health significance. *Ann Emerg Med.* 2006;47(2):170–176.

43. Vlietstra RE, Wagner LK, Koenig T, et al. Radiation burns as a severe complication of fluoroscopically guided cardiological interventions. *J Interv Cardiol.* 2004;17(3):131–142.

44. McManus J, Huebner K. Vesicants. *Crit Care Clin.* 2005;21(4):707–718, vi.

45. Schneider E, Curtui V, Seidler C, et al. Rapid methods for deoxynivalenol and other trichothecenes. *Toxicol Lett.* 2004;153(1):113–121.

46. Zheng MZ, Richard JL, Binder J. A review of rapid methods for the analysis of mycotoxins. *Mycopathologia.* 2006;161(5):261–273.

47. Vojdani A, Thrasher JD, Madison RA, et al. Antibodies to molds and satratoxin in individuals exposed in water-damaged buildings. *Arch Environ Health.* 2003;58(7):421–432.

48. Vojdani A. Antibodies against *Stachybotrys chartarum* extract and its antigenic components, *Stachyhemolysin* and *Stachyrase-A:* a new clinical biomarker. *Med Sci Monit.* 2005;11(5):BR139–BR145.

49. Ngundi MM, Shriver-Lake LC, Moore MH, et al. Multiplexed detection of mycotoxins in foods with a regenerable array. *J Food Prot.* 2006;69(12):3047–3051.

50. Brasel TL, Campbell AW, Demers RE, et al. Detection of trichothecene mycotoxins in sera from individuals exposed to Stachybotrys chartarum in indoor environments. *Arch Environ Health.* 2004;59(6):317–323.

51. Bily AC, Reid LM, Savard ME, et al. Analysis of *Fusarium graminearum* mycotoxins in different biological matrices by LC/MS. *Mycopathologia.* 2004;157(1):117–126.

52. Meky FA, Turner PC, Ashcroft AE, et al. Development of a urinary biomarker of human exposure to deoxynivalenol. *Food Chem Toxicol.* 2003;41(2):265–273.

53. Razzazi-Fazeli E, Böhm J, Jarukamjorn K, et al. Simultaneous determination of major B-trichothecenes and the de-epoxy-metabolite of deoxynivalenol in pig urine and maize using high-performance liquid chromatography-mass spectrometry. *J Chromatogr B Analyt Technol Biomed Life Sci.* 2003;796(1):21–33.

54. Sørensen LK, Elbaek TH. Determination of mycotoxins in bovine milk by liquid chromatography tandem mass spectrometry. *J Chromatogr B Analyt Technol Biomed Life Sci.* 2005;820(2):183–196.

55. Razzazi-Fazeli E, Rabus B, Cecon B, et al. Simultaneous quantification of A-trichothecene myco-toxins in grains using liquid chromatography-atmospheric pressure chemical ionisation mass spectrometry. *J Chromatogr A.* 2002;968(1-2):129–142.

56. Berthiller F, Schuhmacher R, Buttinger G, et al. Rapid simultaneous determination of major type A- and B-trichothecenes as well as zearalenone in maize by high performance liquid chromatography-tandem mass spectrometry. *J Chromatogr A.* 2005;1062(2):209–216.

57. Biselli S, Hummert C. Development of a multicomponent method for *Fusarium* toxins using LC-MS/MS and its application during a survey for the content of T-2 toxin and deoxynivalenol in various feed and food samples. *Food Addit Contam.* 2005;22(8):752–760.

58. Klotzel M, Lauber U, Humpf HU. A new solid phase extraction clean-up method for the determination of 12 type A and B trichothecenes in cereals and cereal-based food by LC-MS/MS. *Mol Nutr Food Res.* 2006;50(3):261–269.

59. Tanaka H, Takino M, Sugita-Konishi Y, et al. Development of a liquid chromatography/time-of-flight mass spectrometric method for the simultaneous determination of trichothecenes, zearalenone and aflatoxins in foodstuffs. *Rapid Commun Mass Spectrom.* 2006;20(9):1422–1428.

60. Zollner P, Mayer-Helm B. Trace mycotoxin analysis in complex biological and food matrices by liquid chromatography-atmospheric pressure ionisation mass spectrometry. *J Chromatogr A.* 2006;1136(2):123–169.

61. Demeke T, Clear RM, Patrick SK, et al. Species-specific PCR-based assays for the detection of *Fusarium* species and a comparison with the whole seed agar plate method and trichothecene analysis. *Int J Food Microbiol.* 2005;103(3):271–284.

62. Halstensen AS, Nordby KC, Klemsdal SS, et al. Toxigenic *Fusarium* sp. as determinants of trichothecene mycotoxins in settled grain dust. *J Occup Environ Hyg.* 2006;3(12):651–659.

63. Llorens A, Hinojo MJ, Mateo R, et al. Characterization of *Fusarium* spp. isolates by PCR-RFLP analysis of the intergenic spacer region of the rRNA gene (rDNA). *Int J Food Microbiol.* 2006;106(3):297–306.

64. Llorens A, Hinojo MJ, Mateo R, et al. Variability and characterization of mycotoxin-producing Fusarium spp isolates by PCR-RFLP analysis of the IGS-rDNA region. *Antonie Van Leeuwenhoek.* 2006;89(3-4):465–478.

65. Li HP, Wu AB, Zhao CS, et al. Development of a generic PCR detection of deoxynivalenol- and nivalenol-chemotypes of *Fusarium graminearum*. *FEMS Microbiol Lett.* 2005;243(2):505–511.

66. Widestrand J, Lundh T, Pettersson H, et al. A rapid and sensitive cytotoxicity screening assay for trichothecenes in cereal samples. *Food Chem Toxicol.* 2003;41(10):1307–1313.

67. Yike I, Allan T, Sorenson WG, et al. Highly sensitive protein translation assay for trichothecene toxicity in airborne particulates: comparison with cytotoxicity assays. *Appl Environ Microbiol.* 1999;65(1):88–94.

68. Hsueh CC, Liu Y, Freund MS. Indirect electrochemical detection of type-B trichothecene mycotoxins. *Anal Chem.* 1999;71(18):4075–4080.

69. Begley P, Foulger BE, Jeffery PD, et al. Detection of trace levels of trichothecenes in human blood using capillary gas chromatography-electron-capture negative ion chemical ionisation mass spectrometry. *J Chromatogr.* 1986;367(1):87–101.

70. Black RM, Clarke RJ, Read RW. Detection of trace levels of trichothecene mycotoxins in human urine by gas chromatography-mass spectrometry. *J Chromatogr.* 1986;367(1):103–115.

71. Koch P. State of the art of trichothecenes analysis. *Toxicol Lett.* 2004;153(1):109–112.

72. Rodrigues-Fo E, Mirocha CJ, Xie W, Krick TP, Martinelli JA. Electron ionization mass spectral fragmentation of deoxynivalenol and related tricothecenes. *Rapid Commun Mass Spectrom.* 2002;16(19):1827–1835.

73. Bloom E, Bal K, Nyman E, et al. Mass spectrometry-based strategy for the direct detection and quantification of some mycotoxins produced by *Stachybotrys* and *Aspergillus* in indoor environments. *Appl Environ Microbiol.* 2007;73(13):4211–7.

74. Jestoi M, Ritieni A, Rizzo A. Analysis of the *Fusarium* mycotoxins fusaproliferin and trichothecenes in grains using gas chromatography-mass spectrometry. *J Agric Food Chem.* 2004;52(6):1464–1469.

75. D'Agostino PA, Provost LR, Drover DR. Analysis of trichothecene mycotoxins in human blood by capillary column gas chromatography-ammonia chemical ionization mass spectrometry. *J Chromatogr.* 1986;367(1):77–86.

76. Sugita-Konsihi Y, Tanaka T, Tabata S, et al. Validation of an HPLC analytical method coupled to a multifunctional clean-up column for the determination of deoxynivalenol. *Mycopathologia.* 2006;161(4):239–243.

77. Smoragiewicz W, Cossette B, Boutard A, et al. Trichothecene mycotoxins in the dust of ventilation systems in office buildings. *Int Arch Occup Environ Health.* 1993;65(2):113–117.

Specific Classes of Poisoners

26 | Medical Serial Killers

*Thomas M. Neer, James McCarthy, Bernard Postles,
and R. Brent Furbee*

INTRODUCTION

The true incidence of homicides committed by medical professionals is impossible to determine. There are, however, numerous examples of healthcare providers preying on helpless patients, such as the notorious cases of Donald Harvey, Kristen Gilbert, Genene Jones, Efren Saldivar, and Charles Cullen. For several reasons, the healthcare system is historically slow to investigate such allegations. Ironically, the failure of healthcare workers to consider a coworker as a murderer has caused delays in the recognition of those deaths as homicides and subsequently delayed the prevention of further murders. When patient homicide is discovered, individuals and institutions are reticent to document it for fear of damage to their reputations and increased exposure to litigation. This chapter will focus on three cases in which the authors were directly involved with the criminal investigation: Michael Swango (Neer and McCarthy), Harold Shipman (Postles), and Orville Lynn Majors (Furbee).

MICHAEL SWANGO, MD

When Michael Swango graduated valedictorian of his Quincy, Illinois, high school class in 1972, no one suspected he would become a notorious doctor and murderer. Although he pled guilty to the poisoning deaths of four hospital patients in New York and Ohio, authorities believe he was responsible for many more, especially when he worked in hospitals in Africa. What makes Dr. Swango's activities particularly disturbing is that despite his history of aberrant behavior, warnings from coworkers, and dismissals from hospitals, he was able to get hired repeatedly by other medical facilities and to continue poisoning. In many cases, the substances he used left no obvious signs of poisoning. In most cases, physical evidence was lacking, due in part to the passage of time from the deaths to the subsequent police investigation and because of the refusal of some families to have autopsies performed.

The first signs of trouble appeared after Swango entered the Southern Illinois University School of Medicine in 1979. Despite the school's rigorous curriculum and demanding schedule, Swango continued to drive great distances to work as a part-time emergency medical technician (EMT). Classmates could not understand why Swango would work while attending medical school, considering that time was precious and he was not exceptionally talented. Because he crammed for examinations, classmates coined the word "swangoing" to describe his study habits. During a class in radiology, Swango asked the professor what a particular mass was on an x-ray. The professor replied, "That's the heart, Mike." In an anatomy lab, Swango drew the attention of his classmates by mangling the section he was required to dissect.

On clinical rotations, several of Swango's patients died mysteriously. Although none was considered homicide, classmates jokingly referred to him as Double-O-Swango, a reference to the James Bond (agent 007) character and his "license to kill." While working on his OB/GYN rotation, faculty caught him falsifying records. To avoid expulsion from school, Swango hired a lawyer and was able to negotiate a compromise, agreeing to repeat his clinical rotation. Still, two classmates felt so strongly about Swango's incompetence that they sent a formal letter to the dean outlining their misgivings about him.

Swango graduated from medical school in 1983. In July, he began a general surgery internship and neurosurgery residency at Ohio State University (OSU). Within months, the staff noticed oddities such as a fascination with Nazis and the Holocaust. Supervisors noted that his medical histories were cursory at best and that he had difficulty performing basic surgical procedures. When criticized, he immediately did push-ups.

In January 1984, supervisors placed him on probation and warned him that his residency in neurosurgery was in jeopardy. Within weeks, several suspicious deaths occurred on the floor where he worked; some were under his care, but others were not. Almost all deaths were preceded by respiratory arrests, and Swango had visited many patients immediately prior to their codes. On several occasions, Swango had been seen next to the patient's intravenous (IV) line. One patient reported that Swango injected an unknown substance into her IV line, which caused intense burning and paralysis. Swango told her that when the substance reached her elbow, she would be dead.

Wary hospital administrators elected to conduct an internal inquiry rather than contact the police. Despite inconsistencies in Swango's accounts to other doctors about the suspicious deaths, he was never formally interviewed about them. When the OSU Police Department was finally called to investigate these deaths 9 months later, Swango had been dismissed from the hospital, and physical evidence was no longer available. Nevertheless, the police conducted a comprehensive investigation for 13 months and interviewed more than 400 people, including 45 doctors and more than 100 nurses. A subsequent review of their investigation by the Franklin County Prosecutor's Office determined that due to a lack of physical evidence, Swango would not be charged.[1]

After Swango left OSU, coworkers recalled an incident during his rotation at the Children's Hospital from April to June of 1984. Swango brought in a box of chicken for doctors. One by one, those eating became violently ill with severe stomach cramps, headaches, and vomiting. At the time, no one suspected Swango might have been poisoning them.[1]

After leaving OSU, Swango worked as a paramedic for the EMS company that had employed him during medical school. Coworkers, apparently unaware of his recent dismissal from OSU, observed a change in his behavior. In addition to volunteering for extra shifts, he seemed obsessed with death, pasting into a scrapbook a number of news articles on traffic accidents and plane crashes. The more gruesome a tragedy, the more excited Swango became. When a gunman entered a McDonald's in San Ysidro, California, and killed several people, Swango complained that someone else always stole his ideas.

In October 1984, concerns intensified when several of Swango's coworkers became ill after consuming doughnuts that he brought them. Their symptoms included severe headaches, gastrointestinal distress, and vomiting. Suspecting that Swango may have poisoned the doughnuts, coworkers searched his locker and found a box of arsenic-laden ant poison. A week later, before leaving to answer a call, a coworker brewed unsweetened tea. Swango was seen in the area. When the coworker and his colleagues returned and found overly sweet tea, they took samples of it. The lab results confirmed suspicions: the tea contained arsenic consistent with Swango's ant poison. A coworker recalled that Swango's ambition was to be a doctor who invented an untraceable poison.

A criminal investigation ensued, and Swango was arrested. A search of his apartment revealed mouse poison, bottles of ant poison, leaf and garden spray, numerous sacks of castor beans, roach powder, needles and syringes, a jug of sulfuric acid, numerous jars of assorted chemicals, a book on satanism, a book on how to extract ricin, and several index cards containing recipes for ricin, cyanide, and botulism.[1] Although Swango maintained his innocence, in August 1985 he was convicted of assault and sentenced to 5 years in prison but was released after serving only half this time.

When news about Swango's interest in ricin was made public, a doctor at OSU recalled the unexpected death of one of his patients. The patient had died of respiratory arrest. What puzzled him was that the autopsy revealed clots in the arteries of the patient's heart and in the vessels of her kidneys, liver, intestines, and lungs. When the doctor learned that Swango had been on duty at the time, he suspected that Swango may have killed his patient with ricin because he believed that blood clots were a telltale sign.[1]

In 1988, after Swango was released from prison, he concealed his conviction and medical degree and moved to Virginia, working at a placement center counseling students applying to medical school. Shortly after his arrival, two workers became ill after they drank coffee; staff contacted the Board of Health to check if the coffee had spoiled but no problems were found. Before suspicion could fall on Swango, he quit and began working as a lab technician at a coal company, marrying a nurse he had dated in Ohio.

Coworkers considered Swango odd because he often talked of serial murder. When several of his coworkers fell ill with headaches and severe abdominal distress, Swango expressed interest in their symptoms, calling some at home to question them. Eventually, coworkers discovered Swango's identity after opening his briefcase and finding news articles about suspicious deaths at OSU Medical School. This led them to suspect Swango of poisoning, and they notified the police. Unfortunately, important physical evidence had disappeared. A search of Swango's residence revealed a variety of books on poisons but no evidence linking him directly to any criminal activity.

Before quitting his job and leaving Virginia, Swango divorced his wife and began dating a local nurse, Kristen Kinney. He applied to work as a physician at a residency program in Sioux Falls, South Dakota, one of the few states that allowed felons to work in hospitals. Using what was described as unusual charm and persuasion, Swango disarmed his interviewers by disclosing his previous criminal conviction, minimizing culpability and concealing incriminating details. His perceived honesty impressed the administrator, allowing Swango to begin work before a thorough background check was performed.

In 1992 problems started. A Sioux Falls hospital across town from where Swango worked complained that he was sexually harassing a nurse. When Swango's employer confronted him about these accusations, Swango apologized, and the matter was dropped.

Coincidently, 2 months later, an ABC news documentary by John Stossel on the previous suspicious deaths at OSU Medical School aired nationally. Officials at the South Dakota hospital promptly contacted OSU for additional details, then fired Swango, who contested his dismissal. Although his fiancée, Kinney, outwardly defended him, privately she had doubts about his innocence after discovering incriminating information in their apartment, including a hidden poison recipe card. Because Kinney complained about stomach problems and migraines, officials later wondered whether Swango may have been poisoning her. The stress of her association with Swango reached a peak when she was found at night wandering naked and confused on the freezing streets of Sioux Falls. Her worried parents eventually persuaded her to return to Virginia.

As Kinney regained control of her life, Swango returned to Virginia and started leaning on her financially and emotionally. In 1993, he was accepted into a psychiatric residency at the State University of New York (SUNY) Hospital at Stony Brook. Although he readily disclosed his assault conviction during his interview, he claimed it was due to a bar room brawl. His new assignment began with a required surgical internship at the nearby Veterans Affairs (VA) hospital in Northport, New York.

VA hospitals often have a large number of elderly and terminally ill patients. It is not uncommon for such patients to request do not resuscitate (DNR) orders. As a rule, after staff members discuss DNR with patients, they seldom raise the issue again unless the patient asks. Swango, however, aggressively tried to persuade patients who had not requested DNR orders to change their minds. He was no doubt aware that hospital personnel who know a patient has requested a DNR are less inclined to question a patient's death.

In at least one instance, Swango entered a DNR order on behalf of a patient without consent. Swango had been pressuring the patient to request a DNR, but the patient refused. Investigation determined that Swango, listed as a first-year resident (R-1), told his supervisor (an R-2) that he had contacted the chief resident via telephone after the patient became unconscious and that they had discussed the need for a DNR order. Swango convinced the R-2 that this conversation with the family constituted a DNR order. During a subsequent interview, the chief resident asserted that he had received no such phone call and would have recalled it. R-1's do not commonly telephone the chief

resident about a routine DNR order. During a subsequent interview, the R-2 conceded that he had probably been tricked by Swango. Incidentally, the R-2 recalled a previous occasion when he dined with Swango at a restaurant and became violently nauseated on the drive home. In several other suspicious deaths at Northport, Swango was observed in patients' rooms immediately prior to their demise.

During Swango's time at Northport, Kinney committed suicide. In her suicide note, she sounded exhausted and depressed but claimed she still loved Swango. Kinney's parents believe their daughter's suicide was caused by the stress of her relationship with him and the chronic headaches and stomach problems she had been experiencing. Before Kinney was buried, her mother clipped off a section of her hair for sentimental reasons. Later, the Federal Bureau of Investigation (FBI) Laboratory determined the hair contained large amounts of arsenic. Swango's longstanding interest in arsenic, coupled with Kinney's chronic headaches and abdominal distress, strongly suggest he was poisoning her, but this suspicion cannot be confirmed. As will be discussed later in this chapter, there is strong evidence that Swango poisoned other acquaintances, although not necessarily to kill them.

When hospital officials in South Dakota learned that Swango was working as a doctor, they contacted VA officials who promptly suspended Swango and initiated an inquiry into suspicious deaths. Without notifying the FBI, the Suffolk County Police Department, or the Suffolk County Medical Examiner's Office, the VA's Office of Inspector General (VA-OIG) conducted a cursory investigation and advised the U.S. Attorney's Office that they could find no evidence of wrongdoing.

During their investigation, the VA rejected requests by Suffolk County homicide detectives to interview Swango, claiming the county had no jurisdiction on federal property.[2,3] The detectives promptly contacted the FBI. When the two agencies arrived, they were shocked to learn that Swango had already been fired and allowed to return to remove his belongings. It seemed that the VA-OIG lacked an understanding of the value of immediate physical evidence. Years later, an FBI agent was shown photographs the VA-OIG had taken of Swango's quarters and was shocked to see bottles, pill containers, notebooks, and binders that might have contained possible evidence of a murder.

Swango relocated to Georgia, legally changed his name to Jackson Kirk, moved in with one of Kinney's friends, and secured a job at a water treatment facility. At that time, neither the FBI nor any other law enforcement agency had sufficient evidence to arrest him for murder. Without eyewitnesses or specific knowledge of the type of substance he used to kill people in hospitals, the FBI continued their investigation.

The FBI obtained an arrest warrant for Swango for falsifying his application for employment at the Northport VA hospital. They exhumed the bodies of five patients who had died under suspicious circumstances. However, before process could be served, he disappeared. Thinking he may have fled the country, the FBI placed a border stop on him. Almost 2 years later, as Swango was returning from overseas, U.S. immigration officials detained him based on the outstanding warrant.

A subsequent investigation revealed that while Swango was living in Georgia, he had quietly applied through the Evangelical Lutheran Church to work as a physician in Africa. To avoid having to explain the suspension of his medical license, he submitted forged documents indicating that he was properly licensed and in good standing.

When Swango subsequently arrived at Mneme Hospital in rural Zimbabwe, he was greeted warmly because qualified doctors were in high demand. Nonetheless, it soon became apparent that Swango's medical skills were lacking, particularly in the area of obstetrics and general surgery. Hospital officials reassigned Swango to Mpilo Hospital in Bulawayo for several months for remedial education and closer supervision.

Swango returned to Mneme Hospital, but nurses and patients complained about his suspicious behavior and abruptness with patients. A pregnant patient awaiting dispatch to the delivery room recalled seeing Swango surreptitiously remove a syringe from his jacket pocket and inject her IV with an unknown substance, practically in front of nurses. She instantly felt an intense burning sensation and paralysis but was able to attract the attention of a nurse who confronted Swango. He adamantly denied injecting anything. A patient, who had undergone

a successful leg amputation and was soon to be discharged, reported that Swango entered the ward late at night and injected him in the buttocks with a substance that immediately caused intense burning and paralysis. After administering the injection, Swango waved "bye-bye" to the patient and left the room. It was noted that Swango was not assigned to this ward, and the patient was not under his direct care.

The symptoms described by these survivors suggest Swango may have injected them with succinylcholine, a muscle relaxant. However, this could not be proven because blood samples were never drawn from these patients.

Thereafter, nurses began noticing an inordinate number of deaths when Swango was around. Hospital officials notified the police who initiated a criminal investigation and found five suspicious deaths and two attempted murders. Their investigation determined that Swango neglected to record treatment or drugs given and failed to swab areas before giving injections. They noted that patients died within minutes of injection and that with the exception of one, Swango certified the deaths himself, avoiding postmortem. All of the patients who died had fully recovered or had undergone successful surgeries. A search of Swango's quarters revealed syringes, medication, and other substances, but before they could be forensically tested, the police lost them. Nevertheless, the hospital suspended Swango, and he promptly hired a lawyer to contest this action. Amazingly, in the interim, he was allowed to work as a volunteer at Mpilo Hospital.[4]

As the criminal probe expanded, Swango fled to Zambia and quietly obtained a position at the University Teaching Hospital (UTH) in Lusaka. It was not long before nurses noticed his indifference to patients. As an adjunct to his regular duties, he earned extra money certifying the deaths of patients brought in dead. When Swango pronounced a man dead without entering the examination room, the family complained to administrators who ordered Swango to show greater sensitivity. Swango then propped up the corpse in full view of the bereaved family, inserted a tongue depressor in his mouth, tapped the deceased's knee for reflexes, and laid him back down, saying, "He's dead."

UTH doctors found Swango's surgical skills lacking. Besides Swango's marginal medical skills, the nursing staff found his hygiene to be so poor that they refused to eat food he brought them. Informed that Swango was suspected of killing patients in Zimbabwe, UTH suspended him. Swango promptly contested the suspension. Although UTH officials were ultimately unable to attribute specific deaths to him, they were wary. In early 1994, when Zambian immigration officials arrived at UTH to question him, Swango climbed out a window and fled to Namibia. In the capital, Windhoek, Swango tried unsuccessfully to obtain a job at a forensic laboratory. Zimbabwean authorities had already disseminated a warning about him.

The police and Interpol turned over to the FBI dozens of Swango's books (many on serial murders), a partial diary, and an address book that, because of weight restrictions, he was forced to leave behind. Contact with the individuals listed in this address book enabled the FBI to piece together Swango's activities in Namibia.

Unable to find employment in Africa, Swango made arrangements to work at a hospital in Saudi Arabia. This required him to return to the United States and obtain a visa. When he reentered the United States, the FBI arrested him based on the sealed fraud indictment. In Swango's possession was a notebook with a reminder to himself to research all available information on serial killers by examining public documents and going to libraries and bookstores. Organized into dozens of short, numbered paragraphs with repeated references to death, murder, and emptiness in life, the writings resembled the beginning of a screenplay whose overall tone was, not surprisingly, somber. The following are some selected excerpts:

He could look at himself in a mirror and tell himself that he was one of the most powerful and dangerous men in the world. . . . He could feel he was God in disguise.[5]

There is, of course, one major disadvantage that dawns on every master criminal sooner or later. He can never achieve public recognition, or at least only at the cost of being caught. He must be content with the admiration of a very small circle. This explains why so many "master criminals" seem to take a certain pleasure in being caught. They are at last losing their anonymity. This

is the irony of the career of the master criminal; unless he is caught, he feels at the end the same frustration, the same intolerable sense of non-recognition that drove him to crime in the first place.[6]

Spin bacteria out of blood samples and mix it with anything, ie cyclosponne [sic] at hospital pharmacy. . . . You think pharmacies don't know anything beyond counting pills . . . but we're scientists; we're chemists. Any fool can use a centrifuge. Pharmacies create compounds; we create things. Pharmacies intent on killing their patients gave them placebos instead of anti-ejection drugs. How simple. Look for a drug that wasn't there...[7]

Swango pled guilty to the single fraud charge (Title 18, USC 1001) and was sentenced to 5 years in a federal prison. This conviction afforded the FBI time to further investigate in Africa and the United States. As part of the investigation, three bodies were exhumed in New York and four in Zimbabwe in hopes of discovering what killed these individuals.

While Swango was serving his sentence in a federal prison, the FBI went to interview him. They learned that he was enjoying high status among inmates, teaching Graduate Educational Development (GED) classes, working in the prison library where he had access to reading materials, living in a dorm with access to cooking facilities, cooking for the other inmates, and receiving regular visits from his half-brother. When the staff discovered him serving refreshments during an awards ceremony, they stopped him because this was a violation of the judge's sentencing order prohibiting Swango from accepting work in prison food service, the infirmary, or pharmacy. FBI agents explained the history of Swango's obsession with poisoning people and the continuing danger he posed. Coincidentally, there was a rebroadcast of an ABC documentary about suspicious deaths attributed to Swango. Prison officials promptly transferred him to a more secure facility. Less than a month after his arrival, an inmate attempted to cut his throat. Swango ducked, and the near fatal wound missed his carotid artery, leaving a scar across his face.

FBI agents visited Swango and outlined their investigative work in New York and Africa. They told him he would stand trial in New York on five capital murder charges and that he if he were acquitted, he would be sent to Africa to stand trial for murders there. The agents made clear they would accompany him to ensure that Zimbabwean investigators and prosecutors had all the information they needed. Swango countered that this was impossible in the absence of an extradition treaty. When the agents produced a recently ratified treaty between the United States and Zimbabwe, Swango indicated he was willing to make a deal. He was flown to New York and in a matter of weeks agreed to plead guilty to three federal murder charges in New York and one state charge in Columbus, Ohio. Swango would be sentenced to life without parole, and charges in Zimbabwe would be dropped.

Considering Swango's lifelong interest in poisons and access to a variety of medicines, it is difficult to determine all the substances he may have used. In New York, Swango used epinephrine and succinylcholine to kill patients. In Ohio, on at least one occasion, he used potassium. Proving potassium poisoning can be difficult because as the body dies, cells release potassium, producing high levels in the decedent. In this case, the patient Swango injected was being monitored with an electrocardiogram (ECG). Physicians were able to review the ECG and identify when the victim's heart reacted to the injection and when she died; the times coincided with Swango's visit.

There appear to be no common characteristics in the poisons Swango is suspected of using except their availability. He has denied singling out victims and described his selection as random. He has claimed that he killed with no emotion. Because he was a doctor, gaining access to patients in hospitals, particularly in Africa, was easy, and he was supremely confident he could talk his way out of any suspicions.

His victims were diverse in race, age, gender, religion, education, and health. Risks that might have dissuaded others from committing a murder, such as the presence of medical personnel, did little to deter Swango, as he often injected poisons with other staff nearby. In fact, those who survived his poisonous injections reported that he would carry a legitimate syringe in one hand while concealing another in his jacket pocket.

FBI agents who investigated Swango for several years believe he enjoyed killing people at whim. He seemed to derive particular pleasure witnessing the surprised reactions of victims as well as the shock and grief expressed by families and hospital staff. Many victims were not patients under Swango's care. For a doctor whose own competence was often called into question and who must have felt increasingly self-conscious because of his inadequacies, he may have been particularly gratified to see the patients of other physicians die, especially if their deaths were unexpected.

Apart from patients and coworkers, there is evidence that Swango routinely poisoned acquaintances, including his girlfriends and landlords. Remarkably, almost no one suspected Swango of poisoning them until they were questioned by FBI agents. Then many recalled experiencing periods of severe and unexplained headaches, abdominal cramps, and vomiting in his company—symptoms that disappeared after Swango left.

Anger appears to be Swango's motivation for poisoning a number of acquaintances, although revenge was sometimes a clear motive. In New York, after arguing with his landlord, he sought to reconcile by giving her a large drink from a local convenience store. Immediately after drinking it, she became violently ill with severe stomach distress, headaches, and double vision—symptoms consistent with arsenic poisoning. He had a landlord in Africa who experienced identical symptoms shortly after Swango rented a room; later, a sample of her hair contained traces of arsenic. At least two girlfriends reported similar illness when they were with Swango. According to many sources in the United States and Africa, Swango frequently carried with him a bag that he guarded carefully. When one girlfriend inquired what it contained, Swango answered "vitamins" and would not allow her to look inside.

In addition to anger and revenge, it seems clear there was a strong sadistic element to Swango's actions. This sadistic quality was evident in a Toastmaster's speech that Swango helped a female acquaintance write in Africa. Describing her own negative experiences with doctors, she asked Swango for help in editing the speech. She was shocked when he wrote an eerie piece about how words can cause miscommunication. In his example, Swango described how a child's accidental death was made all the more tragic because his parents did not understand the medical procedures performed on him. What struck the woman was that Swango's example was not only unrelated to her topic, but that Swango presented it with remarkable coldness. Swango's reference to a child involved in an accident resonated with FBI agents who had met a Zimbabwean doctor who suspected Swango of murdering a child who was recovering from surgery following an accident.

In choosing a career as a doctor, Swango guaranteed himself easy access to the most trusting and unsuspecting of victims and unlimited opportunities to kill them. This access, coupled with his obsession with violence, made him a dangerous individual. The healthcare system in which Swango operated could not have been more conducive to fulfilling his murderous fantasies. It was a system characterized by poor information sharing, incomplete background investigations, reluctance to acknowledge mistakes, fear of lawsuits, aversion to negative publicity, and a need to fill positions.[8] Within this system, Swango found that he could take advantage of people's trust and use his skills of persuasion to overcome people's doubts. His confidence in talking his way out of trouble served him well. Far from feeling worried about allegations against him, he often appeared to relish the attention and the challenge of talking his way out of trouble.

By working long hours in hospitals (and sometimes living in them), Swango was able to monitor the presence of staff and take calculated risks to enter rooms of patients (often ones not under his supervision) and quickly kill them. His nefarious activities were so completely unexpected that it is understandable that staff failed to recognize the demonic swath he was silently cutting through wards to which he was not even assigned. Securing evidence for possible prosecution was not only a matter far from their job description, it was something far from their imaginations. Although exhumations ultimately proved helpful in identifying causes of death, they alone could not prove Swango's guilt. Exhumations require the permission of victims' families, and they are not always willing to provide it. In such cases, or in the case of cremations, potential toxicologic evidence is lost.

Swango was one of those rare individuals whose capacity for evil was nearly unimaginable.

Operating on a higher intellectual plane than most serial murderers, he was smart enough, at least for a while, to avoid detection. He used his intellect, medical training, and charm to con nearly all he knew. With a sense of entitlement and complete indifference to the feelings of others, he exploited people and organizations to satisfy his obsessions and perverse desires. He knew the difference between right and wrong, as evidenced by his efforts to avoid detection, but he chose to pursue a path of violence.

The FBI's persistence paid off by pulling together the work of state, local, and foreign police, medical examiners, toxicologists, pathologists, emergency medicine personnel, laboratory and forensic examiners, behavioral specialists, journalists, television producers, diplomats, prosecutors, and hundreds of witnesses. Swango pled guilty to three murders in New York and one in Ohio. He was sentenced to four consecutive life sentences without the possibility of parole.

HAROLD FREDERICK SHIPMAN

On January 31, 2000, at Preston Crown Court in Northern England, Dr. Harold Frederick Shipman was convicted of the murder of 15 of his patients and of forging the will of one of them. The number of murder counts in the indictment earned Shipman the notoriety of the most prolific British serial killer. But, as investigators knew before his trial, and as a subsequent official inquiry would establish, the 15 murders with which he was convicted were only the tip of the iceberg; it became apparent that Shipman had killed hundreds of his patients in a murderous career that spanned more than two decades.

Shipman was a general practitioner (GP). General practice in the United Kingdom involves a doctor contracting his skills to the National Health Service, maintaining a list of patients in the area, and catering to their medical needs—usually when patients come to his office or clinic with an ailment. Home visits are undertaken but are less popular with doctors given the amount of time they consume. The offices do not have facilities for admitting patients overnight, and appointments typically last for only 10 or 15 minutes.

Unlike other medical personnel who have murdered patients in the enclosed medical setting of a hospital, Shipman primarily murdered his patients in their homes, although there were a few occasions when he murdered them during an appointment. This meant that only rarely did he run the risk of other medical professionals either interrupting him in the act of killing or raising concerns about the number of deaths among patients. A combination of deceit and arrogance were usually sufficient to allay suspicion.

Shipman trained as a doctor at Pontefract General Hospital in the North of England from 1970 until he qualified in 1973. He remained at the hospital practicing as a "junior doctor" until he left in 1974, having obtained employment as a GP at the Abraham Ormerod Medical Practice in Todmorden in the North of England.

While he was at this practice, his fellow doctors discovered that Shipman had forged documentation to obtain the drug pethidine (known as meperidine in the United States) from a nearby community pharmacy for his own illicit use. He admitted to an addiction to pethidine, which he was taking intravenously. Shipman was prosecuted for the offences and heavily fined; his employment was terminated, and he obtained treatment for his addiction. In interviews with detectives, Shipman claimed to have started abusing drugs to escape from the pressure of his work, which he claimed had left him with depression.

In 1975, he moved to Hyde in Greater Manchester and joined the Donneybrook medical practice. He told his fellow doctors of his previous addiction and his criminal convictions. They obviously decided that his addiction and his previous dishonesty were not in conflict with his medical ethics, as they employed him at the practice.

In 1992, following a dispute over funding and the computerization of the practice, Shipman left Donneybrook and set up a solo practice. He took most of his patient list with him. He first came to the notice of the police in March 1998 after another GP expressed concerns to the local coroner.

U.K. doctors are authorized to issue a Medical Certificate of Cause of Death (MCCD) following the death of a patient when there are no suspicious circumstances, when they have treated the individual during the course of the final illness (within 14 days of death), and

when the doctor is confident they know what has caused the death. Once an MCCD has been issued, the death is registered and burial is authorized. When a body is to be cremated, a second doctor from a different medical practice is needed to countersign documentation. Providing the second doctor is content that there are no suspicious circumstances, there is no need to report the matter to the coroner and no need for a postmortem examination or any further investigation of the death.

This procedure allowed Shipman to issue an MCCD for patients whom he had murdered and, if they were to be cremated, the opportunity to persuade a fellow doctor to countersign cremation documentation. In most cases, Shipman went to the Brooke practice that operated from a building opposite his own. At the Brooke practice, there were several doctors, and they took it in rotation to countersign cremation certificates referred to them by Shipman. One of these doctors became concerned by the number of certificates that she and her fellow doctors were asked to countersign. She compared the number of deaths being referred by Shipman with the number generated within the larger community of Brooke, and she found Shipman's numbers alarmingly high. She suspected that Shipman might be killing his patients and contacted the coroner.

The coroner took the doctor's concerns to the police who began an investigation based on an examination of cremation certificates completed by Shipman over the preceding 6 months. Nineteen deaths became the focus of the investigation. The investigation was not thorough, probably because there was a fear that the doctor, the coroner, and the investigators would be proved wrong, and the good name of Dr. Shipman would be besmirched. But perhaps more significantly was the inability of investigators to identify a credible motive for Shipman. The reluctance to believe that a doctor could murder his patients became known as the "credibility gap." The investigation was closed and Shipman continued to practice. No interview of Shipman took place. Nor were postmortem examinations conducted on the bodies of two of Shipman's patients who died during the investigation.

Shipman was eventually stopped in July 1998 when the police were contacted by the daughter of one of his patients. She alleged that Shipman might have been involved in the forgery of a will purportedly made by her mother. The 81-year-old female patient had died suddenly on June 24, 1998, within a few hours of a home visit by Shipman, who was supposedly obtaining a blood sample. She was discovered in the late morning by two friends after she had failed to keep an appointment with them. The door to her house was unlocked, and she was lying fully clothed on a sofa in the living room.

Shipman attended at the house, issuing an MCCD and certifying the cause of death as old age. Although this is an acceptable cause of death in individuals over 70 years, there should be documentation of a prolonged general deterioration in health affecting the major organs. This was not the situation, but the patient's daughter accepted Shipman's explanation of death and believed in his concern for her general well-being.

During the subsequent investigation, it was apparent that Shipman had lied. The patient had been living an active life. She did volunteer work, drove a car, and enjoyed an active social life, having been walking in the nearby countryside earlier in the week and visiting friends the evening before her death. She was not suffering from any life-threatening conditions and was being treated for only minor ailments.

Following burial, a poorly typed will leaving the patient's property to Shipman came to the attention of her daughter. The will had arrived by post at a local solicitor's office on the day of her mother's death and was dated some 3 weeks before the death. The solicitors did not know the patient and had never acted for her. The daughter, after making some initial enquiries, contacted the police.

Realizing that this was the same doctor investigated earlier in the year, the police opened investigations, exhuming the body to perform a postmortem exam. The pathologist did not agree with Shipman's cause of death on the MCCD; thus, muscle tissue was obtained and sent for analysis. Forensic toxicologists soon detected opiates in the tissue that were consistent with the administration of a significant quantity of morphine or diamorphine. The patient had not been suffering from any condition that warranted prescribing or administering morphine prior to her death.

Press interest in the investigation resulted in the reexamination of the deaths of the earlier investigation. This in turn created media interest and resulted in the public expressing concerns that they had harbored for many years about the circumstances surrounding the deaths of family members and friends who had been patients of Shipman. All these reported concerns and the circumstances surrounding the deaths were investigated, resulting in a thorough examination of the 136 deaths of Shipman's patients.

What the investigation found was extraordinary. Many of the deaths shared similarities. Shipman used the same lies and stories to explain deaths to multiple families. It became apparent that Shipman was a consummate liar who forged legal documentation and falsified medical records.

In the course of the investigation, the bodies of 12 of Shipman's patients were exhumed and postmortem examinations carried out by a pathologist. Each of them had had an MCCD issued by Shipman giving a cause of death. In none of them could the pathologist agree with the cause of death as stated by Shipman in the MCCD.

Deep muscle tissue was submitted for examination by forensic toxicologists. In nine cases, substantial quantities of morphine were found in the tissue, consistent with morphine levels in deaths caused by that drug. None of the patients had been suffering from any condition that required the administration of morphine. In fact, investigators deliberately avoided exhuming bodies where evidence existed that morphine had been used therapeutically. The significant issue was that morphine was present at all. In each case, the pathologist concluded that the patient had died as a result of morphine toxicity.

The toxicology and pathology in the other three exhumation cases was inconclusive. Because the bodies had been buried nearly 5 years, body tissue degradation was more advanced, making interpretation difficult for pathologists.

Investigators used the many similarities in the circumstances surrounding different deaths to show that Shipman was responsible for killing patients whose bodies had been cremated and were therefore unavailable for pathologic examination. The lack of a cause of death was seen as a difficulty, but prosecutors were convinced that the similarities among the cases were sufficiently compelling. Shipman was thus charged with six deaths wherein the body had been cremated.

Not all of the murders included in the indictment were exactly alike. In fact, investigators charged Shipman with cases in which some of the similarities were present but new similarities with other cases were identified that could be mapped to other cases. Many of these similarities were present not only in the 15 counts in the indictment but also in the other deaths that were investigated.

These similarities were formed into criteria used to determine whether Shipman was likely to have murdered in any particular case. One salient feature was that the death occurred within a short time of Shipman having visited the patients in their home or administered to them in his office. Usually, death occurred within just a few hours of his consult, but, on occasions, he was discovered in his ministrations by members of the family or friends who had arrived home unexpectedly—after he had administered morphine but before he had had a chance to leave. In such cases, he often told the same lies to family or friends.

In one case, a 77-year-old female patient living alone was in the process of doing her laundry and cooking her lunch when Shipman called at her home to deliver antibiotic tablets. The woman, a ballroom dancer who was fit and active, was suffering from a chest infection, and Shipman had prescribed the antibiotics. While there, he injected her with a massive dose of morphine or diamorphine, causing her to collapse. Before he could leave, the patient's dance partner arrived. Shipman claimed that he had found the patient in a collapsed state and had summoned an ambulance. When the patient failed to respond, Shipman pronounced her dead and went through a charade of canceling the ambulance. Subsequent inquiries with the ambulance service and telephone records failed to validate Shipman's story. Shipman performed this charade on many occasions when he was interrupted while murdering his patients.

Many of Shipman's victims were elderly and living alone, almost always in good health but suffering from minor ailments. These circumstances obviously made it safer for him to carry out murder—he was less likely to be interrupted and had a ready excuse to be in attendance. On occasion, however, he mistakenly believed that patients were alone in their home.

On one such occasion, he attended at the home of an 81-year-old patient who was in discomfort with a hip prosthesis. He murdered her with a lethal injection of diamorphine. The woman's friend was at her home but had gone upstairs just before Shipman arrived. As she was returning through the kitchen, she heard voices in the living room; knowing her friend was expecting the doctor, she waited in the kitchen in silence to afford her friend some privacy. After a few moments, the voices stopped, and a few minutes later, Shipman entered the kitchen. He was somewhat surprised by the friend, but without any difficulty said that the patient had collapsed and died.

Shipman's capacity to lie manifested itself in other ways. He falsified the causes of death on the MCCD, and he lied on cremation documentation in which he said that his victims' relatives had been present at the time of death when they had not been. This deception was obviously to allay the suspicions of the counter-signing doctor.

Shipman forged other documentation to cover his tracks. He kept his patients' medical notes on a computerized system to do so. These were supplemented by paper records containing correspondence and reports from medical experts and specialists to whom patients had been referred as well as written records relating to visits conducted at a patient's home and where Shipman would not have had access to his computer. In many cases, shortly after murdering a patient, he altered the medical record to create a false history of a medical condition that he then used on the MCCD as the cause of death. Most commonly, Shipman falsified symptoms of heart disease or of high blood pressure before then listing the cause of death as a heart attack or stroke.

None of these practices were known to his patients, and many of them regarded him highly. His patient list was extensive, and there was a waitlist to get on it. He was regarded as a good doctor who was plain speaking and had a caring manner. He could be relied upon to spend time with his patients and was willing to attend to the elderly ones in their homes.

He was also prepared to confront those who regulated his practice, especially in relation to curbs on his drugs budget. He regarded them as petty bureaucrats who deprived his patients of the best drugs and most appropriate care, and he seized every opportunity to let it be known. This made him popular with his patients but brought him into conflict with health authorities. He saw those who opposed him as feeble minded and inferior, and he often adopted an aggressive and demeaning attitude toward them.

At a meeting, he took great delight in ridiculing a drug company's representative who perhaps did not know her product, eventually reducing her to tears. He aggressively challenged speakers at medical conferences, almost shouting them down. He was arrogant and aggressive whenever his authority was challenged, and this manifested itself when relatives and friends asked why their perfectly healthy relatives had died suddenly.

His caring manner seemed to disappear on such occasions, and he seemed unable to empathize with the relatives who had suffered a sudden and devastating loss. On many occasions, he would bring the relatives together and "pontificate" about what had been wrong with the patient. He would chastise relatives because they had failed to appreciate how ill the patient had been, implying they had failed to provide the necessary support and care. But he stopped short of suggesting they were to blame for their relative's death.

He implied that he was the only one who recognized the seriousness of the patient's condition and that he had been doing his utmost to treat the patient. This charade was partly to satisfy his desire to appear omnipotent, to revel in the attention he was given, and to enjoy the esteem of others. However, he also needed to provide as full an explanation as possible to ensure that the family would not press for a postmortem examination that might have led to his crimes being discovered.

There is no doubt that Shipman had a conceited view of himself, and there is no better illustration than in the wording of the will he forged that led to his arrest. In it, Shipman wrote (assuming the part of the deceased patient) that he should be rewarded for all the care he had given her and the people of Hyde and that he was sensible enough to deal with any difficulties that the bequest would present him.

When arrested and interviewed, he took exception to the questioning of detectives and attempted to dominate the interview with a combination of tactics, including accusing the interviewer of asking two questions at once, adopting a sneering attitude toward them because of their lack of general medical practice knowledge, and implying that they were intellectually inferior. His arrogance, however, failed to provide him with plausible answers to the questions, and he was consequently charged with the offenses.

Investigators sought to identify how Shipman had obtained the murder weapon—morphine. Early in the investigation, detectives discovered Shipman's previous convictions for obtaining pethidine. Since then, Shipman reported that he had decided not to carry any controlled drugs—including morphine—unless it was an absolute emergency. This decision meant that Shipman was not required to maintain a drug register.

Diamorphine (diacetylmorphine, heroin) is a stronger version of morphine, having about twice its potency. However, after entering the body, diamorphine metabolizes almost immediately into morphine. Consequently, forensic toxicology findings indicated the presence of morphine, although detectives established that Shipman had been illicitly obtaining diamorphine and then administering it to his patients to kill them. The presence of an intermediate metabolite, 6-monoacetyl morphine, may sometimes help identify diamorphine as the original drug if exposure has been recent.

Shipman had been writing out prescriptions for diamorphine for patients who did not need it and, on some occasions, had been writing prescriptions for fictitious patients. He would go to the pharmacy, collect the drug, and keep it himself. On some occasions, he would write prescriptions for patients who had died several days before. On other occasions, he would write a prescription for a patient who needed the drug, collect it, and then deliver only part of the prescription to the patient, retaining the rest. He also obtained the murder weapon by taking the residue of diamorphine from a patient who had died of natural causes (usually cancer) on the pretext of disposing of it in a safe manner.

Although there was no evidence that Shipman had returned to abusing drugs, his methods of obtaining diamorphine to murder his patients were almost identical to those he used to obtain pethidine for self-administration 20 years earlier.

Shipman's home was searched on two occasions. Despite his role as a health authority, the interior of his home was dirty with unwashed clothes and dishes. The officers conducting searches were both surprised and disgusted by their findings, especially when they discovered a quantity of permitted medicines and ointments in the house. Hidden in one of the innocuous medicine boxes were four 10 mg ampoules of diamorphine together with 50 morphine sulphate tablets, which he had taken from the homes of two separate patients some years earlier, supposedly so he could properly dispose of the drugs. This provided evidence of Shipman's practice of hoarding diamorphine.

The condition of Shipman's home was surprising especially because he was married and had four children, three of whom were young adults living in the house. Shipman's wife and children supported him during his medical career and continued to support him after his conviction, refusing to believe that he was responsible for the murders. There is speculation that Shipman was an autocratic individual who did not allow meals to commence until he was present. Shipman must have used deceit to keep his murderous activities from his family. There is no indication that any of them knew he was murdering his patients. However, for that to be the case, he must have lied to them about his whereabouts at times when he was carrying out a murder. It is likely, given the town's size, that his family members knew many of his victims.

It is difficult to identify what motivated Shipman to kill his patients. Except for his last victim, there is no evidence that he attempted to profit financially from his murders. Likewise, there was no evidence to suggest that any of his victims had been the victims of any form of sexual abuse by Shipman before or after death. The victim's clothing was often still buttoned, in many cases with high necklines as one might expect given the age of the victims. This lack of disturbance was surprising because Shipman usually described how he fought to save their lives. There was no evidence of "arranging of the body" except on a few occasions when he placed a magazine or pair of glasses on the victim's knee to suggest death had occurred suddenly during some mundane activity.

To identify Shipman's motivation, it is perhaps necessary to turn to some of the findings of the Public Inquiry, convened after his conviction. At Shipman's conviction, investigators had already provided evidence of a further 23 patient deaths, demonstrating that Shipman murdered them. However, prosecutors wanted to wait until after the trial before dealing with these additional charges. As evidence unfolded in the trial, the British government—particularly the Secretary of State for Health and the Secretary of State for Home Affairs—realized that a GP murdering his patient posed a threat to public safety. Consequently, they announced that a Public Inquiry would be held.

A Public Inquiry requires the appointment of a senior judge of the English High Court who utilizes a team of government lawyers to hear evidence from witnesses and experts to make recommendations for the future safety of the public. In the case of Shipman, the terms of reference required the Inquiry to establish the extent of Shipman's unlawful activities. The Inquiry investigated every death in which Shipman had been involved back to the start of his general practice; in each case, the Inquiry published a finding as to whether Shipman had murdered the patient.[9-14] This was a much wider remit than that of the criminal investigation and involved an examination of more deaths.

The Inquiry concluded that, together with the 15 convicted murders, sufficient evidence existed to establish that Shipman had killed 215 of his patients and that there was a "real possibility" that he had killed another 45. Destruction of documentation and witnesses' fading memories prohibited the Inquiry from making a decision in a further 38 cases, mainly from when he was in Todmorden. The Inquiry examined 888 deaths.

Although not covered by the terms of reference, toward the end of the Public Inquiry, concern was expressed about Shipman's time as a junior doctor at Pontefract General Hospital. The Inquiry decided—as well as it was able, given the passage of time—to examine the deaths Shipman was involved with at the hospital in the early 1970s. The Inquiry was hampered by the passage of time but concluded that there was suspicion about Shipman's involvement in 24 cases of death during his tenure at the hospital.

The Inquiry also examined Shipman's possible motivation and method of selecting his victims. This was a difficult task. Shipman never admitted responsibility for his crimes and refused to cooperate with police, prison authorities, or the Inquiry after his conviction. In fact, a forensic psychiatrist advising the police, who still hoped to gain a full account from Shipman, advised that Shipman was unlikely to remember details of everyone he had murdered and that consequently, he might never be able to provide a full account. There is no indication that Shipman kept written records of his murders. In January 2004, during the Inquiry process, Shipman hung himself in his prison cell.

Of those Shipman murdered, 171 were women and 44 were men. The majority of his victims were murdered in their homes and were elderly. Although most were women, if the opportunity arose, he murdered men. The imbalance in female victims over male victims is perhaps explained by the fact that, in general, women live longer than men and were thus more likely to be living alone in the community where Shipman worked.

Although he tended to choose elderly victims, he occasionally killed younger victims if he felt safe in doing so. His youngest victim was a 41-year-old man who was in the advanced stages of terminal cancer and whose death Shipman hastened with an overdose of diamorphine. His oldest victim was a 93-year-old woman.

The earliest death for which Shipman was responsible occurred in March 1975 and the last, which resulted in his arrest, was in June 1998. The majority of the killings (143) were in a 6-year period while he was operating as a solo practitioner. Over an 18-year period, he killed 72 people while practicing as a GP in partnership. The increasing murder rate as the years passed suggests that there was an addictive element to his murders. This may explain why the close proximity of fellow professionals did not deter him.

However, despite his addictive nature and his extreme self-confidence, he seemed to be aware that he could be caught. There are gaps between murders, sometimes of many months; these long gaps seem to have occurred after he had just escaped detection. On one occasion, as Shipman explained to the daughter of a victim why a postmortem examination was unnecessary, the victim groaned. The woman lived another 24 hours. Shipman may have worried that she would recover and disclose what he had done, but she did not survive. Two months later,

Shipman killed another patient. In that case, a relative complained about the hospital's failings. Shipman may have been concerned that an investigation of that matter would result in his discovery. It did not, but after these two close calls, Shipman did not kill for more than a year.

On another occasion, in February 1994, Shipman gave a patient, suffering an asthma attack, a large dose of diamorphine—an inappropriate treatment that caused her to collapse. The patient's daughter arrived, intervened, and summoned an ambulance. The patient was taken to hospital where she survived in a vegetative state for more than a year before dying from pneumonia brought on by inactivity. Shipman was forced to admit his administration of morphine to ambulance staff and doctors at the hospital. Shipman must have worried that he would be investigated at least for negligence, and he was careful to curtail his murders for some time. The Public Inquiry later criticized the senior medical personnel for failing to report Shipman at that time because they had been made aware of Shipman's actions that, at best, indicated incompetence. The coroner and pathologist were also criticized for their failure to thoroughly examine the true circumstances of this death. If Shipman had been caught at this time, his murderous career would have ended 6 years earlier, and over 100 lives would have been saved.

Early on, Shipman appeared to have selected victims suffering from terminal illness or those who were extremely ill. He may have thought these murders were less likely to attract attention and lead to his discovery. It may also have been that he was able to rationalize the killing of a terminally ill individual as an act of mercy. However, as time passed, he became bolder, selecting patients who had some ailment but were not at imminent risk of death.

Although he still killed terminally ill people, he often singled out those who had been or were likely to become a burden on his practice and a demand on his time—individuals with chronic conditions or those with mild mental health problems who were otherwise physically well. Shipman may have believed he was saving all of them from an unhappy and pointless existence. Possibly supporting this is the fact that when he was called to care for individuals who had suffered a heart attack, rather than treat them, he would give them a lethal injection, perhaps out of concern for their future quality of life. He had even been heard to comment that he did not believe in "keeping them going."

There are also examples of Shipman murdering patients who would not take his advice—particularly in relation to going into elderly residential care. He seems to have taken delight in killing the fitter member of a married couple, thereby ensuring that the less mobile surviving member would be taken into residential care.

Despite outlining Shipman's victimology, it was not possible for the Public Inquiry or anyone else to state what Shipman's motivations may have been. At an impressionable age, he witnessed his mother's decline and eventual death from cancer. In the process, he no doubt witnessed the relief from pain she gained from the administration of morphine. It is impossible to say whether this had any influence on his desire to kill.

Insight into Shipman's motivation can perhaps be gained from the circumstances surrounding his capture. His attempt at forging his patient's will was at best amateurish. The document was ill-prepared and was sent to a lawyer who had no dealings with the patient. Shipman knew the patient well and knew her daughter was a solicitor. He must have realized that the validity of the will would be challenged and the circumstances of its creation investigated. There was little likelihood of him getting away with the proceeds of his patient's estate, estimated at 360,000 pounds. Yet, he pressed on with his scheme, which, given the date of the creation of the will, had taken him some time to plan.

Whatever the motivation for his deeds, Shipman managed to evade detection for over 20 years because the safeguards designed to prevent such events were inadequate. For instance, there was no system for monitoring death rates at a particular practice. Had there been such a system, Shipman's high death rate would have been identified. Also, there was no close examination of the MCCDs, and family members did not have the opportunity to challenge that information. Had they had such an opportunity, they would very likely have discovered that Shipman had lied extensively on the documentation.

Furthermore, there were failings in the control of dangerous drugs such as diamorphine. While controls were in place until a doctor prescribed the drugs, no one effectively monitored the amounts being prescribed by an individual doctor. Nor were there any controls once they had been collected or delivered to the patient in respect to disposing excess drugs. Shipman exploited this flaw to access the murder weapon. Shipman managed for two separate lengthy periods to obtain dangerous drugs in huge quantities without detection.

The Public Inquiry made a number of recommendations in order to close the loopholes that Shipman exploited. However, 3 years after the Inquiry, many of these had still not been implemented.

ORVILLE LYNN MAJORS

A licensed practical nurse (LPN), Lynn Majors joined the Vermillion County Hospital (VCH) staff in the fall of 1993. VCH was a small rural but modern hospital with a dedicated staff. As with most small towns, the members of the hospital staff knew each other well. When the four-bed critical care unit had patients, Majors would be assigned there with a registered nurse (RN) as his supervisor. When the unit was empty, he usually was assigned to pass medications on the medical floor. The annual admission rate in that intensive care unit (ICU) had been consistently close to 350 patients, with about 27 deaths. In 1993 the rate increased almost imperceptibly, but by the spring of 1994, a climb in those numbers began to draw attention. Rumors began to circulate that Majors was associated with that increase. By summer of 1994, the increase in ICU cardiac arrests was clearly noted, and in July, the death rate in the ICU accelerated. There are conflicting stories as to when the hospital administration became aware and what steps were taken. In early 1995, the nursing director of the ICU completed a survey comparing the deaths in the ICU for 1993–1994 with employee time cards. What she found was of grave concern. Of the 147 deaths in VCH's ICU between May of 1993 and December of 1994, 130 occurred when Majors was working. In March, VCH officials notified the Indiana State Police of their concerns. Majors was placed on leave and eventually fired. Thus began the largest criminal investigation in Indiana's history. It lasted four years and cost over two million dollars.

The Indiana State Police assembled an independent medical investigative team consisting of an emergency physician, a registered nurse, two intensivists, two pathologists, a medical toxicologist, a cardiac electrophysiologist, a cardiac pathologist, and an epidemiologist. Over two years, charts were reviewed on all patients who had died during the period in question. The thrust of the investigation was to answer *two* questions for each case:

1. Was the death consistent with the patient's clinical course?
2. If not, was there a person or persons who appeared to be associated with the death?

Within weeks, their review showed that deaths in the ICU followed one of three patterns:

1. Sudden onset of hypertension followed by circulatory collapse and cardiac arrest
2. Sudden loss of consciousness followed by oxygen desaturation, then dysrhythmia
3. Unheralded terminal dysrhythmia with wide-complex tachycardia, then asystole

The investigative team members generally believed that over 100 of the cases appeared suspicious. Majors was in close proximity when death occurred in nearly all of the cases. Seven cases were selected for trial. While many more cases were suspected murders, the prosecution decided that presenting a large number of cases would tend to be confusing to both witnesses and the jury. They chose cases that demonstrated ECG findings consistent with hyperkalemia and that in many cases involved witnesses who saw Majors inject the patient just prior to death.

The investigators determined that Majors had killed the majority of victims with potassium chloride. ECG findings of QRS widening, P-wave changes, and sine-wave patterns were frequently documented. A search of Majors's van revealed eight vials of potassium chloride, two syringes of epinephrine, and three vials of injectable nitroglycerin.

Majors was usually assigned to the ICU, but if the unit was empty, he was assigned to pass medicines on the wards. Investigators believe that when Majors worked on the medicine floor, he injected patients with epinephrine intravenously, causing a hypertensive crisis and eventually ventricular tachycardia. He would then initiate a code, and almost invariably, lidocaine would be ordered as part of the resuscitation effort. It is speculated that Majors would then add

potassium to the lidocaine infusion or inject potassium directly into the intravenous line. The patient would be moved from the floor to the ICU, and Majors moved with them to staff the area with a supervising RN. In the ICU, he would inject the patient with more intravenous potassium. On one occasion, there were three simultaneous cardiac resuscitations in progress in the four-bed ICU. Majors had discovered all three. When Majors took a vacation, the deaths stopped. According to police investigators, of the 33 patients moved from the wards to the ICU, Majors moved 23. None of those 23 survived to discharge.

Some of the victims' family members described unusual behavior in Majors. In one case, he was working with the IV fluid bags when a family member entered. Majors ran from the room, almost knocking down the patient's wife. He sat at the nurses' station staring into the room. Moments later, the patient gasped and fell back on the bed, unconscious and cyanotic. Though the patient survived the initial resuscitation, the supervising RN's notes state that he died hours later after suffering a "respiratory arrest" while on the ventilator.

Despite all of the resuscitations, only one set of electrolytes was ever documented. The potassium was 6.8 mEq/L. In that case, the patient had suffered an arrest on the ward and was moved to the ICU. The records of that "code blue" are bizarre. The initial blood pressure entry was 229/158 mm Hg. Pressure then dropped to 94/57 mm Hg only 16 minutes later. It increased to 209/159 mm Hg 46 minutes later before dropping again to 105/100 mm Hg. Two more peaks hit 224/158 mm Hg and 173/105 mm Hg before the patient became asystolic. These events led the medical investigators to speculate that the patient was receiving intravenous infusion that had been laced with potassium chloride. It also appears that during the code, he received doses of epinephrine causing the marked increases in his blood pressure. Epinephrine shifts serum potassium back into the cells, thus decreasing its effects on the heart. Eventually, if epinephrine is not given, potassium shifts back into the serum resulting in asystole. ECG monitor strips show markedly peaked T waves consistent with hyperkalemia (Figure 26.1). In a different case, tracings demonstrated the sine-wave pattern considered virtually pathognomonic of hyperkalemia (Figure 26.2). Likely because the patients were older and no one suspected anything but natural causes, routine lab work, drug screens, and autopsies were almost never done.

In the state of Indiana, the accused has a right to request that trial proceedings begin within 75 days of arrest. Knowing that this would be a complicated and difficult case to present to a jury, prosecutors delayed Majors's arrest until the case could be presented. As a result of the work of the Indiana State Police investigative team, Majors was arrested on December 29, 1997. Trial began 19 months later.

Because of publicity, the venue was changed to nearby Brazil, Indiana, in Clay County. Jurors were selected from Miami County in north-central Indiana. The prosecution argued that the deaths of the seven patients were not consistent with their clinical course. Furthermore, cardiac rhythms, consistent among the patients, were indicative of either:

1. Massive myocardial infarction
2. Catastrophic saddle embolus (a large blood clot in the root of the pulmonary artery)
3. Injection of potassium chloride

Cardiac pathologist Bruce Waller ruled out a myocardial infarction. Pathologists John Heidingsfelder and Mark LeVaughn showed that saddle emboli were not present in the exhumed bodies. Ruling out the first two, cardiac electrophysiologist Eric Prystowski testified that the only plausible explanation that remained was poisoning with potassium.

In October of 1999, Orville Lynn Majors was sentenced to 180 years in prison for six of the seven murders for which he was tried. Like other serial killers, he had several supporters who saw him as a scapegoat. The prosecution was disallowed the presentation of certain compelling statistics. During the investigation, an intense epidemiologic study of VCH was performed. Time cards, vacation dates, and time and date of deaths were reviewed in a blinded fashion.

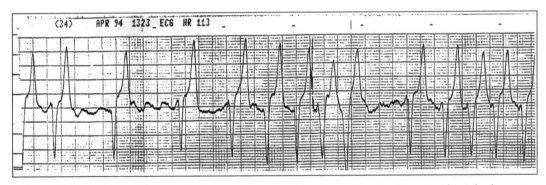

FIGURE 26.1   **This monitor strip shows tall peaked T waves often indicative of marked hyperkalemia.**

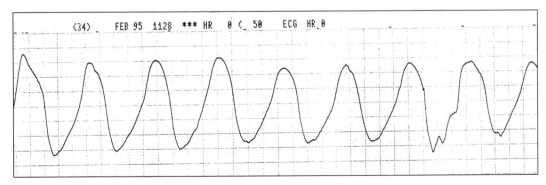

FIGURE 26.2   **Concomitant widening of the QRS and T waves leads to the usually terminal pattern known as "sine wave."**

Stephen Lamm, MD, found that the mortality was of "epidemic proportions" from July to December 1994. He concluded the following:

"Increased mortality occurred in the Intensive Care Unit. . . . One intensive care nurse was uniquely and very strongly associated with that mortality. . . . No other service or service provider shows any association that even approximates in magnitude that of the ICU nurse. . . . The likelihood of someone dying in the Intensive Care Unit was 42.96 times greater than it would be if he were not working."

The statistics also showed that when Majors took a vacation, the deaths essentially stopped[15] (Figure 26.3). Graphs relating time worked to deaths were also ruled inadmissible. One member of the prosecution team remarked that if the jury had been allowed to see those charts, the trial would have been over in half a day. After the trial, they were allowed to review those charts[15] (Figures 26.4 and 26.5). What they saw was chilling. The death rate tripled during Majors's employment. In terms of hours per patient deaths, he had approximately one death per 10 hours worked, while workers who were not part of his team had rates of one death per hundreds of hours. Those graphs were based upon the statistics compiled by Dawn Stirek, the nursing director of the Vermillion County Hospital ICU.[15] In the end, it was her courage in performing the study that sparked the investigation and trial.

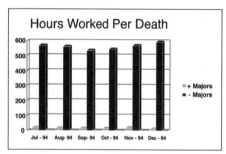

FIGURE 26.3   The graph above compares the hours worked per patient death when Majors was working compared to when he was absent.

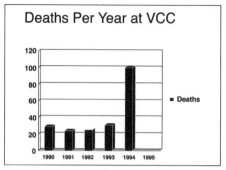

FIGURE 26.4   The graph above represents the number of deaths per year in the Vermillion County Hospital Intensive care unit. Majors was hired in late 1993 and dismissed in spring of 1995.

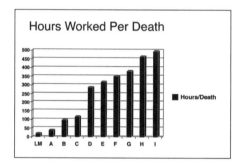

FIGURE 26.5   The graph above represents the hours worked per patient death for each nurse working in the Vermillion County Hospital intensive care unit. Majors is represented at the far left. The three nurses represented to the right of him frequently worked as part of his team.

THE COMMON THREADS IN MEDICAL SERIAL KILLERS

The Poisoners

In most reported cases of medical serial killers, the perpetrator is narcissistic. While they occasionally claim to be euthanizing patients, close scrutiny indicates that there is secondary gain in the form of excitement or superiority. Investigators in the Majors case speculated that he appeared to try to pass himself as a physician, commonly wearing surgical scrubs and no nametag indicating he was an LPN. Donald Harvey characterized his motivation as follows, "I controlled other people's lives, whether they lived or died. I had that power to control. After I didn't get caught for the first 15, I thought it was my right. I appointed myself judge, prosecutor and jury. So I played God."[16]

Another striking characteristic is that the poisoners frequently polarized their coworkers, having a few staunch supporters and an equal number of detractors. Often, they appear to be more knowledgeable than others at their training level and in most cases assume tasks above their capability. They curry favor with their supervisors, providing a shield for their activity and leading to deflection of criticism as jealousy by coworkers. A surprising number are suspected by coworkers. In general, it is the nursing staff that recognizes the problem first. Physicians, nurses, and hospital administrators are often so difficult to convince that more deaths occur after the killer has been identified.

The majority of serial killers in the healthcare system are male. Making up only 7% of all nurses, they account for 33% of the murderers.[17] Surreptitious behavior is often noted by coworkers or family members. Remarkably, killers' bizarre behavior is only noted in retrospect. Equally impressive is how often lethal injections are made with families present yet no one connecting the injection and death.

M. William Phelps, in his account of Kristen Gilbert, *Perfect Poison*, attempts to answer the difficult question of why these people murder: "Adults don't wake up and decide to become serial killers; they are wired at some point—usually during childhood—so that they might later cultivate a malevolence and perpetrate crimes based on what they have been taught."[18]

The Victims

For serial killers to operate in a healthcare setting, selection of victims is important. The very old or very young are often targeted because they are unable to communicate. In some cases, the victims may recognize the perpetrator but are unable to verbalize their fears. Even when

they can, their complaints are disregarded as delusions. In the Majors case, a patient told his family that a nurse was trying to kill him and that if the family did not take him from the hospital that evening, he would not survive until morning. The family disregarded his concerns, and the patient was killed during the night.

When deaths are both sudden and unexpected, they should raise concern. This is especially true when multiple deaths have occurred. Several things shelter the serial killer in this setting, but the greatest is the near refusal on the part of healtcare providers to accept that something as heinous as murder could occur. Thus, these deaths are often accepted as natural, particularly in regard to elderly victims. A common defense for healthcare serial killers is that the patients were old and sick so their death was anticipated. Furthermore, the likelihood of an autopsy being ordered on an 80-year-old is low. When faced with an unexpected death, healthcare workers should bear in mind that even elderly patients almost always have a clinical course that declines prior to death. They might consider how many times they have lost patients when death actually was a complete surprise.

The Methods

Potassium chloride has been a relatively popular drug among serial killers because it is readily available and quick acting. Because of postmortem redistribution, the serum concentration rises rapidly after death. Thus, an elevated postmortem potassium concentration is common and of no predictive value in the determination of the premortem level. In recent years, hospitals have made efforts to avoid accidental administration of potassium chloride. Though very seldom reported in medical literature, potassium overdose and death have been a concern in the healthcare setting.[19] When given surreptitiously, it is unlikely to be treated successfully in resuscitation attempts unless electrolytes are measured. Often overlooked is neuromuscular paralysis that occurs as a result of potassium administration.

Neuromuscular paralytic agents are available in the hospital setting and are not controlled substances. They have rapid onset and appear to induce coma. Patients exposed to these agents can frequently identify their assailants, but they are not always believed. Laboratory detection is possible but not rapidly available in most hospitals. Kerskes et al. described the use of high-performance liquid chromatography-electrospray ionization-mass spectrometry (LC-ESI-MS) for the detection of quaternary nitrogen muscle relaxants such as pancuronium and rocuronium.[20]

Because of its use in homicidal poisoning, the detection of succinylcholine has been the subject of much study. Gao et al. were able to detect succinylcholine to a concentration of 0.25 µg/mL in human plasma, but concentrations may be well below that in postmortem specimens. They applied their method in a patient receiving 1 mg/kg as an IV bolus. The initial plasma concentration of 25.33 µg/mL declined to 0.11 µg/mL in 3 minutes. By 4 minutes, it was undetectable.[21] In postmortem specimens, such attempts at obtaining levels would be of little use.

In 2001, William Sybers, a Florida physician and medical examiner, was found guilty of the first-degree murder of his wife.[22] The conviction was heavily based upon laboratory determination that she had been injected with succinylcholine. A method was described to identify the metabolite, succinylmonocholine, as a marker for the neuromuscular paralytic agent. The metabolite is present for a much longer period and was felt to occur only after exposure to succinylcholine and not as an endogenous compound. In February of 2003, Sybers appealed on the basis that the test for succinylmonocholine was new and not accepted as standard medical practice. His appeal was successful, and a new trial was ordered. He subsequently agreed to a plea bargain and was sentenced to 10 years and a $500,000 fine, though he continued to maintain his innocence. He was released on time served for the original conviction. In November of 2003, LeBeau and Quenzer of the FBI Laboratory in Quantico, Virginia, released results of a small study of succinylmonocholine in patients who had not been injected with succinylcholine prior to death. They were able to identify small concentrations of the compound in autopsy tissue from the six patients they studied. They concluded that, "succinylmonocholine is not an exclusive indicator of exposure to the parent drug, succinylcholine."[23]

While timely supportive care is life saving following lower doses of paralytic agents, little is known about the effects of massive doses. Prolonged paralysis has been reported,[24] but there appears to be other potentially life-threatening effects from paralytic agents such as hyperkalemia, hyperthermia, or cholinergic activity.[25]

Opioids have been widely used to murder. These agents are found throughout hospitals, but they are controlled. Parenteral administration may occur if the drug can be removed and replaced with water or other liquid. Many undocumented reports exist concerning healthcare workers who are discovered diverting opioids when patients complain of pain in the face of repeated or high-dose analgesic administration. Naloxone, if given in adequate doses, will reverse opioid-induced coma. Many healthcare providers are unaware that opiate screens typically only demonstrate the presence of morphine, codeine, or heroin, with 6-acetyl morphine used to distinguish the latter.[26,27] Oxycodone or hydrocodone will occasionally cause positive opiate screens if present in high doses, but synthetic agents such as meperidine, propoxyphene, or fentanyl derivatives will not.

Sedative–hypnotics such as benzodiazepines may be used but seem to be less dependable as lethal agents. Benzodiazepines cause less profound respiratory compromise than opioids or paralytic agents. Veterinary pharmaceuticals may also be used.

Arsenic has long been used in malicious poisonings. Donald Harvey used it to kill patients, and Michael Swango employed it in an attack on coworkers. For serial killers it has the advantage of lacking a recognizable toxidrome. The initial symptoms are similar to gastroenteritis, and the poison can be administered in small doses that have a cumulative and eventually fatal effect. It has the disadvantage of being very detectable, even in exhumations. In living patients, 24-hour urine specimens are the most useful to demonstrate arsenic. Elevated arsenic concentrations may be found in people who have consumed seafood, but speciation of the type of arsenic can help exclude it.[28]

Cyanide was also allegedly used by Donald Harvey and Michael Swango. Many other serial killers have employed it in the past. Humans are capable of metabolizing small amounts of cyanide, but increasing doses cause symptoms such as altered consciousness, tachypnea, tachycardia, and acidosis. Lethal doses rapidly produce respiratory arrest.[29] There are disadvantages to its use as a lethal agent. It is relatively difficult to obtain. Incorrect usage can injure the perpetrator, and it is thought that some people can detect its odor.[30] Laboratory detection is usually available at reference labs but not in hospitals. A concern about cyanide analysis is that whole blood concentrations, while widely employed, may not be as reliable as red cell or plasma cyanide concentrations. Vesey and Wilson reported significant artifactual cyanide formation because acidification during the test caused cyanide production from thiocyanate.[31] Plasma or red blood cell cyanide analysis is therefore recommended when cyanide poisoning is suspected.[29]

Laboratory Studies

Laboratory studies have a limited but critical role in the detection of healthcare serial killers. They also play an important role in their prosecution. A major deficiency is the inaccuracy of postmortem urine or serum concentrations in predicting premortem concentrations. A number of reports of postmortem redistribution of drugs show that many drugs shift from internal organs into central circulation after death. Postmortem blood collected from large thoracic vessels or the heart may be several times higher in concentration than blood collected from the femoral or other peripheral vessels.[32,33]

Blood chemistries also vary. While some electrolytes such as sodium or chloride decline postmortem, potassium begins to climb within an hour after death.[32-36] This information was derived from comparing postmortem electrolyte concentrations with premortem concentrations obtained a short time before death.

Unfortunately, many of the specimens examined in investigations of suspected serial killings are obtained following exhumation. These materials are generally much less revealing of toxins but have some utility. In a review of their experience and of the previous medical literature, Grellner and Glenewinkel cite 40 pharmacologic agents that have been recovered by postmortem sampling in the interval between death and testing.[37] Neuromuscular paralytic agents are among compounds successfully recovered.[38]

A chillingly consistent finding in hospitals where serial killers have operated is the slow response of administrators and physicians to involve the police. This reluctance appears to be due to both a fear of litigation and potential adverse media coverage; sadly, it costs more lives. Healthcare providers and administrators are neither trained nor appropriate to conduct investigations of suspected homicides. Whistleblowers have been ignored, or worse, punished for raising the question of criminal activity. Anonymous reporting has been a fairly common way of contacting police in these cases.

Hospital mortality committees are required to provide surveillance of deaths that occur. Variations in mortality rates must be explored, not simply excused. The following list describes some of the factors that can indicate a potential problem:

- **Deaths occur around meal times:** As Donald Harvey noted, during meals, half the nursing staff is off the unit. The remaining staff members are busy in other rooms, leaving many patients unattended.
- **Deaths occur in 24-hour cycles (same shift):** This was noted with Kristen Gilbert and Orville Lynn Majors. In addition, vacation times often correspond with a cessation of codes and deaths, as seen with Genene Jones and Majors.[16]
- **Deaths do not follow "glide slope":** Prior to typical natural death, a progressive decline in clinical course often predicts the outcome. This decline can be subtle in the elderly or the critically ill. Patients usually show a clinical decline before terminal events, whereas murdered patients have abrupt arrests.
- **Success rates during codes is poor:** The immediate survival rate of in-hospital codes is 44%, with 17% finally living to leave the hospital. Success rates appear to be lower when a serial killer is at work. In a review of 14,720 cardiac arrests in 207 hospitals, Peberdy et al. found the most common causes were cardiac arrhythmias, acute respiratory insufficiency, and hypotension.[39] Resuscitation teams must assume they are working with the most common causes of cardiac arrest. They seldom have the time to determine and correct the cause of the arrest if an unknown toxin is at work.
- **Evidence exists of uncharted injections:** While this factor is very difficult to find during a routine chart review, it still

deserves notation. In-hospital poisonings are generally administered orally or, more often, intravenously. *Because the perpetrator is usually the person charting, injections of unordered medicines are undocumented.* Discovery of needle marks, witness reports of injections, or questionable discarded medications should be checked against physicians' orders and nursing notes.

- **Medications frequently come from the hospital:** In several cases, the hospital pharmacy or medications on the wards serve as the source for the serial killer's poison. These medications are chosen because they are easily procured and because many of them will not show up on routine drug screens. For example, serum potassium concentration increases shortly after death, making it an unreliable indictor of premortem potassium concentration. Neuromuscular paralytic drugs, another frequent choice of poison, will not be found by a drug screen and require specific testing that is generally beyond the ability of most hospital laboratories.

While state laws prescribe certain circumstances that mandate a coroner's case, an autopsy is not necessarily performed even in those instances. Particularly, deaths of elderly patients are considered "natural" simply because of their age. As in the Majors case, out of 140 deaths, none had a postmortem examination unless they were exhumed as part of the investigation. As Harvey put it, "I could have been apprehended with the first one if they had done the autopsy."[40]

If a patient death is not consistent with the clinical course, an autopsy is imperative. If the autopsy is not consistent with the reported medical condition(s), homicide should be in the differential diagnosis. Physicians have an obligation to report concerns to the coroner or medical examiner.

- **Patient complaints are ignored:** Unfortunately, this is almost always found in retrospect. Remarkably, even the victims are often unaware that they are being abused.
- **Employee suspicions are ignored:** Almost without exception, it is the killer's coworkers who discover the criminal ac-

tivity. In case after case, physicians and administrators discount reports and denigrate whistle-blowers. More than half of nurses in one study feared there would be repercussions if they reported a medication error.[41]

- **Communication among hospitals is poor:** Probably the most effective approach to this problem is better communication between hospitals and preemployment screening to look for potential problems.

CONCLUSION

Numerous healthcare professionals have been found guilty of murdering their patients. These perpetrators used a variety of poisons to kill their victims. Even though these murderers were unique in how they killed, a number of common characteristics have been noted regarding these cases that should heighten healthcare workers' and administration's concern of potential foul play (Table 26.1).

TABLE 26.1 Common Factors in Medical Serial Killings

- Deaths occur around meal times.
- Deaths occur in 24-hour cycles (same shift).
- Deaths do not follow "glide slope."
- Resuscitation rate is low.
- Evidence exists of uncharted injections.
- Medications used in the murder frequently come from the hospital.
- Few autopsies are performed.
- Patient complaints are ignored.
- Employee suspicions are ignored.
- Communication among hospitals is poor.

REFERENCES

1. Morgan E. Report to the Prosecuting Attorney, Franklin County Ohio, regarding incidents related to the internship of Michael J. Swango and hospital/police/prosecutor handling of those incidents. Columbus, OH: Franklin County Ohio, Ohio State Police, Assistant Prosecuting Attorney with the Assistance of the Ohio State Police Department;1986.
2. Montaldo C. Profile of Serial Killer Richard Angelo – Angel of Death. About.com: Crime/Punishment. http://crime.about.com/od/serial/a/richardangelo.htm.
3. Geringer, Joseph. Michael Swango: Doctor of Death - Double-O Swango. tru TV – CrimeLlibrary. http://www.trutv.com/library/crime/serial_killers/weird/swango/swango_2.html.

4. Zimbabwe Republic Police, ed. Report of Criminal Investigation Department, Zimbabwe Republic Police, re: Mneme Hospital Investigations: CID Gewru ER 143/95. 1995.

5. Franke D. *The Torture Doctor.* Hawthorn Books, New York, NY. 1975.

6. Wilson C. *Criminal History of Mankind.* Paragon. London, United Kingdom. 1993.

7. Fromer MJ. *Scalpel's Edge.* Berkley Pub Group. New York, NY. 1991.

8. Stewart J. *Blind Eye: How the Medical Establishment Let a Doctor Get Away with Murder.* New York: Simon & Schuster; 1999.

9. Smith DJ. *The Shipman Inquiry, First Report—Death Disguised.* Norwich, England: Her Majesty's Stationery Office; 2002:1–346.

10. Smith DJ. *The Shipman Inquiry, Second Report—The Police Investigation of March, 1998.* Norwich, England: Her Majesty's Stationery Office; 2003:1–169.

11. Smith DJ. *The Shipman Inquiry, Third Report—Death Certification and the Investigation of Deaths by Coroners.* Norwich, England: Her Majesty's Stationery Office; 2003:1–530.

12. Smith DJ. *The Shipman Inquiry, Fourth Report—The Regulation of Controlled Drugs in the Community.* Norwich, England: Her Majesty's Stationery Office; 2004:1.

13. Smith DJ. *The Shipman Inquiry, Fifth Report— Safeguarding Patients: Lessons from the Past - Proposals for the Future.* Norwich, England: Her Majesty's Stationery Office; 2004:1–1178.

14. Smith DJ. *The Shipman Inquiry, Shipman: The Final Report.* Norwich, England: Her Majesty's Stationery Office; 2005:1–92.

15. Turchi DF. Probable Cause Affidavit. Indiana: Vermillion Circuit Court; 1997:1–64.

16. Schechter H. *The Serial Killer Files.* New York: Random House; 2003.

17. Pyrek KM. *Healthcare serial killers: recognizing the red flags.* Forensic Nurse http://www. forensicnursemag.com/articles/391feat1.html. Accessed November 22, 2009.

18. Phelps M. *Perfect Poison.* New York, NY: Kensington Publishing Corp; 2003.

19. Anon. Intravenous potassium predicament. *Clin J Oncol Nurs.* 1997;1(2):45–49.

20. Kerskes CH, Lusthof KJ, Zweipfenning PG, Franke JP. The detection and identification of quaternary nitrogen muscle relaxants in biological fluids and tissues by ion-trap LC-ESI-MS. *J Anal Toxicol.* 2002;26:29–34.

21. Gao H, Roy S, Donati F, Varin F. Determination of succinylcholine in human plasma by high-performance liquid chromatography with electrochemical detection. *J Chromatogr B Biomed Sci Appl.* 1998;718(1):129–34.

22. McGraw S. Notorious murders/not guilty? The Bill Sybers case. In: Bardsley M, ed. *Crime Library:* Court TV; 2005.

23. LeBeau M, Quenzer C. Succinylmonocholine identified in negative control tissues. *J Anal Toxicol.* 2003;27:600–601.

24. Ohata H, Kawamura M, et al. Overdose of vecuronium during general anesthesia to an infant. *Masui.* 2005;54(3):298–300.

25. Otteni JC, Steib A, Pottecher T. Cardiac arrest during anesthesia and recovery period. *Ann Fr Anesth Reanim.* 1990;9(3):195–203.

26. Fehn J, Megges G. Detection of O6-monoacetylmorphine in urine samples by GC/MS as evidence for heroin use. *J Anal Toxicol.* 1985;9(3):134–8.

27. Kintz P, Jamey C, Cirimele V, et al. Evaluation of acetylcodeine as a specific marker of illicit heroin in human hair. *J Anal Toxicol.* 1998;22:425–429.

28. Nixon DE, Moyer TP. Arsenic analysis II: rapid separation and quantification of inorganic arsenic plus metabolites and arsenobetaine from urine. *Clin Chem.* 1992;38:2479–2483.

29. Curry S, LoVecchio F, eds. *Hydrogen and Inorganic Cyanide Salts.* Philadelphia, PA: Lippincott Williams & Wilkins; 2001.

30. Gonzalez ER. Cyanide evades some noses, overpowers others. *JAMA.* 1982;248:2211.

31. Vesey C, Wilson J. Red cell cyanide. *J Pharm Pharmacol.* 1978;30:20–26.

32. Anderson W, Prouty R, eds. *Postmortem Redistribution of Drugs.* Chicago, IL: Yearbook Medical Publishers, Inc; 1989.

33. Coe JI. Postmortem chemistry: practical considerations and a review of the literature. *J Forensic Sci.* 1974;19:13–32.

34. Coe JI. Postmortem chemistries on blood with particular reference to urea nitrogen, electrolytes, and bilirubin. *J Forensic Sci.* 1974;19:33–42.

35. Coe JI. Postmortem chemistry of blood, cerebrospinal fluid, and vitreous humor. *Leg Med Annu.* 1977;1976:55–92.

36. Coe JI. Postmortem chemistry update: emphasis on forensic application. *Am J Forens Med Pathol.* 1993;14:91–117.

37. Grellner W, Glenewinkel F. Exhumations: synopsis of morphological and toxicological findings in relation to the postmortem interval. Survey on a 20-year period and review of the literature. *Forensic Sci Int.* 1997;90:139–159.

38. Andresen BD, Alcaraz A, Grant PM. Pancuronium bromide (Pavulon) isolation and identification in aged autopsy tissues and fluids. *J Forensic Sci.* 2005;50:196–203.

39. Peberdy M, Kaye W, Ornato J, et al. Cardiopulmonary resuscitation of adults in the hospital: a report of 14720 cardiac arrests from the National Registry of Cardiopulmonary Resuscitation. *Resuscitation.* 2003;58:297–308.

40. Burkowski T. *In Our Midst: Donald Harvey.* In: Lock A, ed DH989. Lombard, IL: Commuicorp Television Productions; 1989

41. Schmidt CE, Bottoni T. Improving medication safety and patient care in the emergency department. *J Emerg Nurs.* 2003;29:12–16.

27 | Munchausen by Proxy

David L. Eldridge

INTRODUCTION

Munchausen by proxy (MBP) is an insidious and perplexing condition that often eludes detection. Perpetrators of these cases are deliberately deceptive. Medical personnel involved in the clinical investigation of possible MBP cases need to recognize the red flags that may indicate this diagnosis; such signs can be found in the history, clinical presentation, and characteristics of both the victim and the perpetrator. The victim may present with physical symptoms and history purposefully designed to be nonspecific (e.g., abdominal pain and vomiting) and confusing to the medical team, or the perpetrator may shape the victim's presentation to mimic a particular disease process (e.g., cystic fibrosis). Typically, the victims in MBP will be children and the perpetrator will be a parent—most often the mother.

Although a number of different means may facilitate MBP, poisonings are employed extensively.[1,2] Knowledge of the substances used in previous cases and the pattern of the physical findings and symptoms that these substances may induce is crucial. Awareness of this information can help medical personnel recognize and direct diagnostic testing to reveal the true chemical culprits that have led to each victim's illness.

HISTORIC BACKGROUND AND DEFINITION

Baron von Munchausen was a German who fought with the Russian army against the Turks in the 18th century,[3] but his true claim to fame occurred after this service. The Baron became well known at dinner parties for his ability to spin incredible yarns related to his exploits in Russia.[4] Stories reportedly based on these tall tales were later published by Rudolf Erich Raspe as *Baron Munchausen's Narrative of His Marvellous Travels and Campaigns in Russia.*[4] Fictional exaggeration became synonymous with the Baron's name, leading to its use in medical literature 150 years later.

The term *Munchausen syndrome* (MS) was first coined in an article by Dr. Richard Asher in 1951.[5] In this piece, he described cases in which patients intentionally manufactured medical histories and symptoms (which may be actively induced) in order to obtain medical therapy and hospital admission.[3] MS patients are usually medically savvy and will often take their charades to the point of undergoing invasive procedures.[6] Critical to the diagnosis of MS is that the patient's motivation in carrying on such an elaborate hoax does not involve obvious secondary gain (e.g., avoiding work or receiving money) and does not involve malingering behavior.[6] MS fits under the larger psychiatric category of a factitious disorder because the reported history and physical ailments are voluntarily produced by the patient.[1] The true incentive for these patients is speculative but seems to involve a desire to take on the role of patient and receive the care and attention of a hospital and its staff.[3,6,7]

Munchausen by proxy (MBP) is a different and more sinister disorder. In these cases, the falsified illness is forced by one person onto another vulnerable individual. More than 25 years after Asher's original article, Roy Meadow first reported cases in which false illnesses were ascribed by mothers onto their children.[8] Meadow's case reports described the elaborate deceptions and unbelievable persistence that these mothers employed to convince physicians and hospital staff that their children were ill and in need of hospitalization. Physical findings were falsified, laboratory studies were tampered with, and one child was surreptitiously given large amounts of sodium to continue the charade. So great was the determination of one mother that her child underwent multiple invasive procedures as doctors searched in vain for a diagnosis.

Referring to Asher's original article, Meadow coined the term *Munchausen syndrome by proxy*. These initial case reports by Meadow have since served as the model for recognizing and describing other cases of MBP.[8] Simply put, MBP is a category of abuse wherein a dependent individual—typically a young child—either is made to appear ill or is actually made ill by a caregiver, typically the biologic mother, in order to satisfy a psychological need of the caregiver.[9-11] Because it is a crime of deceit, the exact incidence of MBP is unknown,[9] but in a recent review of the subject, it was estimated to be about 0.4/100,000 in children younger than 16 years old and about 2/100,000 in children younger than 1 year old.[12]

Some have argued that the presence of MBP truly requires two separate diagnoses to be made—one in the perpetrator and one in the victim.[13] The perpetrator's diagnosis is a psychiatric one, involving a pathologic need that is satisfied by the illness he or she projects upon the victim.[11] The perpetrator's reported motivations vary, including the need for attention, the excitement of being in a hospital environment, the satisfaction in being perceived as an ideal parent, the fulfillment of the need to assume the sick role (through the victim), and the challenge of outsmarting and fooling physicians and medical staff.[1,13,14] The American Professional Society on the Abuse of Children (APSAC) has argued to classify this psychiatric disorder as "factitious disorder by proxy" (FDP).[15]

The victims in these cases are forced into the roles of sick patients, and their faux illnesses are sold to physicians through a wide array of deceptions.[9,15,16] These ploys can lead to needless hospitalizations, continued unnecessary medical testing and therapy, and even painful and invasive procedures.[17] This ordeal is clearly a form of child abuse.[12,18] Typically, the victims are younger children and infants.[14] The APSAC recommends that this form of child abuse is most appropriately labeled "pediatric condition falsification" (PCF).[15]

The means of deceit at the disposal of the perpetrator are multiple. The simplest ruse is for

TABLE 27.1 **Profile of the Classic MBP Victim**[16,21-25,28-30]

Characteristics and behavior
- Usually young (<5 years old)
- Symbiotic relationship with suspected caregiver
- May exhibit separation anxiety from caregiver
- May exhibit aggressive, hyperactive, or oppositional behavior
- Passively accepts medical procedure

Illness
- No cause obvious despite extensive investigation—often involving multiple medical institutions
- Recurrent episodes of illness with multiple hospitalizations
- Laboratory data incongruent with physical symptoms or history
- Illness not responsive to appropriate therapy
- Symptoms worsen or recur with caregiver present
- Symptoms improve or resolve with caregiver absent

the caregiver to simulate an illness by exaggerating or falsely reporting symptoms to portray a serious illness.[11] Some repeatedly tamper with a victim's lab specimens and tests to produce concerning or confusing results in order to achieve aggressive medical testing and therapies.[19] Others may withhold nutrition or medications in order to induce illness.[19] Perhaps most concerning, some perpetrators will actively induce symptoms in their victims, most commonly by suffocation and poisoning.[10] PCF may still occur as a form of child abuse separate from MBP if the perpetrator's motivation is not one related to FDP (e.g., malingering for secondary gain).[14] When both diagnoses are present—PCF in the victim and FDP in the perpetrator—most agree that the summary diagnosis is MBP.[13] It is important to remember that intentional harm including poisoning may still occur even outside the psychiatric qualifications of MBP.

PROFILE OF THE VICTIM

Although this form of abuse has been documented in a variety of victims who have suffered a wide range of complaints, some recurring, almost pathognomonic, features may help to identify the MBP victim (Table 27.1). A review of the available literature paints a typical demographic picture of the children at risk for MBP. Although MBP cases have been reported in older children, teenagers, and even adults,[20,21] studies show that younger children are the more typical victims. One such epidemiologic study involving cases from the United Kingdom and Ireland[22] and another study involving cases from New Zealand[23] revealed that a large majority of pediatric cases were diagnosed in those under 5 years old (ranging from 66% to 77%).

The median age at the time of diagnosis was 2.7 years in the New Zealand study[23] and 20 months in the United Kingdom and Ireland.[22] Large literature reviews by Rosenberg[24] and Sheridan[25] of existing cases give somewhat similar data on the victims' ages. Sheridan's more recent review found that 75% percent of cases occur when victims are 6 years or younger.[25] The average age when diagnosed was found to be 48.6 months in the cases reviewed by Sheridan; average age was 39.8 months in the cases reviewed by Rosenberg.[25] All of these articles also report a fairly even gender distribution among victims.[22-25] The exception may be the apparently rare circumstances of a male perpetrator; in such cases, the victims usually tend to be male as well.[25]

The nature of the victim's illness is often an invaluable clue to identifying MBP. A wide variety of presenting medical problems are reported in the literature. The most frequent medical problems in the literature review by Rosenberg included bleeding (44%), seizures (42%), central nervous system depression (19%), apnea (15%), diarrhea (11%), vomiting (10%), fever (10%), and rash (9%).[24] Sheridan's more recent review found the most frequent presentations to be apnea (26.8%), anorexia/feeding problems (26.4%), diarrhea (20.0%), seizures (17.5%), cyanosis (11.7%), behavior problems (10.4%), asthma (9.5%), allergy (9.3%), fevers (8.6%), and pain (8.0%).[25] There is considerable overlap in their findings if not in their rankings. Most significantly, these are nonspecific complaints that will present the victim's physician with a large differential diagnosis. There have also been cases, however, where the perpetrator induces or falsifies symptoms with a particular diagnosis in mind such as cystic fibrosis or diabetes.[26,27]

Perhaps even more important than the specific symptoms seen in the victim is their timing. The physical findings of illness may only be witnessed by the perpetrator.[28] In cases where the perpetrator is actively inducing symptoms in the patient (e.g., by poisoning), the presenting signs and symptoms of illness will worsen in the presence of the perpetrator and improve when he or she is removed.[29]

Finally, there are the behavioral problems that these victims may exhibit. These victims will often passively accept both the harmful actions of the abuser and the tests and procedures performed on them.[21] Some researchers have noted that these children begin to demonstrate a symbiotic relationship with the perpetrator and demonstrate significant separation anxiety.[30] Other behavior problems may develop over time. These children may become very withdrawn or begin to show aggressive, hyperactive, or oppositional behavior.[16]

PROFILE OF THE PERPETRATOR

The features of those responsible for MBP have been extensively studied and reported. Though caution should be used in excluding this diagnosis based on a profile such as that given in Table 27.2, there are some common and consistent characteristics that can help arouse suspicion when faced with a confusing medical presentation.

By and large, a fairly consistent demographic profile has been developed. One classic characteristic rendered in Rosenberg's literature review was that the perpetrator was the biologic mother in 98% of the cases.[24] In the same study, Rosenberg found that the other 2% were adoptive mothers. Although this trend of gender exclusivity persists, there have been cases reviewed that involve male perpetrators. Meadow reported 15 cases of MBP involving male perpetrators.[31] The more recent MBP literature review by Sheridan found the mother to be the perpetrator in only 76.5% of the cases, with the father as the guilty party in 6.7% of the cases.[25] The perpetrator is usually well educated, often with formal medical or nursing training.[6] If not formally educated, they are often literate in medical jargon and procedures.[28] In cases where marital status was recorded, Sheridan also found that most commonly these perpetrators were married.[25] It is a commonly held belief that the majority of these female perpetrators are Caucasian. This detail is not consistently available in case reports, but Sheridan did report that, when the information was available, the victims (and presumably therefore the perpetrators) were white 78.79% of the time.[25] However, the vast majority of the cases reported at this time are from English-speaking, industrialized nations including the United States, Europe, Canada, New Zealand, and Australia.[25,32] This fact could certainly shape the profile of the perpetrator with respect to race.

The perpetrator's behavior in the hospital can often be a useful diagnostic clue. Perhaps most striking is the degree to which perpetrators enjoy and thrive on being in the hospital

TABLE 27.2 **Profile of the Classic MBP Perpetrator** [6-9,12,14,17,19,21,24,25,28,33-35]

Characteristics and behavior
- Biologic mother
- Married
- Some form of medical or nursing education
- Constant presence at victim's bedside
- Enjoys being in the hospital and interacting with staff
- Remains patient and calm even if child's condition deteriorates or if child undergoes painful procedure and test

Perpetrator's medical history
- Similar medical problems to the victim
- Depression
- Personality disorders
- History of abuse

Perpetrator's spouse
- Marital strife often present
- Frequently absent from hospital
- Ignorant of abuse that is occurring

environment.[14] They immerse themselves in the hospital by becoming close with the staff, participating in hospital gossip, and, perhaps most importantly, accepting praise from the hospital staff for their efforts to help their child.[9,12,28] Unlike the stereotype of an abuser, the perpetrator of MBP does not display outward anger or impatience toward the victim. Instead, the responsible caregiver will typically be ardently attached to the child. Typically, the perpetrator will stay in the same room as the child and not leave his or her side.[17] Furthermore, the perpetrator will expect and demand to participate physically in the medical care of the victim.[33] Also striking to those participating in the care of these patients is how remarkably calm and composed the perpetrator will appear despite the child's illness, even when that illness is critical.[9,19] Often the perpetrator will eagerly allow medical personnel to perform painful procedures on the child and display remarkably less distress than expected.[9,34] Even in the face of the medical team expressing profound concern about the health of the victim, the perpetrator will often remain relatively serene, sometimes consoling the medical team.[8,17] On occasion, however, the other extreme is reported; in such cases, the perpetrator berates medical staff and demands therapies that are clearly not indicated.[28]

The past medical history of the perpetrator generally will reveal clues as well.

A substantial number of these caregivers have medical problems similar to their children and may display features of MS.[7,24,25,28] Perpetrators also display a high incidence of depression and personality disorders and, not surprisingly, may have been abused themselves.[7,21,28]

Indirect clues to MBP may be revealed with scrutiny of the other parent (usually the child's father) and this person's relationship to the perpetrator. There is often marital strife.[35] The other parent, especially by comparison, seems both emotionally and physically detached from the situation and rarely visits the child in the hospital.[7] The other parent in most cases appears not to know that the abuse is occurring.[28]

GENERAL INVESTIGATIVE APPROACH WITH MUNCHAUSEN BY PROXY

Because the true origin of the physical illness being portrayed is shrouded in deception, a high degree of clinical suspicion is necessary to make the diagnosis of MBP. Like any form of child abuse, however, it should not be treated as a diagnosis of exclusion,[18] and care should be taken to avoid this mentality. Though MBP will not generally be placed at the top of a differential diagnosis list, it must not be forgotten. If there is a sense of general discord with the history, physical exam findings, and laboratory results, MBP should be considered.[36]

As with any medical dilemma, a thorough history is essential. Careful documentation of all symptoms, signs, and exact quotations from the suspected perpetrator, as well as a precise timeline of events (including clinical occurrences with and without the presence of the suspected perpetrator) is essential.[1] If the child is old enough to communicate verbally and provide a history, the child should be interviewed separately.[24] Such interviews with children must be done carefully, without leading questions, and preferably by a child interviewing specialist.

Besides interviewing the patients, hospital staff should explore other potential sources of information. When possible, multiple members of the family, close friends, officials from school, babysitters, store clerks, neighbors, and the primary care physician should be interviewed without revealing the information already provided by the perpetrator.[24,28,37,38] All details of the history presented by the caregiver should be confirmed in this manner.[16] If MBP is suspected, this information will become critical to the police investigation of the caregiver.

All outside medical records (primary care, emergency department, and other hospital stays) should be tenaciously obtained, thoroughly examined, and carefully compared with the information that has been reported by the caregiver.[28] Warning bells should ring if the suspected perpetrator claims that medical records have been lost or that the physician originally responsible for making an initial diagnosis has moved or is unavailable.[24] Diligence is always required to confirm or refute the existence of an illness when there is clear physical and laboratory evidence to the contrary, and treatment should not be made based solely on the word of a family member.[27] The investigator should not rely simply on summary reports (e.g., discharge summaries) but should also look at the original data, such as nursing notes and biopsy results.[11] One may find repeated hospitalizations with extensive investigation and no definitive diagnosis revealed.[9] All records should be carefully examined to make sure they have not been altered by the caregiver.[38] This painstaking process is crucial, as it may reveal discrepancies in the story presented to the medical team that serve as the initial clue to MBP.[36] From a law enforcement perspective, preservation of such documents will be important during a subsequent police investigation.

A careful family history is also important. Some studies have shown that siblings may be similarly abused in as many as 40% of MBP cases, with 18% having a sibling who had died.[12] Repeated hospital admissions of these siblings may be discovered.[39] Sudden unexplained deaths and other strange illnesses in the family may serve to arouse suspicion.[38] The caregiver in question may also have medical problems mirroring the child (i.e., may exhibit MS) or may have been diagnosed with psychiatric illnesses.[28,39] All drugs that are available in the home, regardless of whom they belong to, should be carefully documented.[39] Other possible family illnesses may serve as clues to available medications even if these illnesses were never directly reported (e.g., a history of bipolar disorder may indicate access to lithium).

Physical exams and laboratory evidence should be gathered with similar care and recorded precisely. The patient must receive a thorough physical exam focused on establishing the presence or absence of findings that support the caregiver's claims.[29] There may be significant incongruity between actual clinical findings and the reported history.[34] One may find that these symptoms and signs are not genuine (e.g., a "rash" that washes off).[17] Focused laboratory testing based on logical suspicion is the best approach. If drugs are being taken by the patient or are available in the household, chemical levels may be obtained.[11] Laboratory testing can be done to confirm or refute symptoms described by parents (e.g., serum electrolytes to investigate the claim of chronic vomiting).[16] Suspicion may be heightened for MBP if available laboratory information does not correlate with the clinical picture.[3]

Multiple strategies must be used during a hospital stay to facilitate the investigation and diagnosis of MBP. Throughout the hospital stay, one should pay careful attention to the timing of any exacerbations of the victim's illness.[29] A critical diagnostic finding is if there is clear worsening or recurrence of symptoms only when the suspected perpetrator is present.[34] In line with this temporal relationship, resolution of the patient's symptoms with sustained separation of the suspected caregiver from the patient is equally important to support the suspicion of MBP.[9] A "separation test" must be administered carefully with strict enforcement, allowing the caretaker only supervised visits and no direct role in the feeding and medical care of the child.[6,11] The collection of laboratory data should be meticulously observed, and only samples obtained solely by hospital staff should be tested in order to prevent tampering.[6,21] By eliminating possible interference by the perpetrator, laboratory abnormalities may also be resolved. Documentation should be made when the application of standard therapies for the given medical condition prove unsuccessful (e.g., anticonvulsants will not prevent recurrence of the patient's reported seizure activity).[17]

Perhaps, the gold standard in detecting MBP is covert video surveillance (CVS). The most well-known initial study of this technique in the investigation of MBP was done by Southall et al.[40] In this study, the investigators were able to prove abuse in 33 of 39 reported cases. This study also resulted in the discovery that four deaths, previously attributed to sudden infant death syndrome (SIDS), were actually homicides based on confessions by the mothers. They also studied this technique and confirmed MBP in 23 of 41 cases. When considering this method, however, the investigator must be aware of privacy and legality issues. Before implementing this technique, therefore, at the very least hospital administration and likely law enforcement should be consulted.[41] Interestingly, in some cases even when perpetrators knew that video recording was in progress, they still revealed their actions.[36]

INVESTIGATIVE APPROACH OF MUNCHAUSEN BY PROXY INVOLVING POISONS

MBP through poisoning has been reported with a variety of agents and described in medical literature. One epidemiologic study looking at a series of 128 cases of MBP found that poisons were used in 44 of the cases (34%).[22] In this same study, prescription drugs were found to have been used 71% of the time, with anticonvulsants and opiates being the two most commonly used. Table 27.3 lists some of the specific drugs, chemicals, and drug classes that have been reported in medical literature to have been used for poisoning children in MBP.[1,36,39,42-44]

TABLE 27.3 **Drugs, Drug Classes, and Chemicals Reported in the Poisoning of Children in MBP**

Acetaminophen	Diuretics
Anticonvulsants	Glucose
Antidepressants	Hydrocarbons
Antihistamines	Insulin
Antipsychotics	Laxatives
Acetone	Lomotil
Arsenic	Methaqualone
Barbiturates	Opioids
Benzodiazepines	Paregoric
Bethenacol	Phenergan
Bleach	Salicylates
Carbon monoxide	Salt
Chloral hydrate	Sulfonylureas
Clonidine	Warfarin and
Caustics	superwarfarins

If poisoning is the method suspected, all the history, physical exams, and available and reliable laboratory evidence should be carefully examined. As thoroughly as possible, an inventory of possible available agents to the perpetrator should be made. Even if this information is not volunteered, indirect indicators of medications available may be gained from the family history (e.g., mother is a diabetic). If the available information supports a possible toxin as an etiology, further diagnostic studies may prove helpful in narrowing the focus. All available data should then be examined as a whole to see if a toxin could explain the clinical picture presented. Additional help in this process may be gained through consultation with a regional poison center or inpatient medical toxicology service.[11]

These cases are typically perplexing diagnostic dilemmas. The same general diagnostic approach used in all MBP cases applies to those involving poisonings, but there are also some special consideration. For one thing, by the time poisoning is considered in the differential diagnosis, urine or blood samples may no longer contain evidence of a foreign substance.[1] Another part of the quandary presenting to the physician or investigator is that literally any drug or chemical compound could be surreptitiously used as a poison. Unfortunately, conventional urine or serum toxicology screens identify relatively few substances—typically amphetamines, barbiturates, benzodiazepines, cocaine, opioids, and cannabinoids.[45] Furthermore, these tests frequently suffer from both false positive and false negative results.[46] Therefore, for drug testing to be most useful, it must be focused on a likely list of suspect substances that is based on the victim's history, physical exam, and other general laboratory and diagnostic testing (e.g., serum electrolytes or electrocardiogram).[1,11] Drug levels of medications that are prescribed to the patient should be checked to assure that appropriate amounts are being given.[11] If specific drug levels or other laboratory evidence is sought, the best possible yield is obtained if blood, urine, or gastric washings are sent when the patient is acutely symptomatic.[17,43] All laboratory samples should be carefully stored for further analysis if retrospective analysis is necessary.[27]

If a poisoning is discovered, there are some indications that the exposure was not accidental. Though accidental poisonings are not uncommon in children less than 5 years old,[47] the physician or investigator should keep the child's developmental level in mind when considering the feasibility of such an exposure. For example, an infant who is only a few months old will likely lack the mobility to reach substances or have the manual dexterity to pick up small objects, such as pills, to ingest them. Furthermore, substances such as salt are unlikely to be accidentally ingested by young children in large enough quantities to cause hypernatremia.[7]

To help illustrate the diagnostic thought process involved, examples of poisons that have been used in reported MBP cases will be discussed to show their initial presentation, disease processes that they may mimic, and diagnostic tests that may help elucidate the true poison culprit (Table 27.4).

Syrup of Ipecac

Syrup of ipecac is one of the most well-reported over-the-counter (OTC) drugs used in MBP with numerous case reports in the literature.[48-59] It has been used as an OTC emetic for home management of accidental poison ingestions since 1965.[60] Ipecac syrup is prepared from the dried roots of *Cephaelis ipecacuanha* and *C. acuminata* with the goal of obtaining the active alkaloids, emetine and cephaeline.[49] Vomiting occurs through stimulation of the areas of the central nervous system that trigger emesis and also through direct gastric mucosa irritation.[61] The onset of vomiting is within 20–30 minutes of ingestion.[62] Chronic administration of ipecac causes unrelenting nausea, vomiting, diarrhea, gastrointestinal (GI) bleeding, serum electrolyte disarray, and, most concerning of all, a myopathy involving both skeletal and cardiac muscles.[63] An elevation of creatine kinase may be seen with this myopathy.[64]

Chronic vomiting with other GI symptoms presents a large differential diagnosis. It becomes easy to imagine why this medication would appeal to the perpetrator of MBP. Cases in the past have been misdiagnosed as gastroesophageal reflux, failure to thrive, and gastroenteritis.[48,54] One study looked to identifying the active ingredients, emetine and cephaeline, in the laboratory.[65] Though the investigators found that plasma levels of emetine and cephaeline will be undetectable within 6 hours, these alkaloids could be detected in urine samples some weeks later.[65] Therefore, urine testing for these active ingredients may be helpful in proving ipecac's causative role. It is wise to consider ipecac intoxication if the patient has repetitive vomiting with other GI symptoms, especially if accompanied by an elevated creatine kinase, muscle weakness, or cardiac failure.[59,63]

Laxatives

Multiple cases have been reported in which laxatives were used in the context of intentional poisoning and MBP.[66-71] Similar to ipecac, the appeal to the perpetrator of MBP is that many of these compounds are OTC and easily available. When given surreptitiously, these compounds will yield what appears to be refractory diarrhea. Again, the differential diagnoses for such a complaint can be vast and likely include malabsorption syndromes, viral and bacteria gastrointestinal infection, and food intolerance or allergy—all considerations that may yield lengthy hospitalizations and extensive diagnostic testing.

Various laxatives exist, and because most are OTC medications, they are at the disposal of the perpetrator of MBP. There are the stimulant laxatives that include a broad group of agents such as castor oil, docusate, bisacodyl, and senna.[72] The exact mechanism varies with each agent but generally involves increasing gut motility, altering

TABLE 27.4 Presentation and Suggested Testing for Some Poisons Used in MBP[59,65,72,73,76,77,83-96,98,99,102-105]

Poison	Possible presentation	Suggested laboratory tests
Syrup of ipecac	Chronic vomiting Gastroenteritis Gastroesophageal reflux Failure to thrive Skeletal muscle myopathy Cardiomyopathy	Elevated CK Blood and urine levels of emetine and cephaeline (ipecac metabolites)
Laxatives	Chronic diarrhea Gastroenteritis Malabsorption Failure to thrive Food allergy	Serum electrolytes Stool electrolytes Stool osmolality Urine and stool levels for specific laxatives
Warfarin/superwarfarins	Gastrointestinal bleed Bleeding diathesis Ecchymoses Menorrhagia Bleeding gums Epistaxis	PT, INR, and PTT Coagulation factor levels Blood warfarin level Blood superwarfarin levels
Insulin/sulfonylureas	Seizures Altered mental status Insulinoma Congenital hyperinsulinism	Blood glucose levels Serum insulin levels Serum C-peptide levels Serum/urine sulfonylurea levels

CK = creatine kinase; PT = prothrombin time; INR = international normalized ratio; PTT = partial thromboplastin time.

electrolyte and fluid transport, or both.[72,73] The bulk laxatives such as psyllium likely act by retaining water and providing liquidity to stools.[74] Another group of drugs that act to retain water in the gut lumen are the osmotic agents, which include poorly absorbable salts such as magnesium hydroxide (milk of magnesia), lactulose, sorbitol, and polyethylene glycol (Miralax).[72] Mineral oil is a commonly used lubricant that decreases water absorption by the gut and subsequently softens stools.[72] Phenolphthalein was long used as an ingredient in OTC laxatives. However, after concerns regarding its role as a possible carcinogen and a subsequent ruling in 1997 by the Food and Drug Administration that it was "not generally recognized as safe and effective," it disappeared from the market in the United States.[75] Phenolphthalein use in MBP, however, is well documented.[66,69]

As expected, if forced to consume or surreptitiously given large amounts of laxative, the victim can be expected to have frequent, large, watery stools.[73,76] Other gastrointestinal symptoms are possible as well. Although diarrhea obviously predominates, alternating periods of constipation are also possible.[77,78] The victim may also suffer from abdominal pain and cramping, bloating, nausea, vomiting, and rectal pain upon defecation.[73,76-78] If this pattern continues for some time, the victim may undergo significant fluid and electrolyte loss as well as malnutrition.[73,76] If severe enough, the child may experience failure to thrive, weight loss, tachycardia, hypotension, lethargy, muscle weakness, or syncope.[73,76]

Overuse of anthraquinone laxatives (e.g., senna) has been associated with some unique physical findings. A telltale physical finding related to these laxatives may be discovered on colonoscopy. A distinct, brown pigmentation of the colonic mucosa, called melanosis coli, occurs with continued use of senna and other anthraquinone laxatives.[73,76] Abuse of oral senna has also led to the discovery of finger clubbing in several case reports.[79-82]

Serum electrolytes may also provide the investigator or physician with some clues. Hypokalemia is a common finding that is due to both stool losses and renal losses caused by a secondary hyperaldosteronism that is triggered by dehydration.[72,73,76] This hypokalemia, then, is proposed to impair gut reabsorption of chloride

and increase renal reabsorption of bicarbonate, leading to a characteristic hypochloremic metabolic alkalosis.[72,76] This process can be helpful in diagnosis, as it is unlike what is expected from a severe and acute diarrheal illness—a metabolic acidosis.[73] Although serum deficiencies in magnesium and calcium may occur,[76] hyponatremia is not often seen.[77] One may intuitively expect electrolyte deficiencies in these cases; however, when the laxatives used are osmotic salts with sodium, magnesium, phosphate, or calcium as component ions, high serum levels of these electrolytes can be discovered.[72]

Besides serum electrolyte testing, there are other studies that may be of assistance (see Table 27.4). Stool samples may provide valuable information. They should be fresh and obtained on multiple occasions (along with multiple urine samples) and stored in order to examine these samples serially with a variety of tests if necessary.[83]

Stool electrolytes may also reveal significant abnormalities. Ingestion of large amounts of osmotic laxative salts containing magnesium, phosphate, or sulfate may leave elevated levels of these electrolytes in stool samples.[84,85] Checking stool osmolality may also be helpful, especially if it is low. An excessively low stool osmolality (generally under 250 mOsm/kg) may indicate active dilution of the sample with water.[83,86] It is important to document the osmolality of urine in these cases as well because dilute urine mixing with the stool could be another explanation.[86] Phenolphthalein, though not commonly available, may still be used. If suspected, placing a suspected stool in an alkaline solution will yield a characteristic red color.[69,71]

Finally, some stimulant laxatives or their metabolites can be detected in urine and stool samples using a variety of chromatographic techniques.[87-89] To increase the yield of these studies, serial morning urine and stool samples should be taken to pick up evidence of laxatives that are only sporadically administered.[83] One study examined the use of a commercially available thin-layer chromatography method for bisacodyl and senna detection in stool and urine samples.[88] Unfortunately, this study demonstrated deficiencies in both sensitivity and specificity, with false negatives being common for senna and false positives for bisacodyl. Therefore, such commercial tests must be interpreted with caution. Another study examined using mass spectrometry combined with gas chromatographic analysis to detect some laxatives or their metabolites in urine samples (e.g., bisacodyl, phenolphthalein, and anthraquinones).[83,90] This technique showed more promise for accurate and dependable detection.

Diagnosing MBP caused by laxatives is difficult because of the common presentation of diarrhea and the variety of causative agents at the disposal of the perpetrator. Recognizing that symptom exacerbation occurs with the presence of the perpetrator (and therefore administration of the laxative) and recedes with this person's absence can be an important clue. Persistent collection of multiple stool and urine samples for analysis (all the while maintaining an appropriate chain of custody to assure that no tampering or substitution occurs) will likely be necessary to clinch the diagnosis.[83] Clinical observation on a normal diet while separated from the perpetrator should also provide further evidence with subsequent resolution of diarrhea.[83]

Warfarin/Superwarfarin

Bleeding is a commonly reported presentation of MBP.[24] Although there are many ways that this symptom can be artificially achieved, one well-documented method is the clandestine administration of the prescription anticoagulant warfarin and its OTC rodenticide cousins, the superwarfarins (e.g., brodifacoum).[91-93] Both warfarin and the superwarfarins promote bleeding by blocking the production of the vitamin-K dependent coagulation factors—factors II, VII, IX, and X.[91,94] Even though they are OTC substances, the rodenticide superwarfarins are more problematic in that they are about 100 times more potent and have vastly greater half-lives (greater than 24 days) than warfarin.[94]

The sustained, increased tendency to bleed that is caused by these chemicals can produce a confusing clinical picture. MBP poisoning victims who are poisoned with these compounds may present with a variety of bleeding complaints including ecchymoses, gastrointestinal bleeding, epistaxis, bleeding diathesis, hematuria, abdominal pain, bleeding gums, and menorrhagia.[91-94] Such symptoms generally require large overdoses of these substances—even with superwarfarins.[91,95]

If suspected, there are diagnostic clues that may lead the investigator or physician down the right path. As would be expected therapeutically, warfarin and superwarfarin ingestion should raise the prothrombin time (PT) and international normalized ratio (INR).[94,96] When large, coagulopathic doses are given, the partial thromboplastin time (PTT) will also increase.[91] At this point, the diagnosis of these poisonings can be supported by checking for coagulation factor deficiencies. If only the vitamin K-dependent factors (II, VII, IX, and X) are deficient, the presence of these compounds is supported.[91,93,94] Unless an explanation for vitamin K deficiency or liver disease exists, or unless a legitimate reason for the patient to be on such anticoagulative therapy is documented, this type of poisoning should be suspected.[94] If vitamin K deficiency is plausible but the coagulopathy continues for long periods despite adequate vitamin K1 therapy, MBP using these poisons should still be suspected.[91] The final diagnostic tool is to use the specific assays needed to detect the presence of warfarin and superwarfarin in the victim's blood while the victim is symptomatic.[94]

Insulin and Sulfonylureas

Another group of poisons that have been documented in multiple cases of MBP are diabetic medications capable of inducing severe hypoglycemia—insulin[27,34,97-100] and sulfonylureas.[99,101,102] The use of these toxins in poisonings is discussed in more detail in Chapter 12. However, their use, specifically in the context of MBP, will be briefly discussed here. Both insulin and sulfonylureas poisonings produce a picture of hyperinsulinemic hypoglycemia that can lead to an extensive diagnostic workup. As surreptitious poisonings, these agents have led to presentations of seizure disorders, altered mental states, inborn errors of metabolism, insulinoma, and congenital hyperinsulinism (i.e., nesidioblastosis or persistent hyperinsulinemic hypoglycemia of infancy).[27,34,97-102] Testing should explore such a differential and will probably require lengthy or repeated hospitalizations to facilitate further studies. These studies might include drawing multiple blood samples for complete metabolic testing, prolonged fasting, lumbar puncture for metabolic studies, and pancreatic venous sampling through direct catheterization of pancreatic veins.[98,99,102] It should be noted that the clinical picture portrayed by this induced hyperinsulinemic hypoglycemia is so convincing that these victims have undergone actual subtotal pancreatectomy to correct it.[98,99] In addition to the simulation of these more extraordinary diagnoses, insulin has also been given repeatedly under the false assertion of preexisting diabetes.[27]

When faced with this sort of a diagnostic dilemma, physicians may find that laboratory studies can help identify an exogenous cause of the victim's hypoglycemia (see Table 27.4). First and foremost, blood must be drawn when the suspected victim is actively symptomatic and hypoglycemic.[43] This sample is the best chance to identify the presence (or absence) of a disorder in metabolism or telltale signs of pharmaceutical interference with the body's handling of glucose.[43,103] Barring this measure, serial blood samples may be drawn, analyzed, and even stored for future analysis. If diabetic agents such as insulin or sulfonylureas are suspected, blood samples should be analyzed for both insulin and C-peptide.[103]

If, in a hypoglycemic state, the victim's blood sample has a higher than expected level of insulin without an accompanying rise in C-peptide (i.e., high insulin to C-peptide ratio), it is indicative of exogenous insulin administration.[98,99,104] In some instances, high-pressure liquid chromatography (HPLC) analysis of blood samples has been used to prove the presence of beef and pork insulin and the absence of human insulin.[98]

On the other hand, if the blood sample has high amounts of insulin and a high C-peptide level, either a metabolic disorder (e.g., insulinoma) or a sulfonylurea may be present.[99,102,103] It is advisable in this situation to check sulfonylurea levels in either blood or urine.[103] A wide range of chromatographic techniques have had mixed success in identifying the variety of sulfonylureas that may be used in these cases.[99,105] One study using liquid chromatography and mass spectrometry was able to identify eight different types of sulfonylureas in blood samples.[105] It is important before sending these samples to know which medications are being searched for and the limitations of the particular laboratory technique.[99] Identifying the presence of sulfonylureas is crucial, as it may prevent further invasive diagnostic procedures and even surgery.

OVERALL MANAGEMENT KEYS

In cases of MBP, the endeavor to make the diagnosis and the management of the patient are intertwined. While in the hospital, some key management strategies must be maintained. The medical team should remain supportive of the patient and his or her family and avoid angering or polarizing them in a way that might prompt premature discharge of the victim or continuation of the abuse at another facility.[36] Even as the diagnosis of MBP is debated, it must first and foremost be remembered that the essential concern is that of child abuse.[3] The motivation of the perpetrator of this abuse is a secondary concern and can be assessed in time.[21] Child abuse is not a diagnosis of exclusion, and performing an extensive workup to "rule out" all other possible causes of illness should not be done if abuse is the true concern.[18] It is important to remember that such an evaluation by a physician may be one of the tools of the abuser.[106] For both the good of the victim and diagnostic purposes, the child must be protected from the abuser—usually by separation or at the very least strict supervision by a third party at all times.[36] Symptom resolution during this separation is highly suspicious of MBP.[9,21] Only hospital nurses and ancillary personnel should provide care (e.g., prepare food and deliver medications) while the patient is in the hospital.[43] All samples taken for analysis (e.g., blood, urine, stool) should be carefully gathered by hospital staff with all practical precautions taken to prevent tampering while maintaining an appropriate chain of custody (not only documenting the procession of samples but also limiting access to such samples).[6,35]

Though cases of MBP are challenging to diagnose from a clinical standpoint, they are also challenging from a legal perspective. In this regard, documentation is critical. All inpatient documentation must be thorough and objective, including any aspect that is relevant in stating the case for MBP and in any future criminal investigation and legal proceedings.[35,39] Physician and nursing notes should be legible and carefully maintained. They should be protected from "chart tampering," as perpetrators have been known to obfuscate data obtained in the hospital in order to perpetuate their elaborate charade.[19,38] At times, it may be necessary to develop a procedure whereby the responsible nurse can record data based on his or her observations separately from information reported by the suspected perpetrator.[38] All such documentation should be detailed and should describe the pertinent verbatim comments by the suspected perpetrator, relevant actions by the perpetrator witnessed by the hospital staff, and behavior toward the victim, spouse, and hospital staff.[9]

Finally, a multidisciplinary approach is needed for the successful management of these cases.[37] Immediate involvement of hospital social work, the local department of social services, legal consult, and law enforcement is necessary when any case of child abuse is suspected.[21,24,39] The early involvement of these specialists will be especially helpful in case the family tries to discharge the victim from the hospital prematurely or if a discharge safety plan (e.g., temporary placement with a relative or foster care) is needed for the victim and siblings.[21,39] The advice and expertise of a child abuse specialist is invaluable in evaluating these cases and navigating the medicolegal waters that await.[18,107] Involvement of child and adult psychiatry, as well as family therapy, should be maintained for the health of the victim and also the perpetrator.[21] Regardless of the method used by the perpetrator, it is only through the cooperation of individuals from these different fields that these cases can be successfully managed.

CONCLUSION

These cases are typically perplexing diagnostic dilemmas. Part of the quandary facing the physician or investigator is that literally any drug or chemical compound could be surreptitiously used as a poison. The impetus that leads a parent or other caregiver to harm a child is psychologically complex and thus often difficult to understand.

The perpetrator's motivation in cases of MBP is especially bewildering. The medical team must at all times remember that these are first and foremost cases of child abuse. Protection of the victim is the primary necessity. Any investigation must be thoughtful and deliberate, with care being taken not to enable the abuse of the victim by putting him or her through painful and needless procedures. Before initiating an extensive diagnostic process, attention must be paid to the many available clues to the diagnosis of MBP. These clues are most readily available

through an objective but skeptical and meticulous appraisal of the caregiver's relationship with the possible victim, the available history, a detailed physical exam, and careful recording and monitoring of the victim's hospital course. This high index of suspicion vastly outweighs even the largest battery of tests.

REFERENCES

1. Holstege CP, Dobmeier SG. Criminal poisoning: Munchausen by proxy. *Clin Lab Med.* 2006;26(1):243–253.
2. Cantor RM, Stork CM. Munchausen's syndrome by proxy in the form of child abuse by poisoning: case reports and review of the literature. *J Toxicol Clin Toxicol.* 2001;39(3):264.
3. Murray JB. Munchausen syndrome/Munchausen syndrome by proxy. *J Psychol.* 1997;131(3):343–352.
4. Fisher JA. Investigating the Barons: narrative and nomenclature in Munchausen syndrome. *Perspect Biol Med.* 2006;49(2):250–262.
5. Asher R. Munchausen's syndrome. *Lancet.* 1951(Feb 10);1(6):339–341.
6. Yonge O, Haase M. Munchausen syndrome and Munchausen syndrome by proxy in a student nurse. *Nurse Educ.* 2004;29(4):166–169.
7. Fulton DR. Early recognition of Munchausen Syndrome by Proxy. *Crit Care Nurs Q* 2000;23(2):35–42.
8. Meadow R. Munchausen syndrome by proxy. The hinterland of child abuse. *Lancet.* 1977(Aug 13);2(8033):343–345.
9. Thomas K. Munchausen syndrome by proxy: identification and diagnosis. *J Pediatr Nurs.* 2003;18(3):174–180.
10. Bartsch C, Risse M, Schutz H, Weigand N, Weiler G. Munchausen syndrome by proxy (MSBP): an extreme form of child abuse with a special forensic challenge. *Forensic Sci Int.* 2003;137(2-3):147–151.
11. Galvin HK, Newton AW, Vandeven AM. Update on Munchausen syndrome by proxy. *Curr Opin Pediatr.* 2005;17(2):252–257.
12. Sharif I. Munchausen syndrome by proxy. *Pediatr Rev.* 2004;25(6):215–216.
13. Schreier H. Munchausen by proxy defined. *Pediatrics.* 2002;110(5):985–988.
14. Schreier H. Munchausen by proxy. *Curr Probl Pediatr Adolesc Health Care.* 2004;34(3):126–143.
15. Ayoub CC, Alexander R, Beck D, et al. Position paper: definitional issues in Munchausen by proxy. *Child Maltreat.* 2002;7(2):105–111.
16. Moldavsky M, Stein D. Munchausen Syndrome by Proxy: two case reports and an update of the literature. *Int J Psychiatry Med.* 2003;33(4):411–423.
17. Meadow R. Munchausen syndrome by proxy. *Arch Dis Child.* 1982;57(2):92–98.
18. Stirling J Jr. Beyond Munchausen syndrome by proxy: identification and treatment of child abuse in a medical setting. *Pediatrics.* 2007;119(5):1026–1030.
19. Bools C. Factitious illness by proxy. Munchausen syndrome by proxy. *Br J Psychiatry.* 1996;169(3):268–275.

20. Awadallah N, Vaughan A, Franco K, Munir F, Sharaby N, Goldfarb J. Munchausen by proxy: a case, chart series, and literature review of older victims. *Child Abuse Negl.* 2005;29(8):931–941.

21. Souid AK, Keith DV, Cunningham AS. Munchausen syndrome by proxy. *Clin Pediatr (Phila).* 1998;37(8):497–503.

22. McClure RJ, Davis PM, Meadow SR, Sibert JR. Epidemiology of Munchausen syndrome by proxy, non-accidental poisoning, and non-accidental suffocation. *Arch Dis Child.* 1996;75(1):57–61.

23. Denny SJ, Grant CC, Pinnock R. Epidemiology of Munchausen syndrome by proxy in New Zealand. *J Paediatr Child Health.* 2001;37(3):240–243.

24. Rosenberg DA. Web of deceit: a literature review of Munchausen syndrome by proxy. *Child Abuse Negl.* 1987;11(4):547–563.

25. Sheridan MS. The deceit continues: an updated literature review of Munchausen Syndrome by Proxy. *Child Abuse Negl.* 2003;27(4):431–451.

26. Orenstein DM, Wasserman AL. Munchausen syndrome by proxy simulating cystic fibrosis. *Pediatrics.* 1986;78(4):621–624.

27. McSweeney JJ, Hoffman RP. Munchausen's syndrome by proxy mistaken for IDDM. *Diabetes Care.* 1991;14(10):928–929.

28. Pasqualone GA, Fitzgerald SM. Munchausen by proxy syndrome: the forensic challenge of recognition, diagnosis, and reporting. *Crit Care Nurs Q.* 1999;22(1):52–64, quiz 90–51.

29. Vennemann B, Bajanowski T, Karger B, Pfeiffer H, Kohler H, Brinkmann B. Suffocation and poisoning—the hard-hitting side of Munchausen syndrome by proxy. *Int J Legal Med.* 2005;119(2):98–102.

30. McGuire TL, Feldman KW. Psychologic morbidity of children subjected to Munchausen syndrome by proxy. *Pediatrics.* 1989;83(2):289–292.

31. Meadow R. Munchausen syndrome by proxy abuse perpetrated by men. *Arch Dis Child.* 1998;78(3):210–216.

32. Feldman MD, Brown RM. Munchausen by Proxy in an international context. *Child Abuse Negl.* 2002;26(5):509–524.

33. Kamerling LB, Black XA, Fiser RT. Munchausen syndrome by proxy in the pediatric intensive care unit: an unusual mechanism. *Pediatr Crit Care Med.* 2002;3(3):305–307.

34. Zylstra RG, Miller KE, Stephens WE. Munchausen syndrome by proxy: a clinical vignette. *Prim Care Companion J Clin Psychiatry.* 2000;2(2):42–44.

35. Lieder HS, Irving SY, Mauricio R, Graf JM. Munchausen syndrome by proxy: a case report. *AACN Clin Issues.* 2005;16(2):178–184.

36. Herman MI, Glass T, Howard SC. Case records of the LeBonheur Children's Medical Center: a 17-month-old girl with abdominal distension and portal vein gas. *Pediatr Emerg Care.* 1997;13(3):237–242.

37. Bryk M, Siegel PT. My mother caused my illness: the story of a survivor of Munchausen by proxy syndrome. *Pediatrics.* 1997;100(1):1–7.

38. Meadow R. Management of Munchausen syndrome by proxy. *Arch Dis Child.* 1985;60(4):385–393.

39. Rogers D, Tripp J, Bentovim A, Robinson A, Berry D, Goulding R. Non-accidental poisoning: an extended syndrome of child abuse. *BMJ.* 1976;1(6013):793–796.

40. Southall DP, Plunkett MC, Banks MW, Falkov AF, Samuels MP. Covert video recordings of life-threatening child abuse: lessons for child protection. *Pediatrics.* 1997;100(5):735–760.

41. Vaught W, Fleetwood J. Covert video surveillance in pediatric care. *Hastings Cent Rep.* 2002;32(6):10–12.

42. Hickson GB, Altemeier WA, Martin ED, et al. Parental administration of chemical agents: a cause of apparent life-threatening events. *Pediatrics.* 1989;83(5):772–776.

43. Lorber J, Reckless JP, Watson JB. Nonaccidental poisoning: the elusive diagnosis. *Arch Dis Child.* 1980;55(8):643–647.

44. Shnaps Y, Frand M, Rotem Y, et al. The chemically abused child. *Pediatrics.* 1981;68(1):119–121.

45. Osterhoudt KC. A toddler with recurrent episodes of unresponsiveness. *Pediatr Emerg Care.* 2004;20(3):195–197.

46. Hoffman RJ, Nelson L. Rational use of toxicology testing in children. *Curr Opin Pediatr.* 2001;13(2):183–188.

47. Lai MW, Klein-Schwartz W, Rodgers GC, et al. 2005 Annual Report of the American Association of Poison Control Centers' national poisoning and exposure database. *Clin Toxicol (Phila).* 2006;44(6-7):803–932.

48. Andersen JM, Keljo DJ, Argyle JC. Secretory diarrhea caused by ipecac poisoning. *J Pediatr Gastroenterol Nutr.* 1997;24(5):612–615.

49. Bader AA, Kerzner B. Ipecac toxicity in "Munchausen syndrome by proxy." *Ther Drug Monit.* 1999;21(2):259–260.

50. Carter KE, Izsak E, Marlow J. Munchausen syndrome by proxy caused by ipecac poisoning. *Pediatr Emerg Care.* 2006;22(9):655–656.

51. Colletti RB, Wasserman RC. Recurrent infantile vomiting due to intentional ipecac poisoning. *J Pediatr Gastroenterol Nutr.* 1989;8(3):394–396.

52. Cooper CP, Kamath KR. A toddler with persistent vomiting and diarrhoea. *Eur J Pediatr.* 1998;157(9):775–776.

53. Day L, Kelly C, Reed G, et al. Fatal cardiomyopathy: suspected child abuse by chronic ipecac administration. *Vet Hum Toxicol.* 1989;31(3):255–257.

54. Feldman KW, Christopher DM, Opheim KB. Munchausen syndrome/bulimia by proxy: ipecac as a toxin in child abuse. *Child Abuse Negl.* 1989;13(2):257–261.

55. Goebel J, Gremse DA, Artman M. Cardiomyopathy from ipecac administration in Munchausen syndrome by proxy. *Pediatrics.* 1993;92(4):601–603.

56. Johnson JE, Carpenter BL, Benton J, et al. Hemorrhagic colitis and pseudomelanosis coli in ipecac ingestion by proxy. *J Pediatr Gastroenterol Nutr.* 1991;12(4):501–506.

57. McClung HJ, Murray R, Braden NJ, et al. Intentional ipecac poisoning in children. *Am J Dis Child.* 1988;142(6):637–639.

58. Schneider DJ, Perez A, Knilamus TE, et al. Clinical and pathologic aspects of cardiomyopathy from ipecac administration in Munchausen's syndrome by proxy. *Pediatrics*. 1996;97:902–906.

59. Sutphen JL, Saulsbury FT. Intentional ipecac poisoning: Munchausen syndrome by proxy. *Pediatrics*. 1988;82(3, pt 2):453–456.

60. Shannon M. The demise of ipecac. *Pediatrics*. 2003;112(5):1180–1181.

61. Manno BR, Manno JE. Toxicology of ipecac: a review. *Clin Toxicol*. 1977;10(2):221–242.

62. Silber TJ. Ipecac syrup abuse, morbidity, and mortality: isn't it time to repeal its over-the-counter status? *J Adolesc Health*. 2005;37(3):256–260.

63. Eldridge DL, Van Eyk J, Kornegay C. Pediatric toxicology. *Emerg Med Clin North Am*. 2007;25(2):283–308.

64. Rashid N. Medically unexplained myopathy due to ipecac abuse. *Psychosomatics*. 2006;47(2):167–169.

65. Yamashita M, Yamashita M, Azuma J. Urinary excretion of ipecac alkaloids in human volunteers. *Vet Hum Toxicol*. 2002;44(5):257–259.

66. Ackerman NB Jr, Strobel CT. Polle syndrome: chronic diarrhea in Munchausen's child. *Gastroenterology*. 1981;81(6):1140–1142.

67. Carlson J, Fernlund P, Ivarsson SA, et al. Munchausen syndrome by proxy: an unexpected cause of severe chronic diarrhoea in a child. *Acta Paediatr*. 1994;83(1):119–121.

68. Epstein MA, Markowitz RL, Gallo DM, et al. Munchausen syndrome by proxy: considerations in diagnosis and confirmation by video surveillance. *Pediatrics*. 1987;80(2):220–224.

69. Fleisher D, Ament ME. Diarrhea, red diapers, and child abuse: clinical alertness needed for recognition; clinical skill needed for success in management. *Clin Pediatr (Phila)*. 1977;16(9):820–824.

70. Lasher LJ, Feldman MD. Celiac disease as a manifestation of Munchausen by proxy. *South Med J*. 2004;97(1):67–69.

71. Volk D. Factitious diarrhea in two children. *Am J Dis Child*. 1982;136(11):1027–1028.

72. Xing JH, Soffer EE. Adverse effects of laxatives. *Dis Colon Rectum*. 2001;44(8):1201–1209.

73. Wald A. Is chronic use of stimulant laxatives harmful to the colon? *J Clin Gastroenterol*. 2003;36(5):386–389.

74. Thompson WG. Laxatives: clinical pharmacology and rational use. *Drugs*. 1980;19(1):49–58.

75. Coogan PF, Rosenberg L, Palmer JR, et al. Phenolphthalein laxatives and risk of cancer. *J Natl Cancer Inst*. 2000;92(23):1943–1944.

76. Baker EH, Sandle GI. Complications of laxative abuse. *Annu Rev Med*. 1996;47:127–134.

77. Oster JR, Materson BJ, Rogers AI. Laxative abuse syndrome. *Am J Gastroenterol*. 1980;74(5):451–458.

78. Vanin JR, Saylor KE. Laxative abuse: a hazardous habit for weight control. *J Am Coll Health*. 1989;37(5):227–230.

79. Malmquist J, Ericsson B, Hulten-Nosslin MB, et al. Finger clubbing and aspartylglucosamine excretion in a laxative-abusing patient. *Postgrad Med J*. 1980;56(662):862–864.

80. Pines A, Olchovsky D, Bregman J, et al. Finger clubbing associated with laxative abuse. *South Med J*. 1983;76(8):1071–1072.

81. Prior J, White I. Tetany and clubbing in patient who ingested large quantities of senna. *Lancet*. 1978(Oct 28);2(8096):947.

82. Silk DB, Gibson JA, Murray CR. Reversible finger clubbing in a case of purgative abuse. *Gastroenterology*. 1975;68(4, pt 1):790–794.

83. de Ridder L, Hoekstra JH. Manifestations of Munchausen syndrome by proxy in pediatric gastroenterology. *J Pediatr Gastroenterol Nutr*. 2000;31(2):208–211.

84. Fine KD, Santa Ana CA, Fordtran JS. Diagnosis of magnesium-induced diarrhea. *N Engl J Med*. 1991;324(15):1012–1017.

85. Phillips S, Donaldson L, Geisler K, et al. Stool composition in factitial diarrhea: a 6-year experience with stool analysis. *Ann Intern Med*. 1995;123(2):97–100.

86. Topazian M, Binder HJ. Factitious diarrhea detected by measurement of stool osmolality. *N Engl J Med*. 1994;330(20):1418–1419.

87. Bytzer P, Stokholm M, Andersen I, et al. Prevalence of surreptitious laxative abuse in patients with diarrhoea of uncertain origin: a cost benefit analysis of a screening procedure. *Gut*. 1989;30(10):1379–1384.

88. Shelton JH, Santa Ana CA, Thompson DR, et al. Factitious diarrhea induced by stimulant laxatives: accuracy of diagnosis by a clinical reference laboratory using thin layer chromatography. *Clin Chem*. 2007;53(1):85–90.

89. Stolk LM, Hoogtanders K. Detection of laxative abuse by urine analysis with HPLC and diode array detection. *Pharm World Sci*. 1999;21(1):40–43.

90. Beyer J, Peters FT, Maurer HH. Screening procedure for detection of stimulant laxatives and/or their metabolites in human urine using gas chromatography-mass spectrometry after enzymatic cleavage of conjugates and extractive methylation. *Ther Drug Monit*. 2005;27(2):151–157.

91. Babcock J, Hartman K, Pedersen A, et al. Rodenticide-induced coagulopathy in a young child. A case of Munchausen syndrome by proxy. *Am J Pediatr Hematol Oncol*. 1993;15(1):126–130.

92. Hvizdala EV, Gellady AM. Intentional poisoning of two siblings by prescription drugs. An unusual form of child abuse. *Clin Pediatr (Phila)*. 1978;17(6):480–482.

93. Souid AK, Korins K, Keith D, et al. Unexplained menorrhagia and hematuria: a case report of Munchausen's syndrome by proxy. *Pediatr Hematol Oncol*. 1993;10(3):245–248.

94. Chua JD, Friedenberg WR. Superwarfarin poisoning. *Arch Intern Med*. 1998;158(17):1929–1932.

95. Isbister GK, Hackett LP, Whyte IM. Intentional warfarin overdose. *Ther Drug Monit*. 2003;25(6):715–722.

96. Isbister GK, Dawson A, Isbister JP. Recommendations for the management of over-anticoagulation with warfarin. *Emerg Med (Fremantle)*. 2001;13(4):469–471.

97. Bappal B, George M, Nair R, et al. Factitious hypoglycemia: a tale from the Arab world. *Pediatrics.* 2001;107(1):180–182.

98. Edidin DV, Farrell EE, Gould VE. Factitious hyperinsulinemic hypoglycemia in infancy: diagnostic pitfalig. *Clin Pediatr.* 2000;39(2):117–119.

99. Giurgea I, Ulinski T, Touati G, et al. Factitious hyperinsulinism leading to pancreatectomy: severe forms of Munchausen syndrome by proxy. *Pediatrics.* 2005;116(1):e145–e148.

100. Mehl AL, Coble L, Johnson S. Munchausen syndrome by proxy: a family affair. *Child Abuse Negl.* 1990;14(4):577–585.

101. Aranibar H, Cerda M. Hypoglycemic seizure in Munchausen-by-proxy syndrome. *Pediatr Emerg Care.* 2005;21(6):378–379.

102. Owen L, Ellis M, Shield J. Deliberate sulphonylurea poisoning mimicking hyperinsulinaemia of infancy. *Arch Dis Child.* 2000;82(5):392–393.

103. Marks V, Teale JD. Hypoglycemia: factitious and felonious. *Endocrinol Metab Clin North Am.* 1999;28(3):579–601.

104. Kaminer Y, Robbins DR. Insulin misuse: a review of an overlooked psychiatric problem. *Psychosomatics.* 1989;30(1):19–24.

105. Hoizey G, Lamiable D, Trenque T, et al. Identification and quantification of 8 sulfonylureas with clinical toxicology interest by liquid chromatography-ion-trap tandem mass spectrometry and library searching. *Clin Chem.* 2005;51(9):1666–1672.

106. Jureidini JN, Shafer AT, Donald TG. "Munchausen by proxy syndrome": not only pathological parenting but also problematic doctoring? *Med J Aust.* 2003;178(3):130–132.

107. Arnold SM, Arnholz D, Garyfallou GT, et al. Two siblings poisoned with diphenhydramine: a case of factitious disorder by proxy. *Ann Emerg Med.* 1998;32(2):256–259.

28 | Drug-Facilitated Sexual Assault

Laura K. Bechtel

INTRODUCTION

D rug-facilitated sexual assault (DFSA) is a worldwide problem.[1-3] Numerous agents have been utilized in such assaults, and the diagnosis of the causative agent can be difficult even for experienced teams. *Sexual assault* is broadly defined as any undesired physical contact of a sexual nature perpetrated against another person. Sexual assault is much broader than the term *rape*, traditionally referred to as forced vaginal penetration of a woman by a male assailant.[4] In 2003–2004, a total of 204,370 sexual assaults were reported to law enforcement agencies in the United States.[5] Because most sexual assaults are not reported, this U.S. average is grossly underrepresented. The National Women's Study documented that 84% of women in a sample population did not report rapes to the police.[6] Among U.S. college students, approximately 25% of women reported experiencing completed or attempted rape.[7] In 2003, approximately 9% of high school students reported having been forced to have sexual intercourse.[8] Current estimates from available data indicate that an astonishing one in six U.S. women will be the victim of a sexual assault at least once in their lifetime.[9]

DFSA is defined as the use of a chemical agent to facilitate sexual assault.[10-13] The reported prevalence of DFSA varies. The U.S. Department of Justice estimates 44% of sexual assaults are perceived to involve the influence of drugs or alcohol.[5,14,15] Often drugs and alcohol are used voluntarily by both the victim and offender.[14] One multicenter study estimates only 4.3% of the DFSA victims examined were surreptitiously drugged and 35.4% of the DFSAs involved voluntary use of illicit drugs.[13] Due to the absence of scientific studies examining the prevalence of DFSAs, the exact number of alcohol- and illicit drug-related sexual assaults is unknown. Yet an increasing number of independent testing programs across the world are performing analyses on urine, blood, and hair samples collected from individuals who claimed to have been sexually assaulted and believed that drugs were involved.[11,13,16-18] These reports are due to an increased awareness of the problem and technological advances in rapid drug analyses.

When presented with a victim of sexual assault, healthcare and law enforcement personnel have encountered numerous problems, including failure to recognize the urgency of medical attention, failure to treat patients as victims, and failure to document all available forensic evidence in a timely fashion. To help alleviate these problems, the Office for Victims of Crime, U.S. Department of Justice, granted funding for sexual assault nurse examiner (SANE) programs. A SANE is a registered nurse who works closely with medical staff and interacts with sexual assault crisis centers, law enforcement officers, prosecutors, judges, forensic lab staff, and child protective service workers to meet the multiple needs of victims and to hold offenders accountable for their crimes.[19,20]

Healthcare and law enforcement personnel may encounter unique circumstances when treating DFSA victims because victims may delay seeking medical attention or because officials may not perceive the patient as a sexual assault victim. The sedative–hypnotic and amnesic properties of the drugs used to facilitate a sexual assault can alter the victim's behavior, increase the victim's susceptibility to sexual assault, and diminish recollection of events surrounding the sexual assault. Often victims are reluctant to report incidents because of embarrassment, guilt, perceived responsibility, or relationship with the assailant. Victims may also be reluctant to disclose the extent of their involvement in drug and/or alcohol abuse or to disclose the identities of friends who may have provided the very drugs that unintentionally rendered them vulnerable to the sexual assault. Numerous reports have documented that victims either do not seek medical attention or delay seeking medical treatment for 3–7 days after the assault.[21-27] Extended delays in collecting specimens from DFSAs may reduce the probability of detecting drugs potentially used to facilitate a sexual assault. Most of the drugs typically used in the facilitation of sexual assaults are rapidly absorbed and metabolized by the body, thereby rendering them difficult to detect in routine urine and blood drug screenings.

The most commonly reported symptoms from victims of DFSA are confusion, dizziness, drowsiness, impaired judgment, anterograde amnesia, lack of muscle control, loss of consciousness, reduced inhibitions, nausea, hypotension, and bradycardia. Victims of sexual assault may present with physical injuries resulting from the assault or clinical effects of the drugs. For example, a victim may present with one or a combination of the following: contusions, lacerations, broken bones, altered mental status, and/or intoxication.[28] The healthcare team will treat the urgent injuries but may not inquire about the possibility of sexual assault. They may mistake the clinical effects of the drug used on the victim for self-induced substance abuse. Providers should be aware that symptoms mimicking alcohol toxicity may "point to" the possibility of a DFSA. Teams evaluating these cases must be aware of the necessity to collect sensitive forensic evidence (i.e., clothing) if the victim decides to report the assault.

FORENSIC LABORATORY ANALYSIS

In all reported sexual assault cases, a "rape kit" is used to test for the abuser's DNA. Care must be taken to ensure chain of custody. Semen, blood, urine, vaginal secretions, saliva, vaginal epithelial cells, hair, and other biologic evidence may be identified and genetically typed by a crime lab.[27,29] The information derived from the analysis can often help determine whether sexual contact occurred, provide information regarding the circumstances of the incident, and be compared to reference samples collected from patients and suspects. The most common form of DNA analysis used in crime labs for identification is called polymerase chain reaction (PCR). PCR allows the analysis of evidence samples of limited quality and quantity by making millions of copies of very small amounts of DNA. Using an advanced form of PCR testing called short tandem repeats (STR), the laboratory is able to generate a DNA profile, which can be compared to DNA from a suspect or a crime scene.[29]

For sexual assault cases suspected of involving alcohol and/or drugs, samples should be sent to forensics for toxicology testing. In addition to DNA testing, collection of urine and blood for forensic analysis is typically performed to identify drugs used to facilitate sexual assault. Hair samples removed from the scalp may be requested for drug analysis when there is a significant delay in reporting a DFSA.[30] Analysis of drugs present in hair can offer several advantages over urine and blood specimens in specific cases. The window of drug detection may be extended from days to weeks and even months, due to the stability of the drug once it is deposited.[31] Analysis of sequential hair segments can provide a "chronicle" of drug use. Because the mechanisms by which drugs are deposited in hair are not well understood, prosecution of sexual abuse offenders based solely on results obtained from hair analysis is controversial.[32] Several factors are known to contribute to the deposition of drugs in hair, including rate of growth, anatomical location, thickness and color (melanin content), and environmental contamination. Drugs in hair are usually present in relatively low concentrations (pg–ng/mg); therefore very sensitive laboratory methods are required for detection.[33-35]

Samples must be collected under strict chain of custody guidelines, which include not only documenting procession of specific evidence but also protecting the evidence in a location where it cannot be contaminated or tampered with (i.e., controlled area with limited access). A three-tier chain of testing may be employed to analyze drugs used to facilitate sexual assault at many U.S. state forensic laboratories. The *first tier* of testing quantitatively screens for ethanol from blood specimens using gas chromatography with flame-ionization detection (GC-FID) or gas chromatography-mass spectrometry detection (GC-MS). The *second tier* quantifies drugs of abuse, such as amphetamines, barbiturates, benzodiazepines, cannabinoids, cocaine, lysergic acid diethylamide, and opioids, using immunoassays and fluorescent polarization assays (e.g., EMIT, by Dade-Behring; TDx, by Abbott). Confirmation assays are performed using GC-MS analysis. The *third tier* employs extremely sensitive and specific methodologies of screening using gas chromatography-tandem mass spectrometry (GC-MS) and/or high-performance liquid chromatography mass spectrometry (HPLC-MS/MS) for analysis of a broad array of compounds such as dextromethorphan, tricyclic antidepressants, antihistamines, non-benzodiazepine sedatives–hypnotics, ketamine and other potential DFSA compounds such as gamma-hydroxybutyrate (GHB) that may not be detected using tier two methods.

In many states, victims perceived to be under the influence of alcohol with a blood alcohol concentration greater than 0.08 are not typically analyzed beyond the level of first tier ethanol testing unless there is specific medical documentation of symptoms of additional drug exposure. Therefore, many drug-facilitated sexual assault cases (other than alcohol) may be undetected under the current screening protocols performed at some state forensic laboratories. Several published reports document that 34–45% of victims of sexual assault are under the influence of drugs of abuse, with 8% under the influence of drugs not typically detected by standard drugs of abuse screening methods.[10,11,13,25,36] Teams must document suspicions of drugs, especially in cases of sexual assault. Documentation of these suspicions will justify drug-specific analyses by the forensic laboratory. These analytic results are mandatory for the prosecution of sexual predators.

The U.S. Drug-Induced Rape Prevention and Punishment Act of 1996 (Public Law 104-305) modified Title 21 U.S. Code, section 841, to provide penalties of up to 20 years' imprisonment and fines for persons who intend to commit a crime of violence (including rape) by distributing a controlled substance to another individual without that individual's knowledge. This act provides specific definitions of controlled substances and crimes of violence that assist prosecutors in maximizing the penalties against sexual predators. Controlled substances are categorized as Schedule I–V drugs by the U.S. Drug Enforcement Administration. Extensive efforts have focused on documenting detection limits for common drugs used to facilitate sexual assault to aid in prosecution of sexual predators.[13] Without the extensive efforts of medical staff, forensic toxicologists, police, and judicial officials, these penalties against sexual assault offenders cannot be implemented.

DRUGS USED IN SEXUAL ASSAULT

A majority of sexual assaults have been linked to the abuse of alcohol.[10,12,36-39] It is commonly accepted that there is a high degree of correlation between alcohol intoxication and the risk of being sexually assaulted.[13] In recent years, however, the literature has paid more attention to people using other drugs to render their victims unconscious or lower their level of resistance to enable sexual assault.[17,24,40-42] In addition to alcohol, the drugs most often implicated in DFSAs are gamma-hydroxybutyric acid (GHB), flunitrazepam (Rohypnol or "roofies"), and ketamine ("special K"), although others, including other nonbenzodiazepine sedative–hypnotics and over the counter medications, are used as well (Table 28.1). These drugs share similar characteristics for producing sedation, hypnosis, and anterograde amnesia. These effects often rapidly incapacitate victims, and the effects can be intensified when they are willingly or involuntarily taken with alcohol. Because of the sedative and amnesic properties of these drugs, victims often have no memory of an assault, only an awareness or sense that they were violated (see Chapter 20).

TABLE 28.1 **Examples of Drugs Used to Facilitate Sexual Assault**

Anticholinergics
Antihistamines
Barbiturates
Benzodiazepines
Chloral hydrate
Dextromethorphan
Ethanol
Gamma-hydroxybutyrate
Ketamine
Marijuana
Nonbenzodiazepine sedatives–hypnotics
Opioids
Oxymetazoline

Drugs used in DFSAs (e.g., flunitrazepam) may only be detectable in a victim's urine for a short period; therefore it is imperative that urine testing occur quickly. In addition, search warrants should be obtained as quickly as possible for the suspect(s) and should include appropriate areas (e.g., residence, vehicle, school locker, work space). Friends, roommates, and associates should be interviewed separately as quickly as possible. Searches should extend beyond looking solely for the drug(s) potentially utilized; items such as publications about drugs, receipts, mortar and pestle to crush pills into powder, and eye droppers for introducing the substance into the drinks of unsuspecting victims should also be sought. Any item seized as a result of a search should be promptly forwarded for testing. Not only will the item aid the healthcare team in determining what occurred during the assault and help in treating the victim(s), but it can be used as supporting evidence for prosecution and for issuing alerts.

CONCLUSION

DFSA is a complex and prevalent problem worldwide. DFSA should be considered in patients following a reported sexual assault who are amnestic to the specific details of the event. The presence of ethanol or a positive routine drug screen in a sexual assault victim does not exclude the potential of another drug's presence. In addition, a negative routine drug screen does not exclude all potential agents that are used in DFSA.

Police should be knowledgeable about these crimes and of the fact that drug evidence in the victim may dissipate quickly. To compensate for this fact, they should use a combination of creativity and proactive techniques to identify a suspect and assemble the evidence necessary for conviction. This may include the testimony of other victims, statements made to witnesses, findings on computers, and the possession of drugs used to incapacitate victims

REFERENCES

1. Bechtel LK, Holstege CP. Criminal poisoning: drug-facilitated sexual assault. *Emerg Med Clin North Am.* 2007;25(2):499–525.
2. Du Mont J, Macdonald S, Rotbard N, et al. Factors associated with suspected drug-facilitated sexual assault. *CMAJ.* 2009;180(5):513–519.

3. McCauley JL, Conoscenti LM, Ruggiero KJ, et al. Prevalence and correlates of drug/alcohol-facilitated and incapacitated sexual assault in a nationally representative sample of adolescent girls. *J Clin Child Adolesc Psychol.* 2009;38(2):295–300.

4. American College of Obstetricians and Gynecologists. Adolescent victims of sexual assault. *ACOG Educational Bulletin.* October 1998;Number 252.

5. National Criminal Victimization Survey, 2003. In: BoJ, ed. *Statistics.* U.S. Department of Justice; 2004.

6. Kilpatrick E, Edmunds CN, Seymour A. *Rape in America: A Report to the Nation.* Arlington, VA: National Center for Victims of Crime and Crime Victims Research and Treatment Center; 1992.

7. Fisher BS, Cullen FT, Turner MG. *The Sexual Victimization of College Women.* Washington DC: Department of Justice (US), National Institute of Justice; 2000. NCJ 182369.

8. Grunbaum JA, Kann L, Kinchen S, et al. Youth risk behavior surveillance—United States, 2003. *MMWR.* 2004;53(2):1–96.

9. Tjaden P, Thoennes N. *Full Report of the Prevalence, Incidence, and Consequences of Violence Against Women: Findings from the National Violence Against Women Survey.* Washington, DC: National Institute of Justice; 2000.

10. ElSohly MA, Salamone SJ. Prevalence of drugs used in cases of alleged sexual assault. *J Anal Toxicol.* 1999;23(3):141–146.

11. Hindmarch I, ElSohly M, Gambles J, et al. Forensic urinalysis of drug use in cases of alleged sexual assault. *J Clin Forensic Med.* 2001;8(4):197–205.

12. Slaughter L. Involvement of drugs in sexual assault. *J Reprod Med.* 2000;45(5):425–430.

13. Negrusz A, Juhascik M, Gaensslen RE. *Estimate of the Incidence of Drug-Facilitated Sexual Assault in the U.S.* U.S. Department of Justice; 2005.

14. Fitzgerald N, Riley K. Drug-facilitated rape: looking for the missing pieces. *Natl Inst Justice J.* April 2000.

15. Anonymous. Personal crimes of violence. In: USDJ, ed. *Criminal Victimization in the United States—Statistical Tables Index.* Bureau of Justice Statistics; 2004.

16. Marc B, Baudry F, Vaquero P, et al. Sexual assault under benzodiazepine submission in a Paris suburb. *Arch Gynecol Obstet.* 2000;263(4):193–197.

17. McGregor MJ, Lipowska M, Shah S, et al. An exploratory analysis of suspected drug-facilitated sexual assault seen in a hospital emergency department. *Women Health.* 2003;37(3):71–80.

18. Questel F, Sec I, Sicot R, Pourriat JL. Drug-facilitated crimes: prospective data collection in a forensic unit in Paris. *Presse Med.* 2009;38(7-8):1049–1055.

19. McGregor MJ, Du Mont J, Myhr TL. Sexual assault forensic medical examination: is evidence related to successful prosecution? *Ann Emerg Med.* 2002;39(6):639–647.

20. Campbell R. Rape survivors' experiences with the legal and medical systems: do rape victim advocates make a difference? *Violence Against Women.* 2006;12(1):30–45.

21. Burgess AW, Fehder WP, Hartman CR. Delayed reporting of the rape victim. *J Psychosoc Nurs Ment Health Serv.* 1995;33(9):21–29.

22. Plumbo MA. Delayed reporting of sexual assault. Implications for counseling. *J Nurs Midwifery.* 1995;40(5):424–427.

23. Adamowicz P, Kala M. Date-rape drugs scene in Poland. *Przegl Lek.* 2005;62(6):572–575.

24. Goulle JP, Anger JP. Drug-facilitated robbery or sexual assault: problems associated with amnesia. *Ther Drug Monit.* 2004;26(2):206–210.

25. Scott-Ham M, Burton FC. Toxicological findings in cases of alleged drug-facilitated sexual assault in the United Kingdom over a 3-year period. *J Clin Forensic Med.* 2005;12(4):175–186.

26. Rennison C. *Rape and Sexual Assault: Reporting to Police and Medical Attention, 1992-2000.* Washington: U.S. Department of Justice; 2002. NCJ 194530.

27. Cybulska BaF, G. Sexual assault: examination of the victim. *Medicine.* 2005;33(9):23–28.

28. Feldhaus KM, Houry D, Kaminsky R. Lifetime sexual assault prevalence rates and reporting practices in an emergency department population. *Ann Emerg Med.* 2000;36(1):23–27.

29. A National Protocol for Sexual Assault Medical Forensic Examinations: Adults/Adolescents. In: *Women of VA.* US Department of Justice; 2004.

30. Rossi R, Lancia M, Gambelunghe C, et al. Identification of GHB and morphine in hair in a case of drug-facilitated sexual assault. *Forensic Sci Int.* 2009;186(1-3):9–11.

31. Kintz P, Villain M, Cirimele V. Hair analysis for drug detection. *Ther Drug Monit.* 2006;28(3):442–446.

32. Cone EJ. Legal, workplace, and treatment drug testing with alternate biological matrices on a global scale. *Forensic Sci Int.* 2001;121:7–15.

33. Negrusz A, Gaensslen RE. Analytical developments in toxicological investigation of drug-facilitated sexual assault. *Anal Bioanal Chem.* 2003;376(8):1192–1197.

34. Negrusz A, Moore CM, Kern JL, et al. Quantitation of clonazepam and its major metabolite 7-aminoclonazepam in hair. *J Anal Toxicol.* 2000;24(7):614–620.

35. Kintz P, Villain M, Ludes B. Testing for the undetectable in drug-facilitated sexual assault using hair analyzed by tandem mass spectrometry as evidence. *Ther Drug Monit.* 2004;26(2):211–214.

36. US Department of Justice; Table 32: percent distribution of victimizations by perceived drug or alcohol use by offender. *Personal Crimes of Violence.* 2004

37. Abbey A, Zawacki T, Buck PO, et al. How does alcohol contribute to sexual assault? Explanations from laboratory and survey data. *Alcohol Clin Exp Res.* 2002;26(4):575–581.

38. Murdoch D, Pihl RO, Ross D. Alcohol and crimes of violence: present issues. *Int J Addict.* 1990;25(9):1065–1081.

39. Krebs CP, Lindquist CH, Warner TD, et al. College women's experiences with physically forced, alcohol- or other drug-enabled, and drug-facilitated sexual assault before and since entering college. *J Am Coll Health.* 2009;57(6):639–647.

40. Ledray LE. The clinical care and documentation for victims of drug-facilitated sexual assault. *J Emerg Nurs.* 2001;27(3):301–305.

41. LeBeau M, Andollo W, Hearn WL, et al. Recommendations for toxicological investigations of drug-facilitated sexual assaults. *J Forensic Sci.* 1999;44(1):227–230.

42. McCauley J, Ruggiero KJ, Resnick HS, et al. Forcible, drug-facilitated, and incapacitated rape in relation to substance use problems: results from a national sample of college women. *Addict Behav.* 2009;34(5):458–462.

Glossary

Aerosolization: A fine mist or spray containing minute particles.

Anaphylactoid: Pertaining to a reaction, the symptoms of which resemble those of the anaphylactic response produced by the injection of serum and other nonspecific proteins or chemicals.

Anaphylaxis: A severe, whole-body allergic reaction.

Anhydrosis: Lack of sweating.

Antecubital: Relating to the region of the arm in front of the elbow.

Antemortem: Preceding death.

Anxiolysis: Stopping anxiety.

Anemia: Decreased red blood cells.

Anorexia: A prolonged disorder of eating due to loss of appetite.

Apnea: A period of time during which breathing stops.

Arthralgia: Pain in a joint or joints.

Asymptomatic: Having no symptoms.

Ataxia: Inability to coordinate voluntary muscle movements.

Axillary: Relating to or near the armpit.

Blepharospasm: Spasm of the eyelid muscle.

Bradycardia: Slow heart rate.

Bradykinesia: Slow movement.

Bronchoconsctriction: Constriction of the respiratory airways.

Bronchorrhea: Airway secretions.

Bruxism: Grinding teeth.

Cardiotoxic: Toxic to the heart.

Chorea: Ceaseless rapid complex body movements that look well coordinated and purposeful but are, in fact, involuntary.

Choreiform: Resembling the rapid jerky movements associated with chorea.

Circumorally: Around the mouth.

Clonus: Alternate involuntary muscular contraction and relaxation in rapid succession.

Coagulopathic: Any disorder of blood coagulation.

Constipation: Irregular and infrequent or difficult evacuation of the bowels.

Cyanosis: A bluish color of the skin and the mucous membranes.

Dehydration: Excessive loss of water from the body.

Diaphoresis: Perfuse sweating.

Dinoflagellates: Any of numerous minute, chiefly marine protozoans.

Diplopia: Double vision.

Disseminated intravascular coagulation: A pathological activation of coagulation.

Dysmetria: An inability or impaired ability to accurately control the range of movement in muscular acts.

Dysphagia: Difficulty in swallowing.

Dysphonia: Difficulty in speaking.

Dyspnea: Difficulty in breathing.

Dysrhythmias: Abnormal heart rhythm.

Ecchymosis: A small hemorrhagic spot.

Eschar: Dry scab.

Fasciculation: A small local involuntary muscular contraction visible under the skin.

Gavage: Forced feeding, typically through a tube passed into the stomach.

Guillian-Barré syndrome: Progressive muscle weakness and paralysis.

Hematochezia: The passage of bloody stools.

Hematuria: The passage of bloody urine.

Hemolysis: The destruction of red blood cells.

Hidradenitis suppurativa: Inflammation of the sweat glands of the perianal, axillary, and genital areas, producing chronic abscesses.

Hyperemesis gravidarum: Excessive vomiting during pregnancy.

Hypertonic: Having increased tone.

Hyperkalemia: Elevated blood potassium.

Hypertension: Elevated blood pressure.

Hyperthermia: Elevated body temperature.

Hypocalcemia: Decreased blood calcium.

Hypochloremic: Decreased blood chloride.

Hypoglycemia: Decreased blood glucose.

Hypomagnesemia: Decreased blood magnesium.

Hyponatremia: Decreased blood sodium.

Hypoproteinemia: Decreased blood protein.

Hypotension: Decreased blood pressure.

Hypotonic: Decreased muscle tone.

Hypovolemia: Decreased circulating blood volume.

Insomnia: Inability to fall asleep.

Insulinoma: An insulin secreting tumor.

Leucopenia: Decreased white blood cell count.

Leukocytosis: Increased white blood cell count.

Keratoconjunctivitis sicca: A dryness of the eye caused by a deficiency of tear secretion.

Keratoses: An overgrowth of the skin.

Melanosis: Abnormally dark pigmentation of the skin or other tissues.

Miosis: Small pupils.

Myalgias: Muscle pain.

Myasthenia gravis: An autoimmune disease that causes muscle weakness.

Mydriasis: Large pupils.

Myoclonus: A sudden twitching of muscles or parts of muscles.

Myocyte: Muscle cell.

Myopathy: Disease of muscle.

Necrosis: The morphological changes of cell death caused by progressive enzymatic degradation.

Neuritis: Inflammation of a nerve.

Neurotoxic: Toxic to nerves.

Nystagmus: Rhythmic, oscillating motions of the eyes.

Obtundation: Reduced level of consciousness.

Odynophagia: Painful swallowing.

Parasthesias: A skin sensation, such as burning, prickling, itching, or tingling, with no apparent physical cause.

Pathognomonic: Denoting a sign or symptom on which a diagnosis can be made.

Perioral: Around the mouth.

Periorbital: Around the eye.

Pharyngitis: Inflammation of the back of the throat.

Postmortem: After death.

Proteinuria: Excessive protein in the urine.

Proteolytic: Breaking down proteins.

Pruritis: Sensation of itchiness.

Ptosis: Drooping of the upper eyelid.

Rhabdomyolysis: Muscle breakdown.

Rhonchi: A coarse rattling sound usually caused by secretions in a bronchial tube.

Saponification: Conversion of a fat into a soap by combination with an alkali.

Sepsis: Bacterial infection in the bloodstream.

Steatosis: Fatty degeneration.

Stridor: Noisy breathing.

Syncope: Passing out.

Synesthesia: A condition in which one type of stimulation evokes the sensation of another, such as when the hearing of a sound produces the visualization of a color.

Tachycardia: Rapid heart rate.

Tenesmus: A painful spasm of the anal sphincter accompanied by an urgent desire to evacuate the bowel.

Thrombocytopenia: Low blood platelets.

Tracheitis: Inflammation of the trachea.

Urticaria: Skin hives.

Vertigo: Sensation of rotation or movement of one's self or of one's surroundings in any plane.

Wheezing: A whistling noise in the chest during breathing when the airways are narrowed or compressed.

Xnthochromia: A yellowish appearance of cerebrospinal fluid.

Index

Figures and tables are indicated by f and t following page numbers.

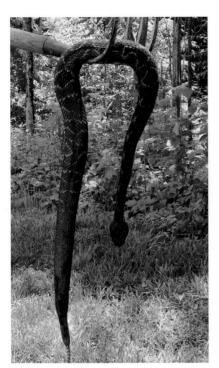

◄ COLOR PLATE 1
Timber rattlesnake (*Crotalus horridus horridus*)

▼ COLOR PLATE 2
Bark scorpion (*Centruroides sculpturatus*)
Adult as seen under Woods lamp lighting with babies on back.

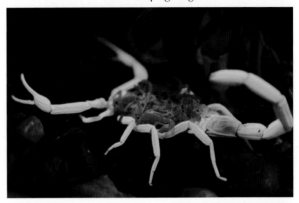

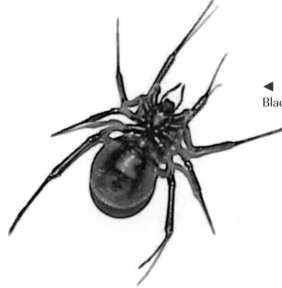

◄ COLOR PLATE 3
Black widow (*Latrodectus mactans*)

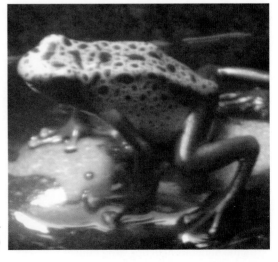

► COLOR PLATE 4
Poison-dart frog (*Phyllobates*)

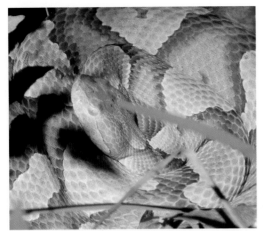

◀ COLOR PLATE 5
Copperhead (*Agkistrodon contortrix*)

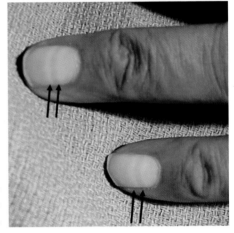

▶ COLOR PLATE 6
Mees' lines following arsenic poisoning. Note the white band traversing the width of the nail at the arrows.

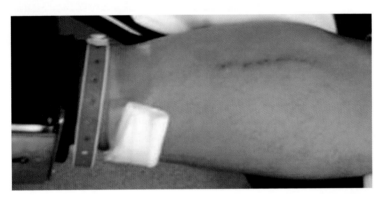

◀
COLOR PLATE 7
Track marks in an intravenous drug abuser

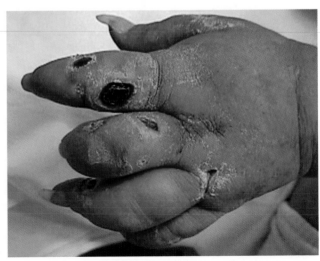

▶ COLOR PLATE 8
Skin popping on a hand of a subcutaneous injecting drug abuser

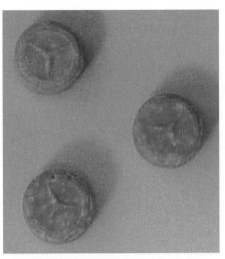

◀ COLOR PLATE 9
MDMA tablets

▼ COLOR PLATE 10
Meth mouth of a chronic
methamphetamine abuser
Used with permission from Dr. John A. Svirksy

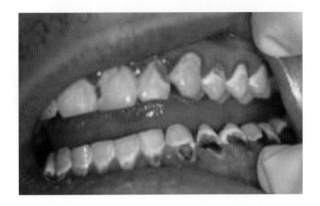

▼ COLOR PLATE 11
Subcutaneous injection of
opioids (*skin popping*) resulting
in multiple ulcers of the legs.

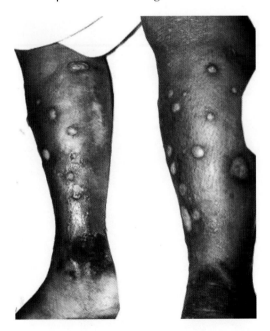

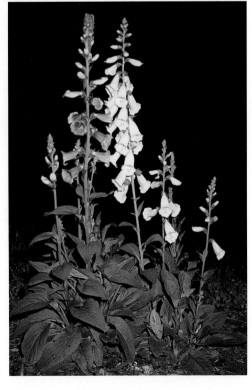

COLOR PLATE 12 ▶
Digitalis purpurea (foxglove)

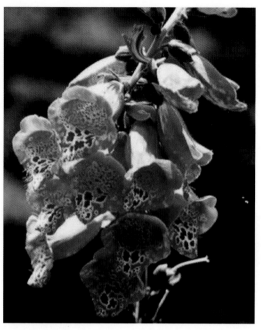

▲ COLOR PLATE 13
Digitalis purpurea (foxglove)

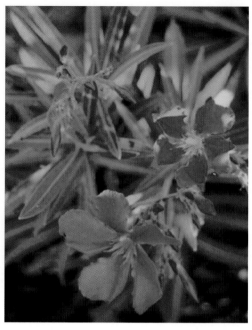

▲ COLOR PLATE 14
Nerium oleander (oleander)

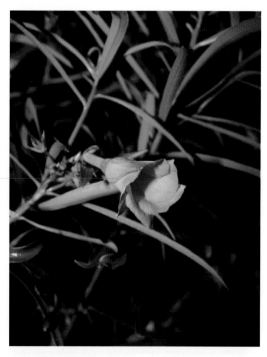

▲ COLOR PLATE 15
Thevetia peruviana (yellow oleander)

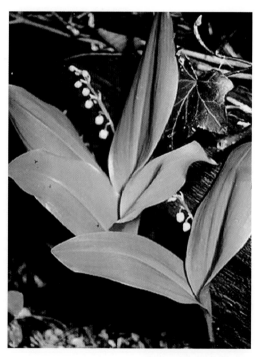

▲ COLOR PLATE 16
Convallaria majalis (lily of the valley)

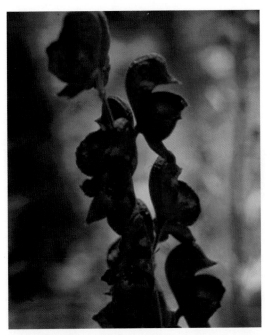

▲ COLOR PLATE 17
Aconitum napellus (monkshood)

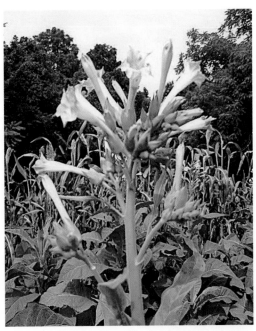

▲ COLOR PLATE 18
Nicotiana tabacum (tobacco)

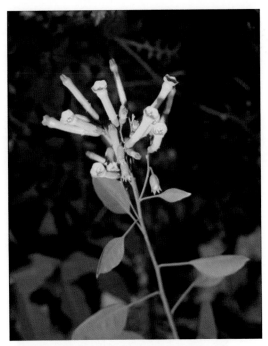

▲ COLOR PLATE 19
Nicotiana glauca (tree tobacco)

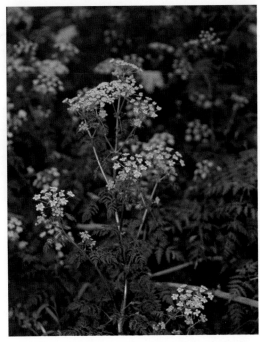

▲ COLOR PLATE 20
Conium maculatum (poison hemlock)

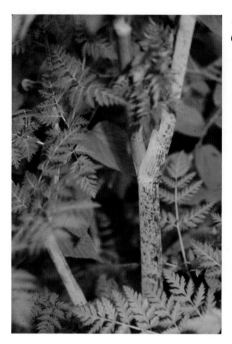

◀ COLOR PLATE 21
Conium maculatum (poison hemlock)

▼ COLOR PLATE 22
Gymnocladus dioicus (Kentucky coffee bean)

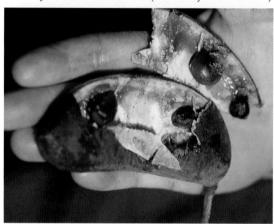

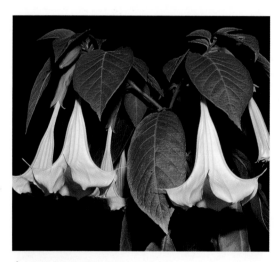

▲ COLOR PLATE 23
Brugmansia spp. (angel trumpet)

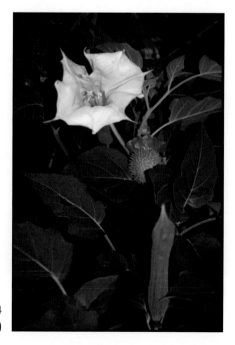

▶ COLOR PLATE 24
Datura meteloides (sacred datura)

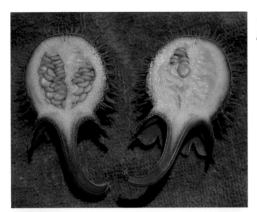

◀ COLOR PLATE 25
Datura meteloides (sacred datura)

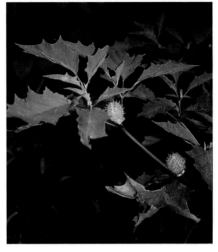

▶ COLOR PLATE 26
Datura stramonium (jimson weed)

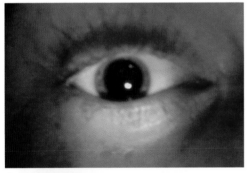

▲ COLOR PLATE 27
Mydriasis (dilated pupil) in a patient
intoxicated with *Datura stramonium*.

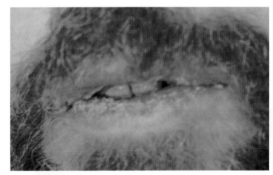

▲ COLOR PLATE 28
Dry mouth in a patient intoxicate with
Datura stramonium.

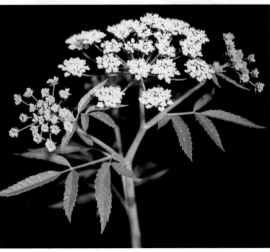

▶ COLOR PLATE 29
Cicuta maculata (water hemlock) flowers